NUTRITION

2ND EDITION

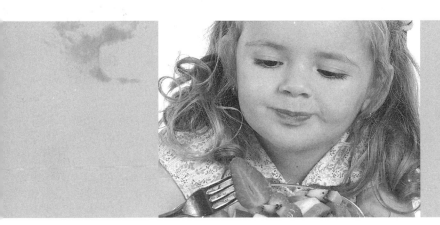

What Every Parent Needs to Know

EDITORS

WILLIAM H. DIETZ, MD, PhD, FAAP

LORAINE STERN, MD, FAAP

American Academy of Pediatrics

DEDICATED TO THE HEALTH OF ALL CHILDREN™

American Academy of Pediatrics Department of Marketing and Publications Staff

Director, Department of Marketing and Publications
Maureen DeRosa, MPA

Director, Division of Product Development
Mark Grimes

Manager, Consumer Publishing
Carolyn Kolbaba

Coordinator, Product Development
Holly Kaminski

Director, Division of Publishing and Production Services
Sandi King, MS

Editorial Specialist
Jason Crase

Print Production Specialist
Shannan Martin

Manager, Art Direction and Production
Linda Diamond

Director, Division of Marketing and Sales
Kevin Tuley

Manager, Consumer Marketing and Sales
Kathleen Juhl

Published by the American Academy of Pediatrics
141 Northwest Point Blvd, Elk Grove Village, IL 60007-1019
847/434-4000
Fax: 847/434-8000
www.aap.org

Cover design by Dan Rembert
Book design by Linda Diamond

Second Edition—2012
First Edition—© 1999 as *The Official, Complete Home Reference Guide to Your Child's Nutrition: Making Peace at the Table and Building Healthy Eating Habits for Life*

Library of Congress Control Number: 2010919006
ISBN: 978-1-58110-321-2

The recommendations in this publication do not indicate an exclusive course of treatment or serve as a standard of medical care. Variations, taking into account individual circumstances, may be appropriate.

Products are mentioned for informational purposes only. Inclusion in this publication does not imply endorsement by the American Academy of Pediatrics. The American Academy of Pediatrics is not responsible for the content of the resources mentioned in this publication. Web site addresses are as current as possible, but may change at any time.

Every effort is made to keep *Nutrition: What Every Parent Needs to Know* consistent with the most recent advice and information available from the American Academy of Pediatrics.

The findings and conclusions in this publication are those of the editors and do not necessarily represent the views of the Centers for Disease Control and Prevention or the US Department of Health and Human Services.

CB0055
9-230   1 2 3 4 5 6 7 8 9 10

What People Are Saying

There is no shortage of nutrition advice out there, but how do parents know what to trust? This book is an invaluable, practical, easy-to-read-and-understand resource for parents, grandparents, child care professionals, and anyone who takes care of children. It is distinguished by providing authoritative advice from the American Academy of Pediatrics about nutrition and feeding and eating behaviors, all together in one place. This is my #1 recommended nutrition book for parents.

> Thomas N. Robinson, MD, MPH
>
> Professor of Pediatrics and Director of the Center for Healthy Weight, Stanford University School of Medicine and Lucile Packard Children's Hospital at Stanford

Parents who wonder—and worry—about what to feed their kids to be healthy now have answers grounded in science and common sense. Drs Dietz and Stern offer practical information that will help guide parents to the nutritious foods that give their children the right start and can help instill healthy eating habits for a lifetime. Every parent—and grandparent—should make this a must read.

> Sally Squires, MS
>
> Director, Health and Wellness Communications, Powell Tate; Adjunct Professor, Tufts Friedman School of Nutrition Science and Policy; and former nationally syndicated Lean Plate Club columnist, *The Washington Post*

As a registered dietitian, I like that this book makes science simple—it outlines practical food tips and offers comforting advice on the subject of feeding healthy children.

> Connie Diekman, MEd, RD, LD, FADA
>
> Nutrition communications consultant and American Dietetic Association Past President

In addition to providing developmentally appropriate nutrition information on what infants and children should be eating, this book includes valuable advice for parents that can help children learn to like and actually eat those foods that comprise healthy diets. The editors provide clear, evidence-based answers to questions and challenges parents face, whether the reader is a first-time parent with a newborn or an experienced parent of school-aged children or adolescents.

> Leann Birch, PhD
>
> Distinguished Professor of Human Development and Director, Center for Childhood Obesity Research, College of Health and Human Development, The Pennsylvania State University

Acknowledgments

Editors

William H. Dietz, MD, PhD, FAAP

Loraine Stern, MD, FAAP

American Academy of Pediatrics Board of Directors Reviewer

Myles B. Abbott, MD, FAAP

Reviewers/Contributors

Steven A. Abrams, MD, FAAP

Robert D. Baker, Jr, MD, PhD, FAAP

Susan Baker, MD, FAAP

Miriam Bar-on, MD, FAAP

Jatinder JS Bhatia, MD, FAAP

William John Cochran, MD, FAAP

Betty Crase, IBCLC, RLC

Stephen Robert Daniels, MD, PhD, FAAP

Evelyn Eisenstein, MD, FAAP

Marianne Felice, MD, FAAP

Carlos Flores, MD, FAAP

Lawrence Gartner, MD, FAAP

Michael Georgieff, MD, FAAP

Elizabeth Gleghorn, MD, FAAP

Peter Gorski, MD, MPA, FAAP

Frank R. Greer, MD, FAAP

Laurence Grummer-Strawn, PhD

Sandra Gibson Hassink, MD, FAAP

Melvin Bernard Heyman, MD, FAAP

Marc Jacobson, MD, FAAP

Tom Jaksic, MD, PhD, FAAP

Desmond Kelly, MD, FAAP

Nancy Krebs, MD, FAAP

Annette Lansford, MD, FAAP

Greg Prazar, MD, FAAP

Peter Rappo, MD, FAAP

Carol Redell, MD, FAAP

Barbara Reid, MD, FAAP

Robert Rothbaum, MD, FAAP

Marcie Beth Schneider, MD, FAAP

Scott Howard Sicherer, MD, FAAP

Janet Silverstein, MD, FAAP

Robert Squires, MD, FAAP

Nicolas Stettler, MD, MSCE, FAAP

Dan W. Thomas, MD, FAAP

Susan Tully, MD, FAAP

John Udall, MD, FAAP

Robert Wood, MD, FAAP

Additional Assistance

Debra L. Burrowes, MHA

Writer

Richard Trubo

To all the people who recognize that children are our greatest inspiration in the present and our greatest hope for the future.

From the Editors

We dedicate this book to the children who have taught us what we really know and the parents who have helped them teach us.

Dr Dietz thanks his wife, Nancy; his children, Jonathan and Sarah, and their spouses, Lauren and Kirk; and the next generation, Jack, Luke, Van, and Hill, whose experiences all contributed to this book.

Dr Stern thanks her patients and grandpatients and her stepdaughter, Tina, who gave her her writing career.

Table of Contents

Please Note

The information contained in this book is intended to complement, not substitute for, the advice of your child's pediatrician. Before starting any medical treatment or program, you should consult with your child's pediatrician, who can discuss your child's individual needs and counsel you about symptoms and treatment. If you have questions about how the information in this book applies to your child, speak with your child's pediatrician.

Products mentioned in this book are for informational purposes only. Inclusion in this publication does not constitute or imply a guarantee or an endorsement by the American Academy of Pediatrics.

The information and advice in this book apply equally to children of both sexes (except where noted). To indicate this, we have chosen to alternate between masculine and feminine pronouns throughout the book.

Foreword

The American Academy of Pediatrics (AAP) welcomes you to the second edition of its popular parenting book, *Nutrition: What Every Parent Needs to Know.*

Giving your child a healthy start with good eating habits promotes his or her lifelong health. The "whys and hows" to do this are tackled in the following pages. Among other things, this book will help parents evaluate food options, prevent food fights, and identify and avoid outside influences.

Pediatricians who specialize in nutrition have extensively reviewed this book. Under the direction of our editors, the material in this book was developed with the assistance of numerous reviewers and contributors. Because medical information is constantly changing, every effort has been made to ensure that this book contains the most up-to-date findings. Readers may want to visit the AAP Web site for parents, HealthyChildren.org, to keep current on this and other subjects.

It is the hope of the AAP that this book will become an invaluable resource and reference guide to parents. We are confident that parents and caregivers will find the book extremely valuable. We encourage its use along with the advice and counsel of our readers' pediatricians, who will provide individual guidance and assistance related to the health of children.

The AAP is an organization of 60,000 primary care pediatricians, pediatric medical subspecialists, and pediatric surgical specialists dedicated to the health, safety, and well-being of infants, children, adolescents, and young adults. *Nutrition: What Every Parent Needs to Know* is part of ongoing AAP educational efforts to provide parents and caregivers with high-quality information on a broad spectrum of children's health issues.

Errol R. Alden, MD, FAAP
Executive Director/CEO
American Academy of Pediatrics

Introduction

Peace at the Table: The Whys and Hows of Healthy Eating Habits

Feeding children should be a shared responsibility: "The parent is responsible for WHAT; the child is responsible for HOW MUCH and even WHETHER."

> —Ellyn Satter, author of *How to Get Your Kid to Eat...But Not Too Much*

One of our favorite cartoons is *Baby Blues,* by Rick Kirkman and Jerry Scott. A young couple have 2 children, a preschooler and an infant. In one strip, the preschooler climbs up on a stool next to her mother and asks, "What are you cooking?"

"Chicken and rice," her mother answers.

The child screws up her face, throws herself on the floor, and writhes, yelling, "Bleah! Yuk! Gaak!"

In the last box, she lies quietly on the floor and asks, "What's that taste like?"

What we hope this book will do, among other things, is help you to be calm and effectual when faced with situations such as this.

Meals: Time to Relax and Enjoy

Nurture means to care for and to feed. As we nurture our children, we often allow food to become an indicator of how well we are doing our job. As a result, food turns into a measure of how much our children love and obey us, rather than a source of energy and nutrients. Food becomes emotionally charged, and mealtimes may become a source of anxiety and tension rather than an opportunity to relax, interact, and enjoy one another.

What food we offer children and what they eat have a great deal to do with their health and growth. But whether they actually eat what we serve depends on more than what we choose to lay before them. Their own tastes and preferences, their moods, and—most important— what they learn from people around them in subtle and not-so-subtle ways determine what and how much they eat.

The title of this introduction includes "peace at the table." Peace is best maintained by wise administrators who know when to intervene and when to hold back, not by a police state. If you turn into food police, our experience is that you may provoke conflict and make the situation worse. As parents and care providers, you are responsible for offering a healthful variety of foods. Your children are responsible for deciding what and how much they want to eat from what they are offered.

Offer Wholesome Choices, Then Stand Aside

Children will not become ill or suffer permanently if they are picky eaters or refuse a meal or two, but parents sometimes act as though such children might shrivel up and die. Parents' fears and concessions have produced toddlers who will eat only white foods such as milk, macaroni, white bread, and potatoes; children who take no food other than milk; or parents who greet each meal with clenched teeth while their toddler rules the family from her booster seat. All of these situations eventually resolve; all of them can be prevented. With infants and young children, your job is to offer wholesome food choices and then step back.

Lois, the mother of a patient, told Dr Stern the following story: Lois's sister and brother-in-law took off for a long weekend, leaving Kristin, their 8-year-old daughter, with Lois. When they dropped Kristin off, they also left a long list of what she would and wouldn't eat. Lois accepted the list and wished her sister and brother-in-law a good time.

That evening at dinnertime, Kristin asked, "What are we having?"

When Lois told her, she screwed up her face and said, "I don't like that."

"Gee, I'm sorry," Lois said. "You don't have to eat it if you don't want to."

Kristin left the main course on her plate, although she picked a little at the side dishes while she pouted. Lois paid no attention and took Kristin's plate away when everyone was through. Kristin probably went to bed a little hungry. However, the next morning, because she was hungry, she relished what was served for breakfast. She made no more complaints and ate well the entire weekend. Of course, we're sure she went back to being picky with her parents when they returned.

After Kelly, a colleague of Dr Dietz, found herself making a separate main course for her 4-year-old every time she cooked something he didn't like, she promised herself this would not happen with her next child. So when 3-year-old Colleen turned up her nose at the fish the rest of the family was eating, Kelly said, "You don't have to eat it. I'll just put it in the refrigerator and you can have it later if you want."

When bedtime arrived, Colleen said, "I think I'd better eat that fish or I'll get hungry."

This tactic works.

Emotions Complicate Nutrition

Parents of young children worry mostly about whether their children are eating enough of the right foods. Among older children and adolescents, however, the most serious nutritional issues are usually obesity and eating disorders, such as anorexia and bulimia. Early experiences, interactions within the family around foods, the influence of peers, the media, and lifestyles that reduce the time children spend eating with the family all probably contribute to these diseases. In addition, a teenager who is preoccupied with weight and body image may literally and symbolically slam the door when worried parents try to discuss issues of food and weight. Every pediatrician has the experience of seeing unexpected tears on a teenager's cheeks when the subject of weight arises during a checkup. In these families, everyone is upset—parents, because everything they do seems to make matters worse; adolescents, because they want their parents' help but only on their own terms.

This situation is not very different from food issues with younger children. The nutrients in food are only part of the concern. Emotional, behavioral, and psychological issues are equally important.

Nutrition: A Long-range Issue

In this book, we emphasize healthful food choices, but we do not emphasize rigid fat and calorie counting. Nutrition is a long-range issue, and one day or week does not make or break good health. Rather, we want you to develop a perspective on how to feed your children a wholesome diet and maintain a healthful lifestyle, how to allow for individual styles and preferences, and how to make shared mealtimes enjoyable as well as stress and guilt free.

This book reflects not only the writers' and editors' experience and opinion but also information reviewed by many experts. Although we have included personal anecdotes from our practices, this book represents the consensus of the 60,000 pediatrician members of the American Academy of Pediatrics. Members include pediatricians, pediatric medical subspecialists, and pediatric surgical specialists.

Nutrition: What Every Parent Needs to Know is designed to be useful at various points in your children's lives and to help solve particular problems that may arise. Because we know it may not be read straight through, some sections may be repetitious. This is deliberate. We want to make sure that a parent, grandparent, or any care provider consulting us from time to time will not miss important points that are covered in other parts of the book.

Peace, and bon appétit!

> William H. Dietz, MD, PhD, FAAP
> Loraine Stern, MD, FAAP
> Editors

Chapter 1

What's Best for My Newborn?

Like many new parents, you're probably eager to do what's "right." We want to stress at the outset that you're embarking on one of life's greatest and most rewarding adventures—namely parenthood. Usually there is no right or wrong way; instead, it's a matter of deciding what works best for you and your baby. So relax. Enjoy getting to know your new baby and trust your own sense of what's right for you.

When Laura and Jim Hawkins brought baby Emily home from the hospital, they were overjoyed and overwhelmed. "We were absolutely delighted to finally have a baby," Laura recalls, "but neither of us knew anything about infant care. Since I planned to breastfeed, I figured I'd instinctively know what to do. It didn't take long for reality to set in!" Nurses at the hospital helped Laura start breastfeeding and showed her such baby care basics as diapering and bathing. But in just 2 days, the Hawkinses were on their own at home. "For weeks we called our pediatrician almost daily with questions," Laura recounts.

Not surprisingly, many of these questions dealt with Emily's feedings. "How often should I feed her?" "How can I tell whether she's getting enough milk?" "Should I give her supplemental formula 'just in case'?" "Does she need extra iron and vitamins?" "What about water?" "Her stools are runny and yellowish. Does she have diarrhea?" "I have a bad cold. Is it safe for me to breastfeed?" "What should I do if I'm unable to nurse for a few days?"

Common Concerns

Many if not most new parents have similar concerns. In fact, parents ask pediatricians more questions about how and what to feed their babies than about any other aspect of early child care. Although this book is intended to answer the most frequently asked questions, it's important to remember that no 2 babies are exactly alike. What's good for your baby isn't necessarily good for your sister's or your neighbor's. Your pediatrician is your best source of advice about what's best for your baby, and you should not hesitate to discuss any concerns with him or her.

Decisions, Decisions

Even before your baby's birth, you need to decide how you want to feed her. Will you feed your baby breast milk or formula? The American Academy of Pediatrics (AAP), the American Dietetic Association, and other organizations concerned with health and nutrition of newborns, infants, and children advocate exclusive breastfeeding for a minimum of 4 months but preferably for 6 months (about the time your baby's diet begins to include solid foods), and to continue breastfeeding until the baby is 12 months old or as long as baby and mother want to continue.

The AAP has always advocated breastfeeding as the best way to nourish babies. Breastfeeding is best for the health of babies and mothers alike. In addition to numerous benefits, it is economical and convenient.

Breastfeeding guidelines recommend that health insurers cover necessary services and supplies. They emphasize the importance of providing workplace facilities where working mothers can pump and store milk to save for their babies.

Even though breastfeeding is a natural function, most women need help getting started. Prenatal classes often include breastfeeding instruction. Some doctors' offices and most maternity centers have lactation consultants—specially trained nurses or other health professionals—who teach the basics of breastfeeding. Maternity nurses and physicians also help teach new mothers.

In an ideal world, you should deliver your baby at a hospital whose staff can help you with breastfeeding. Unfortunately, the trend toward 24- to 48-hour hospital stays following delivery often doesn't allow enough time to ensure that all is going smoothly before going home. If problems arise after you leave the hospital, don't give up on breastfeeding and switch to bottle-feeding at the first sign of difficulty. Your pediatrician can give advice and may recommend a lactation consultant. Many of these lactation experts make home visits. There are also support groups and telephone hot lines for nursing mothers. Relatives and friends may be able to provide help as well. (See Appendix I).

THE SPECIAL HEALTH BENEFITS OF BREASTFEEDING

Pediatricians and nutrition experts agree that human milk is the ideal food for newborns and young babies. It's also inexpensive, and breastfeeding has emotional and physical benefits for the mother. Here are some of the reasons it is ideal.

- Human milk is uniquely tailored to meet almost all of your baby's nutritional needs for about the first 6 months of life. Its composition changes as your baby's needs change. For example, during the first few days the breasts secrete colostrum, which is especially rich in antibodies to protect against infections. It also contains substances that get your baby's digestive system working.

- Babies can digest human milk more easily than formula.

- Research shows that breastfed babies have fewer allergies, intestinal upsets, ear infections, and other common childhood problems than their formula-fed counterparts. If there is a family history of asthma, eczema, hay fever, or other allergies, breastfeeding is especially important in reducing the risk of allergy developing later. The longer you nurse, the better.

- The benefits of breastfeeding appear to extend beyond infancy. Studies also show that children who were breastfed have lower rates of diabetes, obesity, and certain other chronic illnesses—benefits that tend to persist into adulthood.

- Breastfeeding is cheaper and more convenient than formula.

- Because the tastes of what the mother eats appear in human milk, breastfed babies adapt more readily to new foods when they are introduced.

- A baby's suckling prompts the release of oxytocin, a pituitary hormone that, in addition to triggering the flow of breast milk, causes the uterus to contract and regain its pre-pregnancy size more quickly.

- Women who breastfeed have lower rates of certain types of breast and ovarian cancers, heart disease, and diabetes, and fewer hip fractures later in life.

HOW MANY WOMEN BREASTFEED?

A recent survey found that 80% to 90% of pregnant women wanted to breastfeed. In 2005–2006 about 77% of American mothers started nursing their babies. This figure has increased from 60% in 1993–1994 and markedly improved over the all-time low of 26.5% in 1970.

Getting Started

The offspring of any mammal instinctively seeks out a nipple and begins sucking within minutes of being born. Similarly, most human babies are alert and eager to suckle shortly after birth, provided there are no medical problems. Mothers who breastfeed while still in the delivery room typically describe a deep sense of pleasure and satisfaction. The earlier breastfeeding starts, the easier it is for mother and baby. However, if the first attempt is delayed, breastfeeding can still be initiated successfully later. Olfactory bonding—through which a baby learns to recognize his own mother's scent—develops while the mother holds her baby, even if he is not suckling. Mothers allowed to breastfeed their baby soon after delivery have their milk come in sooner than mothers who do not.

The first time you breastfeed your baby is a time when you can discover how the baby can find your nipple and start to breastfeed. One way to do this is to put the baby on your abdomen or chest using what is called *skin to skin,* where the baby's skin is in direct contact with yours. You may find it helpful to open or remove your gown so that you have nothing in the way between you and your baby. With the baby facing you, you may notice that she will start to move her body and start sucking while moving toward your nipple. Once at your nipple, the baby will begin to breastfeed. Don't worry if it takes a little time for your baby to find your nipple.

A CALM, SOOTHING ENVIRONMENT

Many mothers think that they should be able to handle everything and that breastfeeding their baby should come instinctively and immediately. But Dr Stern recalled an incident in which she was called by nurses at the hospital nursery because a newborn's blood sugar was dropping and the nurses wanted to feed her a supplemental bottle. When she arrived, she entered the room filled with relatives elated at the new addition to the family. But the new mother was exhausted—she had been up all night in labor and had delivered mid-morning. She had gotten no rest and had no time to relax and put her baby to the breast properly. The pediatrician politely asked the relatives to leave and return the next day, and once mom and baby were in a quiet room (and mom had a snack), she began breastfeeding the baby without problems. The baby's blood sugar problems vanished in no time.

At some point, you may need help positioning your baby comfortably and getting him to latch on properly. To do this, with your baby in front of you, lying on his side, belly to belly, bring his head up to your breast until his nose is level with your nipple. Hold your baby with one arm and use the other hand to support the breast. Gently stroke his lips with your nipple to stimulate his rooting reflex and interest in nursing. Position the nipple toward the upper portion of the baby's mouth (Figure 1-1). You also may try squeezing out a few drops of milk, then lightly brushing the nipple against your baby's lower lip; this will further stimulate his desire to nurse and prompt him to open his mouth wide. When his mouth is fully open, quickly bring your baby to the breast with his lips around the areola and the nipple deep in his mouth (Figure 1-2). When your baby is ready, let him position his lips around the areola with the nipple deep in his mouth. Make sure your baby's face is not at an angle to your nipple but facing straight on to your breast. Your baby's chest and abdomen also should be facing directly toward your chest and abdomen. His neck should be straight and not turned.

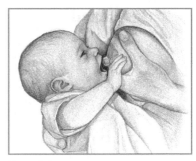

Figure 1-1

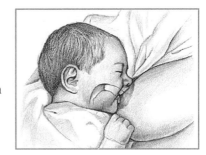

Figure 1-2

NURSING CRAMPS (ALSO KNOWN AS AFTER-BIRTH PAINS)
For a few days after delivery, many women have cramping pain in the abdomen at the start of each feeding. This is because breastfeeding stimulates the release of hormones that help shrink the uterus back to its normal size. You can ease nursing cramps by emptying your bladder before you start to breastfeed (a full bladder will make the cramps more intense). You can relieve the nursing cramps by not lying flat on your back; instead sit up "pretzel style" with your legs folded in front of you. This helps bring your uterus forward and relieves the pressure. You can also take a prescribed pain medication.

Latching On

It's important to position the nipple far back in your baby's mouth so that it touches the roof of her mouth and she is able to compress the *areola,* which is the dark area around your nipple (Figure 1-3).

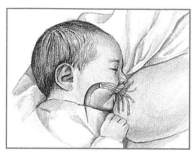

Figure 1-3

If she latches on to only the nipple, milk can dribble out the side of her mouth. In addition, sucking on the nipple alone can make it sore and cracked, leading to excessive pain during nursing. You'll soon be able to feel whether your baby is suckling properly; in the beginning, check that the nipple and most of the areola are inside your baby's mouth, with her nose and chin just touching the breast and the lips looking like her mouth is wide open. Her jaws should move up and down, and she should swallow after every few sucks. If you have continuing pain, take your baby off the breast and reposition her. If your breasts are large and your baby's nose is buried, draw her bottom and legs closer to your midsection and lift your breast up a bit from underneath to let your baby breathe from the sides of her nose as she nurses.

When your baby stops nursing, gently break the suction by inserting a finger in the corner of her mouth. This lets in some air and encourages your baby to let go. To prevent injury to the nipple, do not pull your baby off the breast while she is still suckling and tightly attached.

Finding the Right Position

Almost all nursing mothers describe breastfeeding as a highly pleasurable experience, but to make it so, you need to find a position that is comfortable for you and your baby. Experiment with the following positions until you find what works best for you at various times:

Lying Down (Figure 1-4)

You and your baby lie on your sides facing each other. Bring the baby toward your breast and allow her to latch on. Place a pillow under your head and another behind your back so you can be comfortable. A pillow between your knees is also comfortable. Women recovering from a cesarean delivery often find this the most comfortable position; it's also good for night feedings. After the feedings, put your baby back in his crib. It's the safest place for him to sleep. Keep your baby's crib as close to your bed as possible. This will make it easier to breastfeed during the night.

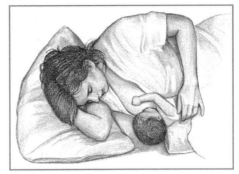

Figure 1-4

Cradle Hold (Figure 1-5)

Sit in a comfortable chair or in bed with pillows tucked behind your back, under your arm on the nursing side, and on your lap to support your baby. Position your baby on his side with his tummy close to yours, his head cradled in the crook of your arm with his face next to your breast, his back resting along your forearm, and his bottom supported by your hand. In this and other positions, he should be able to latch on without turning his head. If your baby is very small or has a weak sucking reflex, try supporting the back of his head with your other hand rather than placing it in the crook of your elbow. (This is sometimes called the modified cradle or transitional hold.)

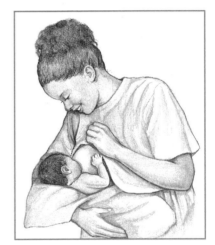

Figure 1-5

Clutch, Side, or Football Hold (Figure 1-6)

Sit in a comfortable chair (a roomy rocker is ideal) with a pillow on your lap to bring your baby up level with your breast. Position him with his legs under your arm and his head resting on your hand. If your arm gets tired, support it on a pillow or your thigh (bend your knee and place your foot on a stool or low table).

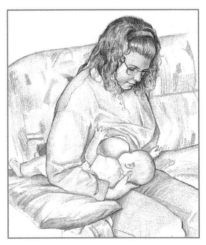

Figure 1-6

The side position works especially well if you have large breasts or flat nipples, or after a cesarean delivery.

Breastfeeding and Intelligence

Several studies of children's development reveal some intriguing findings about the relationship between breastfeeding and intelligence. Children who had been nourished on human milk did slightly but consistently better on standard tests in school than those who were fed formula. The longer they were breastfed, the better they did. What's more, the advantages persisted well beyond early childhood. The breastfed children were more likely to complete high school irrespective of their family income, education, and standard of living, among other factors. Thus, breastfed babies appear not only to be healthier but also to do better in school.

Breast milk's nutritional factors, its effect on lower rate of illnesses, and its psychological effects may also help explain breastfed children's better performance in school.

Vitamins for Breastfed Babies

Human milk provides sufficient amounts of vitamins, except for vitamin D. Vitamin D helps absorb calcium and is needed to build healthy bones and teeth. Although human milk contains small amounts of vitamin D, it is not enough to prevent rickets (softening of the bones). Your pediatrician should prescribe a vitamin D supplement for your breastfed baby; in fact, the AAP recommends that *all* breastfed babies receive 400 IU of oral vitamin D drops, starting during the first few days of life and continuing until they are drinking vitamin D-fortified formula or milk (500 mL or about 17 oz). Most commercial formulas are fortified with vitamin D and other vitamins to ensure that babies get enough of these essential nutrients.

A mother who follows a vegan diet, which excludes all foods of animal origin, should talk to her pediatrician about her baby's vitamin needs. A vegan diet lacks vitamins D and B_{12}. A vitamin B_{12} deficiency in an baby's diet can lead to anemia and nervous system abnormalities.

For many years, some doctors have told parents that babies in highly allergic families may react to certain foods the mother eats that then pass into the breast milk, such as the protein from cow's milk or cheese, or from eggs, seafood, and nuts. However, the AAP has concluded that at this time, there is no evidence that dietary restrictions in a nursing mother can play a significant role in preventing allergic diseases such as eczema, food allergy, or asthma. In rare cases, such as certain metabolic diseases, a baby may not be able to tolerate human milk and will need a special formula. A physical abnormality that makes it difficult for a baby to suckle normally, such as a cleft palate, may make breastfeeding impossible (see "Cleft Lip" and "Cleft Palate" on page 22). Mothers should remember that their pumped milk should be the first choice for any baby that needs a supplemental feed.

Formula Feeding

Breastfeeding has many advantages (see "The Special Health Benefits of Breastfeeding" on page 3), but there are instances in which it is not possible (for example, when a baby has a condition such as classic galactosemia, also known as GALT deficiency, which is a rare, inborn inability to digest a type of sugar [lactose] in milk). A mother may also be advised not to breastfeed when she is HIV positive or has a serious disorder, such as hepatitis B or tuberculosis, that could be passed in the breast milk, or takes medication that might harm her baby (see "Why Some Women Should Not Breastfeed" on page 15). Personal factors may make nursing impossible, and some women or their partners are not comfortable with the idea or harbor mistaken notions about what it entails (see "Common Myths About Breastfeeding" on page 24). At any rate, learn as much as possible about breastfeeding well before your due date and talk over the pros and cons with your obstetrician and pediatrician to make the best decision for your baby and yourself.

There are many kinds of infant formulas; most are based on cow's milk, but there are also several formulas available for babies who cannot tolerate cow's milk. Regular cow's and goat's milk, as well as canned condensed or evaporated milk, should not be given during the first year of life. Young babies cannot digest the protein in cow's milk. Regular cow's milk also doesn't have enough iron and other vitamins or the right amounts of the minerals that are essential for proper growth and development. A child may lose blood through the stools because cow's milk can damage the intestine.

PRACTICAL BOTTLE-FEEDING TIPS

- Bottle-feeding can be a warm, loving experience—cuddle your baby closely, gaze into her eyes, and coo and talk to her. Never prop the bottle and let your baby feed alone; not only will you miss the opportunity to bond with her while she feeds, but there's also a danger that she'll choke or the bottle will slip out of position. Propping the bottle also increases the risk of ear infections. We do not recommend devices to hold a bottle in a baby's mouth—they could be dangerous.

- Although some babies will drink a bottle straight from the refrigerator, most prefer milk warmed to room temperature. You can warm a bottle by placing it in a bowl of hot water for a few minutes. Sprinkle a few drops on your wrist; it should feel lukewarm. If it's too warm, wait for it to cool a bit and test again.

  Note: *Never* warm a bottle of formula or human milk in the microwave. The bottle itself may feel cool while the liquid inside can be too hot. Microwaving also heats unevenly. Even though a few drops sprinkled on your wrist may feel OK, some of the formula or human milk may be scalding. The composition of human milk may change if it is warmed too much, as well.

- Make sure the nipple hole is the right size. If your baby seems to be gagging or gulping too fast, the nipple hole may be too large. If your baby is sucking hard and seems frustrated, the hole may be too small.

- Try different nipple shapes to see which your baby prefers. There is no correct shape.

- Angle the bottle so your baby isn't sucking in air. Burp your baby a couple of times during the course of a feeding.

- Encourage your partner to give your baby a bottle now and then, perhaps one of the late-night feedings. This not only allows you some extra rest, but it also fosters bonding with your baby.

- Don't let your baby fall asleep sucking on a bottle of milk, especially if she is beginning to cut teeth. Milk pooled in your baby's mouth can cause serious tooth decay, known as nursing-bottle caries. After feeding and before putting your baby to sleep, gently wipe any milk residue from her gums. If she needs to suck herself to sleep, give her a pacifier instead of a bottle.

- Repeated sterilization may distort nipple openings. Test to make sure milk flow through the nipple is adequate.

A baby may have a problem that requires a special formula as the primary food or as a supplement to human milk. For example, premature or low birth weight babies may need special formulas to supply the extra energy and nutrients they need for growth. In these small babies

---

INFANT FORMULAS COME IN 3 FORMS

- The ready-to-use types are the most convenient—all you need to do is pour them into a clean bottle—but they are also the most expensive.

- Concentrated liquid formulas are mixed with an equal amount of water; these are not as costly as the ready-to-use type, but you must make sure that the water is clean.

- Powdered formulas are the least expensive; they also require the most preparation.

---

the sucking reflex may not be fully developed, in which case they will be fed with a special tube or by bottle. Still, a premature baby can benefit from the antibodies and other unique components of human milk. Mothers of premature and other high-risk babies are usually encouraged to express their breast milk, which may be fortified with the additional nutrients needed and fed to her baby. When the baby is ready to breastfeed directly from mother, the switch can be made.

What's in It for My Baby?

Although no formulas on the market even come close to matching the hundreds of known ingredients in human milk, most provide a comparable balance of fat, protein, and sugar. Formulas are also supplemented with various vitamins and minerals, especially calcium, iron, and vitamins C, D, and K. Should you choose not to breastfeed, your pediatrician can advise which formula is most suitable for your baby. Regardless of which formula you use, it's critical that you prepare it according to instructions. It is especially important not to add more or less water than recommended.

Families who are short of money may be tempted to add extra water to make the formula go farther. Formulas are designed to provide the energy (about 20 calories per ounce) and nutrients that a baby needs for proper growth. If the formula is diluted, your baby will be underfed and may have stunted growth and develop serious nutritional deficiencies. Formula that is too concentrated can also be dangerous. Not adding enough water can result in dehydration, kidney problems, and other potentially serious disorders.

Sterilizing and Warming Bottles

Parents and pediatricians today are not as concerned with sterilizing bottles and water as they were a generation ago, but many are now having second thoughts in light of recent reports of contaminated city water supplies and increased concern over food safety. For starters, always wash your hands before handling baby bottles or feeding your baby. If you use disposable plastic bottle liners and ready-to-use formula, you still need to make sure the nipples are clean. Scrub them in hot, soapy water, then rinse to get rid of all traces of soap; some experts recommend boiling them for 5 minutes. Always wash and thoroughly rinse and dry the top of the formula can before you open it; make sure the can opener, mixing cups, jars, spoons, and other equipment are clean.

If you use regular glass bottles and concentrated or powdered formula, you must make sure that the bottles and water added to the formula are germ free. You don't need to boil the bottles; you can put them, along with mixing cups and other equipment used to prepare formula, in a dishwasher that uses heated water and has a hot drying cycle. Or you can wash the bottles in hot, soapy water and rinse thoroughly. This alone should kill most germs.

Water for mixing infant formula must be from a safe water source as defined by the state or local health department. If you are concerned or uncertain about the safety of tap water, you may use bottled water or bring cold tap water to a rolling boil for 1 minute (no longer), then cool the water to room temperature for no more than 30 minutes before it is used. Warmed water should be tested in advance to make sure it is not too hot for the baby. The easiest way to test the temperature is to shake a few drops on the inside of your wrist. Otherwise, a bottle can be prepared by adding powdered formula and room-temperature water from the tap just before feeding. Bottles made in this way from powdered formula can be ready for feeding because no additional refrigeration or warming would be required. Prepared formula must be discarded within 1 hour after serving a baby. Prepared formula that has not been given to a baby may be stored in the refrigerator for 24 hours to prevent bacterial contamination. An open container of ready-to-feed, concentrated formula, or formula prepared from concentrated formula, should be covered, refrigerated, and discarded after 48 hours if not used.

Supplemental Bottles

Many breastfeeding mothers use an occasional bottle of expressed, frozen breast milk or formula because they need to be away from the baby. In unusual cases, a pediatrician may

HOW TO STORE AND PREPARE YOUR EXPRESSED MILK

Follow these safe storage and preparation tips to keep your expressed milk healthy for your baby.

- Wash your hands before expressing or handling your milk.

- Be sure to use only clean containers to store expressed milk. Try to use screw-cap bottles, hard plastic cups with tight caps, or special heavy nursing bags that can be used to feed your baby. *Do not use ordinary plastic storage bags or formula bottle bags because these can easily split and leak.* Do not store human milk in ice-cube trays.

- For a normal, healthy baby at home, use sealed and chilled milk within 24 hours if possible. Discard all milk that has been refrigerated for more than 96 hours. For newborns who are hospitalized, follow hospital guidelines for human milk storage.

- Freeze milk if you do not plan to use it within 24 hours. Frozen milk is good for at least 1 month in a freezer attached to a refrigerator or for 3 to 6 months if kept in a 0° deep freezer. Store it in the back of the freezer where the temperature is coldest, not in the door. Also, keep the freezer full to maintain lowest temperatures. Be sure to label the milk with the date and time that you expressed it. Use the oldest milk first. Keep in mind that the fats in human milk begin to break down with storage, so using frozen human milk within 3 months is desirable.

- Freeze about 2 to 4 oz of milk per container to avoid wasting milk after you thaw it. You can always thaw an extra bag if needed.

- Do not add fresh milk to already frozen milk in a storage container.

- You may thaw milk in the refrigerator or by placing it in a bowl of warm water.

- Do not use microwave ovens to heat bottles because they do not heat them evenly. Uneven heating can scald your baby or damage the milk. Bottles can also explode if left in the microwave too long. Excessive heat can destroy important proteins and vitamins in the milk.

- Previously frozen milk that has been thawed in the refrigerator must be used within 24 hours or discarded.

- Do not refreeze your milk.

- Do not save unfinished milk from a partially consumed bottle to use at another feeding.

recommend a combination of breastfeeding and formula if the mother is returning to work or if she is ill or exhausted. It is commonly—though often wrongly—thought that supplemental bottles are given because the mother does not have enough milk. As stressed earlier, almost all mothers produce more than enough milk to meet their babies' needs, even for twins. When there appears to be a problem of supply and demand, your pediatrician may encourage you to see a lactation consultant.

If supplemental bottles are given for the sake of convenience, experts advise waiting until your baby is 3 or 4 weeks old. This allows time for your milk supply to become well established and for you and your baby to get used to breastfeeding. To obtain the benefits of human milk, it is best if you express your breast milk and store it for bottle-feeding as needed. Expressing breast milk also helps maintain your milk supply. Formula can be fed while you continue breastfeeding as often as possible. Use the formula your pediatrician recommends. Don't be surprised if your baby doesn't immediately take to a bottle.

DISCARD ANY LEFTOVERS

A Note of Caution: If your baby does not drink the entire bottle, discard what's left over. Germs and enzymes from your baby's mouth can enter the bottle and spoil the milk.

Breastfeeding Problem Solving

Many women breastfeed with nary a problem, but others may encounter difficulties. Many initial problems are due to an incorrect latch that, when corrected, relieves the difficulty. Fortunately, most problems are easily solved. If the measures outlined as follows don't work, talk to your doctor or a lactation consultant.

Inverted or Flat Nipples

Inverted or flat nipples do not rule out nursing and in many cases can be corrected. After the baby is born, you can do exercises or use an electric pump (for a few pumps before a feed) to help the nipples lengthen. Once the nipples lengthen, your baby will be able to latch on easily. Other devices are sometimes recommended, but they often don't work and can make the breasts sore and promote infection. Nipple shields may be recommended under certain circumstances, but only if your pediatrician or lactation consultant agrees.

Engorgement (Overfilled Breasts)

This usually occurs in the first few days when milk first comes in or when you cut back on nursing, resulting in overfilled breasts. Engorgement usually can be prevented by frequent nursing and draining the breasts. Make sure your baby is suckling properly. If your breasts are producing more milk than your baby can consume, try placing the baby in a more upright position, which may decrease the flow of milk. Or you may need to express the excess before he latches on. If pain is hindering your milk flow (letdown), taking a warm shower or applying a warm compress before nursing may help. Some women find that cold compresses or ice packs provide more relief. Occasionally using a breast pump may also help. Experiment to find what works best for you. But above all, don't cut back on your breastfeeding; this will only worsen the problem. Regular, frequent breastfeeding is the best way to prevent and relieve engorgement.

WHY SOME WOMEN SHOULD NOT BREASTFEED

Doctors advise women not to breastfeed under the following conditions:

- If they have certain infectious diseases, a positive HIV test or AIDS, human T-cell leukemia virus infection, or untreated tuberculosis that could be passed on to their babies.

- If they must take medications—such as cyclosporine, antithyroid medications, or drugs that suppress the immune system—that pass into the breast milk and are harmful to babies. Most medicines prescribed by your physician are likely to be safe for breastfed babies, but it's best to ask your physician to check them. If you're breastfeeding, always check with your pediatrician before taking any nonprescription, herbal, folk, or natural remedies.

- If they use marijuana, cocaine, heroin, amphetamines, or other illegal drugs.

- If their breasts lack enough glandular tissue to make milk. This is very rare and is unrelated to breast size (women with small breasts can produce as much milk as large-breasted women).

- Women who have chronic or debilitating medical conditions may be advised not to breastfeed.

- Some doctors think that women with silicone breast implants should not breastfeed, but there is no evidence that implants harm children.

Cracked or Sore Nipples

First, try to find out the cause. Most often, it turns out that the nipple is incorrectly placed in the baby's mouth. The best treatment is making sure that the baby does place the nipple and dark area around the nipple into his mouth, as this will prevent cracked or sore nipples. If soreness develops in the first few weeks of breastfeeding, check to make sure your baby is latching on properly, with most of the areola in his mouth. He may be chewing or gumming on the nipple, or perhaps his lower lip is turned inward, which can lead to soreness and even cracking.

Keep in mind that a few seconds of sharp pain at the onset of nursing is normal for the first week or two. But if this pain persists throughout the breastfeeding session, contact your pediatrician.

To heal the nipples, try expressing a few drops of colostrum or mature milk and rubbing it gently into the sore area. Allow the milk to dry on the nipples. Wash them with plain water and avoid using soap, which promotes cracking by removing protective skin oils. Don't use ointments or creams unless specifically recommended by your doctor. Ultra-purified anhydrous lanolin may promote healing and does not need to be removed from the nipples before nursing.

Poor Milk Letdown

Letdown is the automatic release of milk stored in breast tissue into the milk ducts, allowing it to flow more easily into your baby's mouth. Suckling stimulates the letdown reflex; infrequent nursing or a poor latch on to the breast can hinder it. Stress, pain, fatigue, anxiety, nicotine, alcohol, and certain medications are among the many factors that can inhibit letdown. In most instances, you can solve letdown problems by frequent nursing and properly positioning your baby on the breast. You should also try to reduce stress and avoid alcohol and caffeine. Before breastfeeding, try massaging your breasts, gently rubbing your nipples, applying warm compresses, or taking a warm shower. When using a breast pump, mental images of your baby nursing can also trigger release of the hormone (oxytocin) that prompts letdown. In some women, just hearing a baby cry triggers letdown. If none of these tactics work, ask your doctor or lactation consultant for advice.

Leaky Breasts

Leaking is most common in the early weeks of breastfeeding, but it's not unusual for it to continue for weeks or even months. Sometimes leaking occurs when you're not breastfeeding. Also, some women leak without a letdown, just from continuing overproduction, which can be alleviated by expressing some milk. Many women leak milk when their breasts are stimulated during sexual activity. Wearing breast shells too long can also promote leaking. Cotton nursing pads tucked into your bra help minimize staining. Change pads frequently and avoid using plastic coverings, which can promote bacterial growth and skin problems. You can also stop the milk flow by using the bottom of your hand to apply pressure to your nipples.

Plugged or Caked Milk Duct

A sore breast lump and decreased milk flow without a fever or other symptoms of mastitis (see below) may indicate an obstructed or plugged duct. Possible causes include infrequent nursing, incomplete softening or draining of the breast, and engorgement. To dislodge the plug, try applying a warm compress and then massaging the breast to stimulate milk flow just before breastfeeding. Breastfeed frequently on that side to clear the plugged area. Place the baby's nose or chin in the direction of the plugged duct; this will help drain that area more effectively. If symptoms continue, see your physician.

Mastitis

Mastitis is caused by a bacterial infection in the breast. It typically develops in only one breast and starts with fatigue, achy muscles, fever, and other flu-like symptoms, followed by breast inflammation and pain. Mild cases may require only rest, frequent nursing (or pumping) to drain the breast, and warm compresses to relieve pain. If you develop a fever, make an appointment to be checked by your health care professional. More severe cases can be cleared up with antibiotics. Breastfeeding can and should continue in nearly all cases. If an abscess forms, it may have to be drained. See your doctor promptly if you develop symptoms or signs of mastitis.

Baby Problem Solving

Like most new mothers, Jasmine felt a bit overwhelmed by the responsibility of caring for a brand-new baby, even though her husband was supportive and both of them had prepared thoroughly at parenting classes. Four days after they brought their baby home, Jasmine was worried that she wasn't producing enough milk. Responding to her pediatrician's questions at an office visit, Jasmine told him that the baby nursed vigorously every 2 to 3 hours and slept after each feeding. Her breasts felt full before feedings and softened after the baby nursed. The baby had passed 2 loose stools each day since they came home, and Jasmine was changing wet diapers about 6 times a day.

"There's nothing to worry about," the pediatrician told Jasmine. "You're doing a great job and your baby is beautiful. Call me if you have any questions."

Wet diapers are an important guide to whether babies are feeding well. However, the absorbent qualities of some of the newest, stay-dry disposable diapers can make it hard to tell if a baby has urinated. It may be best to avoid superabsorbent diapers for the first few weeks until you and your baby have settled into a routine.

Spitting Up

Most babies spit up varying amounts of milk or formula, often for no apparent reason and with no health consequences. Spitting up, or *reflux* of some stomach contents back into the esophagus, should not be confused with vomiting—the forceful expulsion of a large amount or most of the stomach contents. Reflux becomes a problem if the baby develops esophagitis, which causes pain. In adults, this pain is called heartburn. A baby with esophagitis becomes irritable shortly after feedings begin. The baby may appear hungry and start to feed eagerly

---

WARNING ON WATER

Healthy babies do not need extra water. Human milk or formula provides all the fluids they need. A small amount of water may be needed in very hot weather, but check with your pediatrician about how much is safe. The American Academy of Pediatrics warns that during the exclusive nursing period (a minimum of 4 months but preferably for 6 months), giving a lot of water carries a risk of water intoxication and may interfere with human milk intake. With the introduction of solid foods, water can be added to your baby's diet.

but then begin to cry or fuss as if in pain. If your baby has these symptoms or becomes fussy during feedings, consult your pediatrician. You probably don't need to worry about spitting up so long as your baby is growing normally, wetting at least 6 to 8 diapers a day, and having normal bowel movements. To reduce spitting up, hold your baby quietly upright for a few minutes after each feeding. In bottle-fed infants, intolerance to an ingredient in the formula or a response to supplements may trigger vomiting but not spitting up. If you suspect a problem, consult your pediatrician. (Also see Chapter 9, Spitting Up, Gagging, Vomiting, Diarrhea, and Constipation.)

Gas

When 2-week-old Alex cried hard after feedings, drew his knees up, and passed gas repeatedly, his mother called her pediatrician. "Is it colic? My mother warned me about it."

After a few questions, the pediatrician was able to reassure this mother that her baby wasn't colicky. Alex was calmer after passing gas, he spat up very little, and he was sleeping well between feedings.

"Alex's digestive tract is getting used to food. It's developing a balance of the normal bacteria we need for digestion. The gas is a normal part of this process; it shows that your baby is adapting well to life on the outside."

Colic

Dr Stern's rule for recognizing colic: "You know your baby has colic when you have an irresistible urge to get him his own apartment." Colic is marked by long periods of crying that seem to come from abdominal cramping and discomfort, and the baby cannot be comforted. The spells, which have no apparent cause, typically occur at about the same time every afternoon or evening. Colic usually develops between 2 and 6 weeks of age and disappears in 3 or 4 months. In contrast to simple gas, the crying does not stop after the baby passes gas. While colic lasts, parents and baby suffer. No one knows what causes colic. It occurs more often in bottle-fed babies but can also appear in breastfed infants; it is also more common in first babies. Sometimes, but not very often, changing the mother's diet helps (see Chapter 15, Alternative Diets and Supplements). You might try eliminating cow's milk from your diet as well as other sensitizing foods such as wheat, peanuts, eggs, and seafood. You're more likely to be successful in calming your baby if you experiment with soothing tactics such as rocking, walking, playing music, gently massaging, or going for a car ride. You should consult your pediatrician to make sure the crying is not caused by a medical problem.

Constipation

Some breastfed babies go for several days without having a bowel movement. As long as the stool is soft and easily passed and your baby is growing normally, there's no need for concern. But you should consult your pediatrician if the stools are hard or your baby's tummy is hard and distended.

Some babies cry or even scream, tighten up their legs, and seem as though they were being tortured—and then pass a normal, soft stool, after which they relax. This is not constipation but rather part of normal development. This phase tends to end in a week or two. As long as the stool is soft when it comes out, do not worry.

Diarrhea

Loose stools do not necessarily mean diarrhea. If your baby has no other symptoms and is gaining weight normally, her runny stools may be what are normal for her. But if she has large, frequent, watery stools; a fever; or other symptoms, call your pediatrician. If your baby is dehydrated, she may need a rehydrating solution. In most cases, breastfeeding or bottle-feeding can continue until the problem clears up, but follow your pediatrician's instructions.

Sleepy Baby

Most babies are born alert and eager to feed in the first hour or so of life. Experts recommend feeding a newborn for about 30 minutes. Typically, a baby will then fall asleep and wake up every 2 or 3 hours to nurse. But some babies are sleepy in the first day or two. They often need to be awakened to feed, and even then they may fall asleep after only a few minutes of nursing. Often, cooling your baby down by removing some clothing or a blanket will help wake her up. Or try talking or singing to her, stroking her head, rubbing her buttocks or back, or wiping her face with a damp cloth. It's important that you get her to nurse for long enough to get the milk she needs for proper growth and to drain your breasts to ensure steady milk production. If you have problems keeping her awake to feed, consult your pediatrician.

Fussy Eater

Babies, like everyone else, have taste preferences. If your baby has been feeding normally and suddenly seems unhappy with your milk, suspect something you've eaten. The tastes of onions, garlic, cabbage, and other strong-flavored foods can pass into your milk, and the first time may surprise your baby. Most babies get to like new tastes; babies may even like the taste of garlic. If your baby stays fussy, try eliminating possibly offending foods one at a time for a week. Then eat the eliminated food again. If it provokes a reaction, eliminate the food until you stop nursing.

Breastmilk Jaundice

Many newborns have a yellowish tinge to their skin, which is known as *jaundice.* The yellowing is caused by excess blood levels of bilirubin, a pigment normally eliminated by the liver. For unknown reasons, something in breast milk triggers jaundice in susceptible babies. In nearly all cases, breastfeeding should continue, but your pediatrician will monitor your baby's bilirubin level. If it is very high, you may be advised to stop breastfeeding for a day or so to lower the bilirubin level. During this time, you can keep up the milk flow with a breast pump until your baby is ready to breastfeed again. Interrupting breastfeeding for a day or so promptly results in a decrease in jaundice and you may safely resume breastfeeding. Sometimes, your doctor may advise you to continue breastfeeding and place your baby under special lights to reduce the bilirubin level.

Weak Suck

Most babies are born with a strong rooting reflex and have no trouble suckling, even when they are only minutes old. Occasionally, however, a baby has difficulty sucking. Some premature babies have a weak suck. Also, even though babies born at 37 weeks may not be officially considered premature, they can have some of the same problems including a weak suck.

Telltale signs of a weak suck include losing hold of the breast, possible choking or gagging, and milk leaking from your baby's mouth. Sometimes a weak suck in a newborn is caused by medications given to the mother during birth; if so, it should disappear as the medicines clear from your baby's system. Changing position to give your baby a better latch on may help. But if the problem persists, your pediatrician should evaluate your baby for a possible physical problem or illness.

Growth

Breastfed babies have a different growth pattern than formula-fed babies. In general, exclusively breastfed infants tend to gain weight more rapidly in the first 2 to 3 months. From 6 to 12 months breastfed infants tend to weigh less than formula-fed infants. This is normal and no cause for concern so long as the length increases are steady. (See growth charts in Appendix C.)

Tongue Abnormalities

Rarely, a baby is born with a tongue abnormality that prevents proper latching on or suckling. Your pediatrician can advise you how to handle the problem.

Cleft Lip

Babies born with a cleft lip can usually suckle normally, although the split in the lip will allow some milk to leak from your baby's mouth. You may have to experiment with positions to help your baby latch on; a nurse or lactation consultant can help you get started.

Cleft Palate

A cleft palate prevents a baby from effective suckling, but there are techniques to help babies feed. For example, a baby may be fitted with an appliance to temporarily seal the hole in the palate and make suckling easier. Breast milk is particularly beneficial for babies with cleft palate because it reduces the risk of ear and lung infections, to which they are especially susceptible.

IS YOUR BABY CRYING FROM HUNGER?

All babies cry, some more than others. The reasons are usually hunger, pain, discomfort, or loneliness. They may also cry when they are tired or overly stimulated and need to release tension. There may be fussy periods during the day when nothing you do calms the baby down, but after that fussy period passes, the baby will become calm on her own and may go to sleep. At first you may respond by trying to feed her every time she fusses, but that can lead to overfeeding, especially if the baby is bottle-fed. If you are breastfeeding for the first time, you may think that you do not have enough milk to satisfy her.

After a long sleep, your baby will wake up hungry and you will get to know the quality of that cry. If it is not time for a feeding, try soothing techniques such as rocking, swaddling, singing, walking, burping, or talking in a low voice. Despite what some people say, you will not spoil your baby by holding her when she needs it.

Crying patterns change in the first few months of life; babies cry more often in the first 6 weeks and then crying slows down. The peak time for crying in the second month seems to be in the early evening (what Dr Stern calls the "unhappy hour"). This is also the end of your day and you may be tired and frustrated. If you cannot soothe your baby, allow her some alone time in the crib to see if she can learn to soothe herself. That does not mean you should leave her for an hour, but give her 10 minutes or so to calm down. By 4 months of age, she may stop crying as soon as you enter her room—a dead giveaway that she just needs your presence—or she may have learned that this means she is going to be fed. You will know the difference.

The point is that not all crying is from hunger. You will learn the differences in your baby's cries over the first few weeks—the high-pitched shriek of pain and distress versus the hunger cry.

Is Milk Really Enough?

Yes, for about 4 to 6 months of life. Pediatricians now agree that other foods should not be given until about this time. Still, many well-meaning grandparents, aunts, and others who reared their children in the 1960s and 1970s advise earlier feeding of different foods.

When Gladys Evans became a mother in 1970, her obstetrician discouraged her from breastfeeding and her pediatrician respected her decision to use formula. Her baby, Sally, was healthy and active and at her 8-week checkup, she had gained 3 pounds since birth. At that point, her pediatrician recommended starting Sally on rice cereal thinned with

COMMON MYTHS ABOUT BREASTFEEDING	
MYTH	**FACTS**
You can't get pregnant while breastfeeding.	While it's true that breastfeeding prevents ovulation in some women, it is not a reliable form of birth control. Talk to your doctor about an acceptable form of contraception. Avoid estrogen-containing birth control pills.
You need to toughen your nipples before your baby is born.	Your body naturally prepares for breastfeeding. Tactics to toughen them may actually interfere with normal lactation.
Small breasts don't produce as much milk as large ones.	Breast size has nothing to do with the amount of milk they produce.
Breastfeeding will ruin the shape of your breasts.	Most women find that their breasts go back to their pre-pregnancy size and shape after they stop nursing. Age, the effects of gravity, and weight gain have more effect on breast size than nursing. Breasts will always change in consistency after pregnancy.
Sexual arousal while breast-feeding is abnormal.	Many women experience sexual arousal while nursing. Breast stimulation is an important aspect of sexual activity, so it stands to reason that nursing can also arouse sexual feelings. In addition, oxytocin—the hormone released during breastfeeding—is also released during orgasm, another reason why nursing can be sexually stimulating.
All babies should be weaned before their first birthday.	When to stop breastfeeding is a highly personal decision and varies considerably according to custom and individual preferences. The American Academy of Pediatrics recommends breastfeeding for a minimum of 4 months but preferably for 6 months (about the time your baby's diet begins to include solid foods), and continue breastfeeding until the baby is 12 months old or as long as baby and mother want to continue.

formula and progressing to pureed and strained fruit a week or so later, followed by strained vegetables a couple of weeks after that.

"At first, Sally simply spit out most of the cereal," Gladys recalls, "but then I tried putting the food way back on her tongue so she had to swallow it. After that, I didn't have any problems getting her to eat."

Now that Gladys is a grandmother, it's understandable that she is worried about the way Sally is feeding her own baby. "He's almost 5 months old and he's still on nothing but breast milk," Gladys explains. "Is this really enough?"

Changing Views

As Gladys's example shows, views on infant feeding have changed over the last few decades. Pediatricians and nutrition experts now know that giving foods other than human milk in the first few months of life is detrimental for several reasons.

- Until babies are at least 4 months old, their digestive systems have trouble breaking down the starches and components of other foods.
- An immature digestive system may allow whole proteins to be absorbed, thus setting the stage for an allergic reaction, especially if there is a family history of allergies. By 4 months, the digestive system can break down proteins into their amino acid building blocks, which are less likely to provoke allergies.
- When a spoon touches a young baby's tongue, it triggers an automatic reflex, in which the tongue thrusts forward and prevents swallowing. This reflex is called the extrusion reflex; it disappears at about 3 to 4 months of age.

Human milk provides all the nutrients that a healthy baby needs for about the first 6 months of life. Breastfeeding also benefits the mother (see "The Special Health Benefits of Breastfeeding" on page 3).

Eating for 2

During pregnancy and while breastfeeding, you are eating for yourself and your baby. Indeed, your health and nutrition during pregnancy are big factors in determining your baby's nutritional needs. Ideally, sound infant nutrition begins even before conception. It's a good idea to have a thorough pre-pregnancy checkup to make sure you are not anemic or don't have hidden nutritional, metabolic, or other problems. Your doctor will advise you about what supplements you need during pregnancy and how much weight you should gain, as well as foods and substances you should avoid. Be sure to tell your doctor if you follow a vegetarian diet or one that excludes certain foods. It may be advisable for you to take a vitamin supplement during pregnancy and the same one while breastfeeding.

As part of your plan to breastfeed, you should continue eating a healthful diet that provides the extra energy and nutrients you need to make milk. In the past, breastfeeding mothers were advised to consume an extra 400 or 500 calories a day and to drink at least 8 glasses of water and other fluids. Doctors now recognize that there are no set rules—some women may need an extra 500 calories, while others will gain unwanted pounds by eating this much. The best rule is to eat and drink enough to satisfy your hunger and thirst. Follow the *Dietary Guidelines for Americans* (www.cnpp.usda.gov/DietaryGuidelines.htm) with ample fresh or lightly processed fruits and vegetables to provide essential vitamins and minerals. Nursing mothers eating a balanced diet do not require any added calcium. If there is a family history of allergies, they may prefer to minimize drinking cow's milk while nursing so that their babies are not exposed to excess cow's milk protein.

Certain strongly flavored foods and spices can affect the taste and composition of breast milk and may cause digestive problems in babies. A common culprit is cabbage. Most babies develop a liking for garlic and onions after the initial surprise. Garlic and spices need not be avoided unless your baby continues to react negatively to them. Excessive caffeine (more than 5 cups a day of coffee or other caffeinated beverages, such as tea and sodas) may make your baby jittery and fussy. In addition, caffeine and nicotine decrease milk flow. A cup of coffee in the morning probably will not have an effect; still, if something in your diet seems to upset your baby's appetite or disposition, eliminate it for the time being. You may, however, need to keep a food diary to identify the offending food.

Important No-nos

Because much of what you eat and drink can enter your breast milk, it's important that you avoid any substance that can harm your baby. Here are a few commonsense rules to follow.

Always Check With Your Pediatrician Before Taking Any Medication, Prescription and Over-the-counter Products, as Well as Herbal or Natural Remedies

Although most medications can be taken while breastfeeding, some medications that are not recommended during breastfeeding include some blood-pressure–lowering medications, certain antibiotics, antithyroid medications, and cancer chemotherapy drugs. Many people mistakenly assume that over-the-counter drugs and herbal remedies have no adverse effects; this is not true. Even aspirin in human milk can cause problems in a baby. Herbal remedies can be toxic, especially to babies. However, most over-the-counter products sold to relieve common symptoms such as headache and indigestion are acceptable, although you should check with your doctor before taking them.

If You Smoke, Now Is the Time to Stop

Not only does nicotine enter your breast milk, but it also lowers the amount of milk you produce. If you can't quit, at least cut down as much you can. And if necessary, smoke immediately after breastfeeding so that the nicotine levels in the breast milk will be as low as possible. Remember, too, that secondhand smoke is especially dangerous for your baby. Don't allow smoking in your house or car and certainly not around or near your baby.

Avoid Alcohol While You Are Breastfeeding

Doctors agree that substance abusers (those who use drugs such as marijuana, cocaine, heroin, and amphetamines) should not nurse at all. Alcohol and these other substances pass into human milk and are harmful to your baby. On occasion, one glass of wine or beer is considered safe as long as the mother waits 2 to 2½ hours per drink before breastfeeding.

Avoid Environmental Toxins as Much as Possible

In some parts of the country, breastfeeding mothers are advised not to eat freshwater fish because they may contain polychlorinated biphenyl (PCB), a potent cancer-causing chemical. Mercury is another concern when eating certain seafood, as are contaminants such as dioxin.

ISSUES PARENTS OFTEN RAISE ABOUT BREASTFEEDING

I'm afraid of what's going to happen once I take my baby home from the hospital. What if I'm having problems breastfeeding and my baby isn't getting enough to eat?

If you have concerns after you leave the hospital, call your physician or your baby's pediatrician. He or she will be able to answer your questions and may suggest the help of a lactation consultant. Many of these counselors make home visits. Your doctor may also refer you to a support group for nursing mothers. (See page 4 for more about breastfeeding instruction.)

How will I know when my baby is ready to start breastfeeding?

Like all other baby mammals, newborn humans are almost always alert and eager to suckle shortly after their birth. Provided there are no problems, your baby should be put to the breast immediately after birth. You'll soon learn the cues that tell you she's hungry! (See "Getting Started" on page 4.)

Does breastfeeding make a difference to children's health in the long term?

Breastfed babies have fewer allergies, intestinal upsets, ear infections, and other common child-hood illnesses than formula-fed infants. Not only that, but children who were breastfed as babies have lower rates of diabetes and other chronic disorders long after infancy. (See "The Special Health Benefits of Breastfeeding" on page 3.)

I hoped to breastfeed my baby, but my doctor says I shouldn't because I have to take medication for a chronic condition. Does this mean it'll be harder for me to bond with my child?

Only a handful of medicines are not compatible with nursing. Tell your pediatrician what medications you're taking and ask whether yours are acceptable while breastfeeding.

If your medicines prohibit you from breastfeeding, you can still bond with your baby. Like millions of other parents you'll find bottle-feeding a warm, loving, and fulfilling experience. Cuddle your baby, gaze into her eyes, and coo and talk to her as you feed her. This is all part of bonding. (See "Practical Bottle-feeding Tips" on page 10.)

If my baby doesn't finish a bottle of formula, how long is it safe to keep the leftovers?

Never keep leftover formula or breast milk. Germs and enzymes from your baby's mouth normally enter the bottle and can spoil the formula. Use a fresh bottle for every feeding. (See "Sterilizing and Warming Bottles" on page 12.)

Nevertheless, fish are a good dietary source of beneficial fatty acids called docosahexaenoic acid (DHA) and eicosapentaenoic acid (EPA). Thus, seafood should be part of a healthy diet, concentrating on those that contain little mercury, including salmon, pollack, catfish, canned light tuna, and shrimp. Avoid shark, swordfish, tilefish, and king mackerel.

Pesticides also can enter human milk. Always wash fresh fruits and vegetables before eating them.

Chapter 2

Expanding Your Baby's Diet

Most infants make the transition from human milk or formula to eating other foods between 4 and 6 months of age. Whenever it's practical, the whole family should eat together. This helps your baby develop an eating pattern that lets him interact with other family members at mealtime. In addition, children in families that eat meals together have healthier diets and may have fewer behavioral problems as they grow older.

After some initial difficulties relieved by a discussion with a lactation consultant, Maria and Jose Lopez eased into the breastfeeding routines of their infant Ricky and developed confidence in their abilities to know when he was hungry and how long he should nurse.

"I thought I had a system that worked," says Maria. "But when it came time to introduce solid foods at around 6 months, I didn't have a clue." And she found advice from friends and family more confusing than helpful. "Everyone had different advice to offer, about everything from when I should start offering solid foods to Ricky, to how much I should expect him to eat—even what those first foods should be."

Shifting Views

Not only does personal advice vary, but professional advice has shifted over time. Before 1920, solid or supplemental foods were seldom recommended for infants until 1 year of age. In the 1950s, the tables turned and the trend was to introduce solid foods as early as possible; some even advocated within the first few days of life. Today, the American Academy of Pediatrics (AAP) recommends exclusive breastfeeding for a minimum of 4 months but preferably for 6 months and gradually adding solid foods while continuing breastfeeding until at least the baby's first birthday. The 6-months rule is the age beyond which babies need the extra nutrition that solids can provide.

At the same time, keep in mind that each child's readiness depends on his own rate of development. Whereas one child may be ready mentally and physically to take on new foods at 4 months of age, another may not be ready to take on the task until 6 months. Yet both children are in the normal range of development. Even after introducing solid foods, breastfeeding can and should continue.

How to Know if the Time Is Right

You may worry that you are putting your child at risk of overeating if you introduce other foods too soon, or that she's developmentally delayed if she's not ready until well past 4 months of age. Such fears can be made worse by well-meaning advice from friends and family members. Though advice from those more experienced than you can sometimes be helpful, the best advice is to know your own child so you'll be better able to recognize clues that she's ready for you to introduce her to supplemental foods. Don't be in a rush. Some infants like to take their own sweet time accepting new foods, and forcing the issue will only make the transition more stressful for you and your baby. Above all, relax and allow your growing infant to experiment and develop her own eating patterns and rituals that become familiar and comforting—in short, something she looks forward to.

By 3 to 4 months of age, your child will lose the *extrusion reflex,* which makes an infant instinctively push his tongue out when anything other than liquid is placed in his mouth. You can expect that by 5 to 6 months of age, most children will be able to express their desire for food. For example, until recently you've probably been able to eat your own food without attracting much attention from your child. But now he's likely to show more than a passing interest in what's on your plate, leaning forward, drooling, and even opening his mouth. He may also seem persistently hungry even if you've increased the frequency or length of breastfeeding sessions. Waiting until your child is ready before introducing solid food makes the process easier on everyone. Not only will he accept solid foods more readily in the beginning, but it may also make the transition to family foods easier and shorter. (See "When Is a Child Ready for Solid Food?" on the next page.)

WHEN IS A CHILD READY FOR SOLID FOOD?

Here are some guidelines on how to determine when your infant is ready to start eating solids.

Can she hold her head up?

Your baby should be able to sit in a high chair, feeding seat, or infant seat with good head control.

Does he open his mouth when food comes his way?

Babies may be ready if they watch you eating, reach for your food, and seem eager to be fed.

Can she move something from a spoon into her throat?

If you offer a spoon of rice cereal and she pushes it out of her mouth and it dribbles onto her chin, she may not have the ability to move it to the back of her mouth to swallow it. It's normal. Remember, she's never had anything thicker than breast milk or formula before, and this may take some getting used to. Try diluting it the first few times, then gradually thicken the texture. You may also want to wait a week or two and try again.

Is he big enough?

Generally, when infants double their birth weight (typically at about 4 months) and weigh about 13 pounds or more, they may be ready for solid foods.

THE FIRST SOLID FOODS ARE SEMILIQUIDS

Solid foods for babies are not really solid at all. By tradition, the first solid food is usually a semiliquid ground rice cereal. However, one also needs to consider culturally based or ethnic-based foods. After your child has mastered that, he can move up to strained or mashed foods and, somewhere between 7 and 10 months, finely chopped table foods. At this stage, all foods should be ground or finely chopped, or otherwise have a texture that readily dissolves in the mouth. Foods that need to be chewed rather than gummed are likely to cause choking until the child has the teeth and muscular coordination to deal with such foods. The transition is a gradual process that varies greatly from one baby to another. If your baby was premature, you may find the transition particularly slow and difficult. Some children have an especially hard time adjusting to the new textures of foods and may cough, gag, or even spit up when you try to introduce new foods. If that's the case, you'll need to introduce foods much more slowly, making the addition of solid foods a longer-than-usual process. But eventually, even children with such oral sensitivity come around and are ready and willing to eat when it's time for a meal.

Step by Step, But Not Set in Stone

It's not always a smooth transition from your child's first taste of supplemental food to the time he's eating the same food as the rest of the family.

SOLID FOODS DON'T MAKE BABIES SLEEP LONGER

If your chief reason for introducing solid foods is to get your night owl of a child to sleep through the night, think again, because it won't work. Despite the widespread belief that a bit of food in her stomach will do the trick, research doesn't back it up. Your baby will be able to sleep for extended periods only when she has reached the right level of developmental maturity and is capable of comforting herself when awake and not hungry.

Each infant is unique and has her own opinion about what you're trying to get her to eat. Some children enthusiastically embrace the idea of solid foods, almost as if to say, "What took you so long?" Others may take weeks of gentle prodding with a loaded spoon before they'll venture into unfamiliar territory. Once you've decided that you and your baby are ready for the feeding challenge, keep the following 3 basic points in mind:

1. **Which Food to Introduce First?** Rice cereal is traditionally recommended because it is considered to be well tolerated and to have less potential for allergy. However, its value over other single-grain cereals as a first feeding has not been supported by scientific study. The cereal should be mixed with human milk or warm formula and made thick or thin, depending on your child's eating skills. In general, use about 1 teaspoon of cereal mixed with 4 to 5 teaspoons of human milk, formula, or warm water. By 6 months of age, your baby's natural iron stores are depleted. The extra iron in infant cereals provides about 30% to 45% of your baby's daily requirement for iron. Iron from cereal is well absorbed and should bring your baby's iron stores back to where they need to be. Infant cereals also provide significant amounts of thiamin, riboflavin, niacin, and vitamin B_6. While there are also high-protein infant cereals to choose from, a healthy infant who is growing normally has no need for the extra protein they provide. A single-grain, iron-fortified infant cereal (eg, rice, oatmeal, barley) is the best choice. There are better sources of iron for infants than iron-fortified cereals, including red meat, which should be introduced to the infant's diet sooner rather than later.

2. **How Much Food Should Be Offered?** Give your infant small servings. If the 1 or 2 teaspoons he eats seem like a minuscule amount, don't worry; it's fine for his first few times. You don't want him to eat so much solid food that it replaces the breast milk or formula he needs. At this point, solid food is merely an addition to his breast milk–based diet. Even an experienced 6-month-old may eat only about 3 to 4 tablespoons at a meal. The rest of his nutrient needs will be met by breast milk and formula, at least for a while. Your baby's calorie needs vary depending on how fast he is growing and how active he is. Infants aged 6 months to 1 year need about 50 calories per pound, for a total of about 850 calories a day from a combination of solids, breast milk, or formula. It's important to remember, however, that babies don't eat calories; they eat food, and they regulate their energy intake according to their needs.

3. **How Quickly Should New Foods Be Introduced?** By tradition, new foods are introduced one at a time, which allows for the infant to adjust to each new food. If you offer something new at every meal, it may be difficult to identify adverse reactions to specific foods, should they occur. Give your baby time to experiment with new tastes and textures by introducing a new food every few days.

    Although certain foods are more likely to cause problems, any food has the potential to trigger food allergy or food intolerance. If you or other family members suffer from food allergies, the chances are greater that your child will too. But true food allergies, which set the immune system into action, are rare. It's more likely that your child will experience intolerance to a particular food or ingredient. Food intolerance can cause diarrhea, bloating, and gas, and is often mistaken for a food allergy, but unlike food allergies, it does not involve the immune system. By tradition, foods associated with food allergy such as wheat, egg whites, nut products, and cow's milk have been avoided during the first year of life. However, there is no scientific evidence to indicate that this practice prevents food allergy. In fact, there is a small amount of evidence (for wheat especially) that suggests

---

A NEW ROLE FOR DAD

When introducing solid foods, Dad can help by feeding the baby. Encourage him to share in your infant's discovery of new foods.

that allergy to foods may be prevented by earlier rather than later introduction of the food. In any case, check ingredient labels of foods carefully.

If your child appears to have a reaction to a particular food, remove it from her diet for 1 to 3 months before offering it again. The basic rule here is, if at first you don't succeed, try again later. If the food provokes a reaction on a subsequent try, eliminate it for several months. Research suggests that by 1 year of age, most babies are able to tolerate foods that had earlier caused a reaction.

NO SOLIDS IN BOTTLES

Don't let well-intentioned advice lead you astray. One common piece of advice says, if you can't get your child to accept solid food readily, you should put a little watered-down rice cereal in a bottle with some human milk or formula. Widen the hole in the nipple, they say, and you've got a no-fuss way to give your child solid food. But this teaches the infant nothing about the mechanics or social aspects of eating solid foods. Also, it risks overloading your child with calories.

SPOON-FEEDING YOUR BABY

When it's time to start spoon-feeding, use the following suggestions to make the process as enjoyable and successful as possible:

- Although your goal should be to feed your baby at regular times each day, start out by feeding her when she's hungry and shows signs of wanting to eat.

- Make sure he is sitting up straight in his high chair to reduce the chances of choking, and sit directly in front of him.

- While holding a spoonful of food about 12 inches in front of her, wait until she turns her attention to the food. When she opens her mouth, guide the spoon in.

- Talk to him while he's eating, but avoid making him excited.

- Feed her at the pace she prefers, whether fast or slow, and let her continue eating for as long as she wants to.

- When he shows signs of having had enough, don't try to feed him more.

Adapted from www.ellynsatter.com/to-months-feeding-your-older-baby-i-29.html

Symptoms such as diarrhea, skin rashes, wheezing, nausea and vomiting, cramps, or hives suggest a true food allergy. (For more information on food allergies and food sensitivities, see Chapter 16.)

When Your Infant Says "When"

Ramiel, at 6 months, took to cereals, fruits, and strained carrots like a duckling to water. But when his mother, Naïma, offered him strained broccoli, Ramiel screwed up his face, gagged, squawked, and spat it out. Naïma went back to the tried-and-true for the next few meals, then mixed a little broccoli puree with Ramiel's favorite strained carrots. After a couple of successful mixed feedings, Naïma again served strained broccoli. This time, Ramiel devoured the vegetable. Naïma realized that Ramiel's facial expressions didn't mean he disliked the food; it was just new and different, and he needed to get used to it gradually. You may have to try the same new food several times (sometimes 10 or more times) before concluding that your child does not like that particular food.

START THE MEAL WITH SOLIDS

Save the bottle until your baby has finished eating the solids. He'll be hungriest at the start of the meal and more willing to try new foods. Remember, in the beginning, solid foods are an addition to—not a replacement for—human milk or formula.

FIND A COMFORTABLE SPOT

Though what to feed your child is the major issue, where to feed her can sometimes be just as perplexing. If your child is sitting up, it's time to bring out the high chair. However, if she's ready to eat but has not yet mastered the skill of sitting upright and unsupported for any length of time, you'll need to pick a spot that's comfortable for both of you. You may find it works just fine if she sits in your lap (put all breakables out of reach), or you might try an infant carrier or motionless swing. She may be slightly reclined, but she should be upright enough to eat and swallow without choking. Whatever eating spot you choose, remember it's for a very short time. As soon as she's able to sit on her own, a high chair at the family dinner table is the best feeding spot. And be sure to use the chair's safety straps at all times.

You may get some mixed signals about whether your child likes what you're feeding him. Sweet foods, like applesauce, are usually accepted with a look of satisfaction. But a puckered-up face in response to a new vegetable isn't necessarily a sign that he doesn't want more. It may just be a reaction to a new and unexpected taste or texture. Offer it again—if he opens his mouth, he wants more, despite what his facial contortions may suggest. If it's still a no-go, give it a rest and try again a few days later. Parents often unconsciously give signals for liking or disliking foods, especially when they try to feed children foods they themselves don't like. Try not to let your expression influence your child when serving a food you don't enjoy.

Eventually you'll learn your child's signals that he's had enough—he may lean back, close his mouth tight, or turn his head. When his eye-to-hand coordination improves, he may even try to knock the spoon out of your hand. That's your signal to stop feeding. Don't expect him to have the same appetite at every meal. The appetite of any healthy baby will vary. Sometimes he'll surprise you at just how much food he can hold, while other times he'll leave you frustrated over his lack of interest in food.

There are no hard-and-fast rules about when to introduce new foods to your baby's diet, but the chart below offers some basic guidelines. Notice that the time frames overlap to allow for the wide range of developmental stages among babies of the same age.

MAKING THE TRANSITION	
4 to 7 months	Introduce fruits, single-grain cereals, and vegetables.
7 to 10 months	Offer strained or mashed fruits and vegetables like bananas or applesauce, egg yolk, and some textured table foods (in no particular order); finely cut and chopped meat or poultry.
9 to 12 months	Introduce soft combination foods such as casseroles, macaroni and cheese, and spaghetti; yogurt, cheese; beans.
After 12 months	Give low- or reduced-fat (1%–2%) cow's milk, if indicated.

When Your Baby Can Feed Herself

For Trudi, the first few weeks of baby Hannelore's life were a delight. Hannelore fed well, slept when she wasn't feeding, and looked like a porcelain doll tucked tightly in her bassinet. However, when Hannelore began to show a more demanding personality, Trudi found the baby trying. As Hannelore grew used to solid foods, she would reach for the spoon or plunge her hands into her bowl if Trudi left it within reach. A very neat housekeeper, Trudi would interrupt the meal to wash the baby and change her clothes. By the time they resumed the meal, Hannelore was screaming, hungry, but too upset to eat, while Trudi was angry with the baby not only for making a mess but also for refusing the food that she had prepared. One day Trudi screamed at the baby, "I have better things to do than feed you and clean up after you all day long!"

Noting Trudi's tension and Hannelore's fretfulness at the next checkup, their pediatrician carefully probed until he got to the root of the problem. He sympathized with Trudi; it is difficult, he agreed, to put up with messes and disruptions when you are used to a calm, orderly routine. But he also pointed out that Hannelore was quite advanced for a baby not quite 1 year old, and she shouldn't be expected to act like a big girl for a long time yet.

The doctor explained that the sooner Hannelore was allowed to make a little mess, the sooner she'd learn to be clean, but it wouldn't happen overnight. He suggested that Trudi feed Hannelore in the kitchen instead of the dining room and spread newspapers or a sheet of plastic under the high chair to catch the mess. He urged her to give Hannelore finger foods as well as a spoon and unbreakable bowl so she could learn to feed herself, as she wanted to do. If Trudi found herself getting tense and angry, perhaps her husband would give the baby her evening meal, or Trudi could ask a friend or neighbor to sit with her and help feed the baby during Hannelore's midday meal.

Somewhere around 7 to 9 months of age, infants learn to put objects in their mouths and, given the opportunity, will try to feed themselves. Once your child has a well-developed pincer grasp and can pick up objects between her thumb and forefinger, any food she can pick up and bring to her mouth can be considered a finger food. Foods that dissolve easily, like baby crackers, pieces of bread, plain cookies, sliced cheese, finger sandwiches, and dry cereals, are good first choices. This is also a good time to let your baby gradually get used to handling a spoon. You can let her play with a spare while you do the feeding. And when she finally decides to go it alone, be prepared for cleaning up to take almost as long as the meal itself.

About this same time, you may want to try allowing your infant to take a few sips from a cup with your help. Many breastfed babies never use a bottle and instead move directly to the cup. A 2-handled plastic sippy cup is a good first choice, though until your child is about 10 to 12 months old, more liquid may end up on her and the floor than in her mouth. Still, it's important to remember that play and experimentation are part of your child's mealtime

BABY'S DIET PLAN	
By the end of the transition from all human milk or formula to regular food with human milk or reduced-fat (2%), low-fat (1%), or nonfat (skim) milk (typically between 12 and 18 months), your child's daily intake should look something like this.	
Food	**Servings**
Milk	16 to 24 oz
Fruits and vegetables	4 to 8 tablespoons
Breads and cereals	4 servings (a serving equals ¼ slice of bread or 2 tablespoons of rice, potatoes, pasta, etc)
Meat, poultry, fish, eggs	2 servings of about ½ oz or 1 tablespoon each

SENSITIVE MOUTHS AND COARSER TEXTURES

Some babies find it hard to get used to coarser textures, especially if they come across a lump in a smooth food. A typical offender is a lump or strand of fruit pulp in yogurt. These children may have unusually sensitive mouths; some are also oversensitive to loud sounds and bright lights. Be patient and work on introducing new sensations gradually. Try to make sure that familiar foods don't hide unwelcome surprises. In time, your sensitive eater will accept a wide variety of textures. Only a minority of children have true oral aversions. In these cases, feeding specialists help children adjust to different textures.

and are essential to her growing independence. Follow her lead and tune in to clues that she's still hungry or that mealtime is over. If you try to force-feed her, she may throw her food or "pouch" it, holding it in her cheeks without swallowing. Prodding her to eat more when she's had enough also can cause gagging. But above all, remember never to leave your child alone and unattended at mealtime. She doesn't know her own limitations and could easily choke from eating too fast or stuffing too much food in her mouth at one time. And if you have older children in the house, make sure they don't try to feed your infant what they're eating.

After 1 year you'll make the switch from human milk or formula to regular milk. Between 12 and 24 months your child's doctor may recommend reduced-fat (2%) milk if your child is obese or overweight or if there is a family history of high cholesterol or heart disease. Check with your child's doctor or dietitian before switching from whole to reduced-fat (2%) milk.

Grocery Shopping for Your Baby

One of the first decisions you'll have to make before you mark the calendar for your baby's first solid meal is whether to make it yourself or buy prepared baby food in jars. There is no correct answer; it depends on your budget, your lifestyle, and your concerns. Here are your main choices.

Homemade Foods

One advantage to preparing your baby's food is that he gets used to what your family normally eats, instead of a jar of some commercial combination that you would never serve your family. Cooking and mashing simple foods like carrots, potatoes, squash, and bananas are easy. But preparation may require a little forethought and time as your child's tastes and eating skills expand to include foods such as peas, corn, green beans, peaches, and pineapple, which must be pureed or blended to transform them to textures your child can easily handle. A hand-turned food mill with disks for different textures is inexpensive and easy to use.

For healthful nutrition, bake, broil, or steam foods. When boiling vegetables, use very little water to preserve nutrients. Try to cook fresh vegetables within a day after you buy them. Vitamin C and several B vitamins can be lost while fresh produce sits in the vegetable bin in your refrigerator. If you're using the same foods as the rest of the family, separate your baby's portion before adding salt. And when buying canned or frozen foods, buy those with no or low salt and no added sugar or fat. If time is of the essence and convenience is a top priority in your household, making it yourself may not always be the best option. Some parents prefer to make baby foods for home use and keep a stock of commercial jars for traveling and emergencies. If you make foods yourself, be sure to take food safety precautions (see "Food Safety Tips for Your Baby's Meals" on page 44) when handling and preparing your baby's food.

PREPARING PORTIONS

Remove and warm as much food as you think your baby will want to eat at a meal. If you prepare too much, throw out the leftovers. If you put leftovers back in the jar, it's an invitation for bacteria to grow, and any enzymes from your baby's saliva will thin out the food.

Warm baby foods only to body temperature. If you're using the microwave, remove the container's cover and heat for only a few seconds at reduced power. Be careful not to overheat. Microwaving can create hot spots in the food that can burn your child's mouth. Moreover, thick foods like strained meats and egg yolk, if warmed while still in the jar, can easily overheat in the microwave and splatter or explode. To be safe, remove the food from the jar and place it in a microwave-safe dish—or don't warm it in the microwave at all.

Commercial Foods

Ready-to-eat baby food in jars is convenient. There's no fuss, it's portable, and the food comes in a wide variety of flavors and ingredients. Baby foods today range from simple strained fruits to exotic tropical fruit dessert and organic lentils and rice dinner. You won't have to worry about the sodium content because salt is no longer added to commercially prepared baby foods. Some dinners and desserts do, however, have added sugar or modified food starch. While both ingredients are safe, they take the place of more nutritious ingredients. Most baby food manufacturers categorize their products according to age-appropriate stages, usually 1, 2, 3, and toddler foods, with finely pureed foods for first-timers and thicker and more textured foods for older babies. But instead of making your choice more simple, these stages can sometimes be confusing, as manufacturers don't use standardized ages and stages. Two rules apply across the board: begin with stage 1 foods for beginners, and don't offer your child toddler foods, which often contain chunks, until he is an experienced eater.

Until now your baby has required little or no fluids in addition to breast milk or formula. But now that solid foods are becoming a regular part of his diet, so should additional fluids. Water is the best choice for quenching thirst without adding extra calories, particularly in hot weather. You may wish to offer water at feeding time so that your infant gets all the fluid he needs.

Organic Foods

Organic baby foods, available in some supermarkets and health food stores, have grown in popularity as people have become increasingly concerned about the effects of pesticides and other agricultural chemicals on children's health. Organic crops are grown in soil fertilized with manure and compost instead of synthetic chemicals. Organically produced foods, including meats, are from sources free of added hormones, antibiotics, dyes, waxes, and other additives. (See Chapter 13, Food Safety.) There is no evidence that organic foods are safer, although some recent evidence suggests that they have a higher nutrient content.

While some parents are concerned that children's exposure to pesticides, especially from fruits and vegetables, may be great relative to their size, the levels of pesticides found in produce are typically well below the safety levels set by the Environmental Protection Agency. Moreover, the processing involved in making baby food reduces pesticide residues to such a degree that the final product has no detectable residues. Experts warn that the risks of not including fruits and vegetables in children's diets are far greater than any potential risk from currently allowed levels of pesticides.

Should you feed your baby organic foods? That's a decision only you can make based on your lifestyle and your pocketbook, as commercial organic baby food—or organic produce for making baby foods at home—generally costs considerably more than standard brands.

NO HONEY FOR BABIES

Although honey may seem like a healthy food to feed your infant, don't do it. Honey is linked to infant botulism, an illness that can be fatal. The American Academy of Pediatrics does not recommend honey for infants younger than 12 months. That's because spores of *Clostridium botulinum* can sometimes grow and produce toxins in the infant's intestinal tract, causing a potentially fatal illness. An adult's intestinal tract has the ability to prevent the growth of the clostridium spores.

Tips for Using Commercial Baby Food

- Check the "use by" date on the container to make sure the date hasn't passed.

- Store unopened jars in your kitchen cabinet at room temperature.

- Make sure the vacuum seal button on the lid is down. If it has popped up, discard the jar.

- When you open a jar, listen for a whoosh or pop. If the center of the lid pops up, that's your sign that the seal is good and the food is safe for your baby.

- Remove as much food from the jar as you think your baby will eat. Never feed from the jar. After a jar has been opened, refrigerate the unused portion of the jar immediately. Leftovers should stay fresh for 1 to 2 days.

- Most manufacturers warn against freezing regular baby food. Though it is safe to do, it changes the texture. (Some manufacturers offer lines of frozen baby foods that are specially prepared to preserve texture and flavor.)

Food Safety Tips for Your Baby's Meals

- Keep tools and work spaces as clean as possible. Cutting boards, sponges, and dishrags are well-known breeding grounds for bacteria that can cause food-borne illnesses.

- Wash hands thoroughly with hot, soapy water before preparing—and between handling—raw and cooked foods. Dry your hands with disposable paper towels or freshly laundered, dry cloths.

- Cook meat to a temperature of at least 160°F (the US Department of Agriculture recommends using an instant-read meat thermometer for preparing all meat because meat can appear done at lower temperatures).

- Don't store cooked food for more than 2 days.

Whether you make your own baby foods or buy regular or organic commercial foods, the same basics apply. Here are some specific examples of foods to help you follow the general timeline suggested in "Making the Transition" (page 38).

Cereals

You may wish to start off with plain single-grain cereal. After 6 months, you may want to try a cereal and fruit combination. You can buy ready-made combinations such as rice and

---

WHOLE WHEAT VERSUS WHEAT: WHAT'S THE DIFFERENCE?

Whole wheat bread offers a nutritional advantage over white bread, which is also marketed as "wheat" bread. Both are made from wheat flour; the key is to know the difference. Whole wheat bread contains the fiber-rich outer bran layer and the nutritious inner germ of the wheat kernel, which delivers vitamins B_6 and E, folic acid, copper, magnesium, manganese, and zinc. By contrast, in wheat bread made from refined wheat flour, the bran and germ are eliminated. Whole wheat and wheat bread are fortified with niacin, thiamin, iron, and folic acid. You need to read labels carefully to make the right choice. Don't be misled by the terms "wheat," "made with whole wheat," "unbleached wheat," or even "multigrain." Instead, look for 100% whole wheat as the first ingredient listed.

CHANGES IN BOWEL MOVEMENTS

Don't be alarmed if you notice a change in the color and odor of your infant's bowel movements after he starts eating solid food. Vegetables such as beets, carrots, spinach, and peas are especially likely to cause changes in color. Yellow, green, or red bowel movements are not unusual. What your baby eats can also affect the texture and consistency of his bowel movements. Banana stools come out looking like tiny worms, pear stools like small stones. Rice cereal may cause hard stools, in which case switching to a different kind of cereal (eg, oatmeal, barley) may be a good idea. If your baby has a lot of gas, diarrhea, or stomach upset after eating a specific food, stop feeding it for a few weeks, then try again.

---

bananas or prunes and oatmeal, or you can mix your own. The thickness and texture should depend on your child's eating skills.

In the beginning, your infant is likely to eat only a few teaspoons, but eventually she should be eating about half a cup of iron-fortified cereal a day. If no other iron source is provided, an iron-fortified cereal should be a part of your child's diet until about 18 months of age. Other excellent sources of iron include red meat, beef or chicken liver, tofu, lentils, and wheat germ. However, if your child is drinking an iron-fortified formula, taking a multivitamin with iron, and eating meat, she may be getting too much iron. Talk to your pediatrician to be sure you're giving your child the right combination of iron-containing foods and supplements.

Breads

When you introduce your infant to breads and cereals, you're also introducing him for the first time to wheat, a potential allergen. If he's older than 4 months, it's probably OK, and some evidence suggests that introducing bread before 7 months of age prevents gluten allergy. Wheat-free breads and cereals include rice crackers or corn or rice cereals. Read labels carefully. Wheat may be a hidden ingredient. If wheat is not a problem, offer small pieces of whole wheat bread, pita bread, or bagels. Unsweetened cereals are good finger snacks.

Fruits

All ready-to-eat baby fruits in jars are fortified with vitamin C and provide about 35% to 45% of your baby's vitamin C needs per serving. If you choose commercial varieties, start off with single-ingredient fruits before progressing to 2- or 3-fruit combinations, and then fruits with added tapioca or rice. Soft, easy-to-mash canned fruits usually work well. If you go with regular canned fruits, be sure to include a good source of vitamin C such as vitamin C–fortified juice in your child's daily diet. Fresh fruits like peaches, pears, plums, or bananas can be mashed, diced, or cut into chunks, depending on your child's level of skill.

Juices

Fruit juices, such as orange, apple, and pear, tend to become favorites, sometimes to the exclusion of other foods. While they are moderately nutritious—all baby juices are fortified with vitamin C—it's easy to let your child go overboard. The fruit juice of choice for infants and children is 100% juice rather than the 10% juices that contain lots of extra sugar.

However, don't make the common mistake of offering unlimited access to fruit juice. Not only does it dampen your child's appetite at mealtime, but drinking too much juice can also cause cramping and diarrhea (see Chapter 9, Spitting Up, Gagging, Vomiting, Diarrhea, and Constipation). Research suggests that pear juice is the worst offender, followed by apple and grape juices, which are the most common ingredients in infant juice mixtures. If you offer your child juice, dilute it half-and-half with water. Limit servings to no more than 4 oz (½ cup) per day. Steer clear of regular bottled or canned vegetable juices, which are often

---

CHANGE IS ONE THING YOU CAN COUNT ON

This is a time of rapid transition for your baby. Don't expect to keep to any particular feeding routine for very long. The one thing you can count on during this time is change. Let your infant set the pace. Follow her cues as to what she's ready to try, and you'll have fewer feeding problems.

---

high in sodium. Water is always a good choice for quenching your child's thirst. Getting your infant used to the taste of plain water is a healthy habit that will last a lifetime.

Vegetables

If you make your own baby foods, be aware that home-prepared spinach, beets, turnips, carrots, and collard greens are not good choices during early infancy. They may contain enough nitrates to interfere with the transport of oxygen in the blood. Commercially prepared vegetables are safe because manufacturers test for nitrates. Peas, corn, green beans, squash, mixed vegetables, and sweet potatoes are better choices for homemade baby foods.

Meats

Somewhere between 7 and 10 months of age, your baby will probably be eating 3 meals a day. As solid foods begin to make up more of his intake, human milk or formula intake decreases. That's when it becomes important to feed him protein from other sources, such as ground or very finely chopped meat or poultry.

You may also find out that meat is generally at the bottom of the list of your baby's favorite foods. It probably will be better accepted if it's pureed, warmed slightly, and mixed with a food that your baby likes, such as his favorite vegetable. (At this age, infants still tend to gag and do not have molars for chewing. Even finely chopped meats may be hard to handle and cause choking.) If your child is not getting another good source of iron, it's important that he have some iron-rich meat in his diet, although he doesn't need meat every day. A 2½-oz jar of a commercially prepared, age-appropriate meat dish provides about 50% of an infant's recommended daily protein allowance. It also provides significant amounts of riboflavin, niacin, and vitamin B_6, as well as iron. Though in the past egg yolks were recommended as a good source of iron, the iron they contain is not easily absorbed. Iron-fortified cereals and meat are the best iron sources for your infant.

Mixed Foods

Last on the list of additions to your baby's diet, mixed foods can range from tuna casseroles and macaroni and cheese to toddler "dinners" in jars and frozen entrees. The so-called infant dinners in jars are more appropriate as vegetable servings than as meat servings. That's because most contain small amounts of meat and some vegetables along with starch fillers and seasonings. The ingredients in these dinners vary widely, so read ingredient labels carefully if your child has a food allergy or food sensitivity.

Desserts

If you offer your novice eater desserts, chances are she'll readily accept them and even want more. But offering desserts at this stage is not a good idea. Many commercially prepared baby desserts offer little valuable nutrition but lots of sugar. Stick with fruit or yogurt for a sweet taste to top off your baby's meal.

Vitamin and Mineral Supplements

Human milk provides complete nutrition, except for vitamin D, for about the first 6 months of life. Infant formulas are developed with your infant's complete vitamin and mineral needs in mind when exclusive breastfeeding is not possible. After your baby begins the weaning process, however, your pediatrician will check that he's getting enough of the nutrients he needs. The decision of whether or not to give a multivitamin or mineral supplement is one you should discuss with your pediatrician. Before you decide, here's what you should know.

Vitamin and mineral products for infants come in liquid drops that typically contain vitamins A, D, and C with or without iron, or vitamins A, D, E, and C and the B vitamins thiamin, riboflavin, niacin, and B_6 with or without iron. Recently, vitamin D drops alone have become available for infants, and these are essential for the breastfed infant. Vitamin drops can be purchased without a prescription. All infants, including those who are breast-fed, as well as older children should receive their requirement of 400 IU of vitamin D a day, beginning soon after birth.

The mineral *fluoride* is another important nutrient. It is critical for the formation of your child's teeth. If you live in an area where the water is not fluoridated, if you give your child only bottled water, or if your drinking water is filtered through a process called reverse osmosis, the AAP recommends giving a fluoride-containing supplement between feed-ings after 6 months of age. Fluoride supplements are available by prescription only, alone or in combination with vitamins. Call your local water company to find out if your water contains fluoride. In some areas, fluoride occurs naturally but the levels may be too low to benefit children's teeth. If your local water is not fluoridated, ask your pediatrician about fluoride supplements.

A healthy infant who is consuming human milk or formula along with a variety of solid foods, including good sources of iron and vitamins A and C, shouldn't need supplemental vitamins and minerals, except for vitamin D. If, however, your infant is at risk for nutrient deficiencies because of chronic health problems that affect her ability to eat, or if her appetite is poor, you should ask your pediatrician whether a supplement is advisable.

ISSUES PARENTS OFTEN RAISE ABOUT THE TRANSITION TO SOLID FOODS

My pediatrician says to wait to start giving my baby solid foods, but my neighbor's baby is exactly the same age and he's already eating solid foods. Is my baby behind?

In general, your baby can start solids at 4 to 6 months of age. However, follow your pediatrician's advice. While one child may be ready for solids at 4 months, another may not be ready at 6 months or even older. Both babies are in the normal range, and your pediatrician will advise you about introducing solids, depending on your baby's rate of development (see page 33).

At 4 months, my baby still isn't sleeping through the night and my mother-in-law says that giving her solid foods will fix the problem.

Your mother-in-law means well, but research doesn't back up her opinion. Your baby will be able to sleep for extended periods only when her digestive and nervous systems are mature. Be patient. Your baby will soon be sleeping through the night and switching to solid foods. (Read more on page 34.)

Why is rice cereal the one that's usually recommended for starters?

Rice is free of gluten, a protein in some grains that can trigger allergic reactions. However, using rice cereal as a starting food is based on tradition rather than science. Different cultures introduce their own foods and one needs to respect that. A child may also be sensitive to rice cereal, but this is rare.

How many calories does my baby need?

Your baby's calorie needs vary according to how fast he's growing and how active he is. It's important to remember, however, that babies don't eat calories; they eat food, and they regulate their intake according to their needs. (See page 35.)

Is it really important to introduce foods just one at a time?

If you offer a new food at every meal, it can be difficult to identify reactions to specific foods, should they occur. One new food every few days is a safe approach for getting started. (See page 35.)

When my baby switches to cow's milk, can she go straight on to skim?

Between 12 and 24 months your child's doctor may recommend reduced-fat (2%) milk if your child is obese or overweight or if there is a family history of high cholesterol or heart disease. Check with your child's doctor or dietitian before switching from whole to reduced-fat (2%) milk. (See page 41.)

Chapter 3

The Toddler Years

A toddler may gain no more than about 3 to 5 pounds over the whole of his second year, although he probably gained that much in only about 4 months during the first year. From now on, your child will grow at a slower, steadier rate until he reaches the other big growth spurt at puberty. Because he's growing more slowly, he doesn't need to eat as much as he did during his first massive burst of growth.

David and Helen Chu thought they had feeding all figured out when baby Andrew smoothly crossed over to solid foods. In fact, by the end of his first year, Andrew was eating any food they offered him and could drink from a cup as if he'd been doing it all his life. He had moved easily from purees to more chunky textures, and now most of his meals were well-chopped servings of what his parents were eating.

Suddenly, however, Andrew had become a toddler and he just wouldn't eat anymore. David and Helen encouraged ("One for Daddy…one for Mommy…"), pleaded ("Just 2 more bites?"), and threatened ("No cookie if you don't eat up your broccoli!"). No matter what they tried, Andrew always started playing with his food long before the plate was empty. Feeling desperate, they asked their pediatrician, "Where did we go wrong?"

"Relax," the doctor assured them. "This drop in appetite is a normal stage in development and—at 13 months—Andrew is right on schedule.

"Try giving him smaller portions, with a second helping only if he seems to want more. Don't bargain over foods—if you're serving fruit or yogurt for dessert, just make it part of the meal and let Andrew eat it if he wants to.

"Finally, when he starts playing with his food, he's letting you know that eating time is over. That's your cue to clear the table and go on to the next activity."

Catch-down Growth

It's normal to feel alarmed when you see a sharp drop in your child's appetite, which may start around 9 months of age. Soon after reaching the 9-month to 1-year milestone, most children are literally toddling everywhere, developing new skills, and getting into all kinds of mischief as they explore their expanding world. So it's logical to think that an active toddler would need extra food to power this nonstop activity. As if to balance these giant leaps in development, however, the growth rate slows.

Pediatricians refer to this phase as *catch-down growth*. It's a process that may start at about 6 months and is usually complete by 18 months. Catch-down growth is most clearly seen in a high birth weight (9- or 10-pound) baby whose parents are of average size. While some children can be considerably taller and heavier when compared with their parents' size at similar ages, most conform to a general family pattern of growth and size. So after an initial period of fast growth, the child slows down and settles at a level appropriate to the genes he's inherited. Catch-down growth is the opposite of catch-up growth, which occurs when a child makes up for a setback caused by illness. Less often, the child's birth weight and subsequent growth differ from what would be predicted based on family genes due to a baby's medical condition or during pregnancy. An example would be a baby who weighs more than predicted due to his mother's gestational diabetes.

Who's in Charge?

When you serve food to your children, the responsibility for dealing with it is split 2 ways. You are in charge of deciding what to offer, and your child is in charge of deciding whether or not to eat it—in other words, "parents provide, children decide." The mother of Dr Stern's 3-year-old patient often tried coaxing her child by saying, "Have one more bite for Mommy! One more bite for Mommy!" One day, her daughter said, "I will eat no more bites for ME!"

In many families, what frequently happens is that the parent announces what's for dinner and the child protests. Then the parent—anxious that the child doesn't eat enough—backs down by asking what the child would like to eat. This line of behavior leads to several outcomes, all of them negative. First, when the parent asks the child what she'd like, it puts the child in the inappropriate role of choosing food for the family. Children don't have the knowledge necessary to make such important choices; it's unfair to expect them to decide what's good for themselves or their families. Second, if more than one child is involved and each has a different request, the parent turns into a short-order cook: "Hamburger for this one…spaghetti for that one…who gets the omelet?" If your child turns up her nose at what's served, you don't have to apologize or make excuses. All you need to say is, "This is what we're having today." It's a mistake to encourage, persuade, or bribe a child to eat. Research has shown that such efforts have the opposite effect from what's intended, and the child may actually end up eating less than if left alone. If your child refuses the meal you offer, it's not your job to provide an alternative. You probably worry that if your child doesn't eat, she'll get hungry. Of course she will! And when she's hungry, she'll eat. There's no better stimulus than hunger for getting a child to try something new. However, if your toddler misses a meal of her own free choice, it won't make her sick and she'll probably be ready to eat at the next regular meal or snack time. (Or if not the next, then the one after that.)

It's Food, Not Law Enforcement

Keep your priorities in perspective. It's your job, as the adult, to help your toddler learn a healthy eating pattern. This means that you should provide healthful meals at regular times. You also need to prepare the food in forms and textures that he can learn to eat by himself. And you should keep him company during mealtimes so he learns to eat in a safe and socially acceptable way. But you're the food provider, not the food police. At every age, it's up to your child to choose what he wants from the food that's offered, and to decide how much or how little to eat at a meal.

What parents should do is provide appropriate servings of a healthy selection based on principles from the *Dietary Guidelines for Americans* (www.cnpp.usda.gov/DietaryGuidelines.htm) and respect the child's limits. If he says he's had enough, he knows what he's talking about. Don't insist on "just one more mouthful," or make him finish everything.

LOVE ME, LOVE MY FOOD?

When your toddler turns down food, she's not rejecting you. If you stop and reflect for a moment, you'll see that her negativism shows you're doing a good job. Your child trusts you enough to say "No," confident that this refusal won't change your love for her. Accept what she tells you.

It's natural to worry that your child isn't getting enough to eat when she seems to turn down every dish you offer. It's also understandable that you feel let down if your toddler refuses the food you've lovingly prepared.

Whether your toddler just turns her head away from the food or makes a mess with it, keep *your* comments to a minimum and don't beg or bargain with her. Clean up the mess, offer bread and whatever else is already on the table as an alternative, and if she turns it down, let her know that mealtime is over. If you ask what she wants or leave the table to whip up something on the spot, you're only setting yourself up for battles that you can't win.

Of course, you should respect your child's likes and dislikes. It's not fair to insist on serving textures and flavors that make her gag. At any given meal, place a reasonable selection on the table, with whole-grain bread or crackers as an option if the main dish doesn't appeal to her. However, if your child often gags, it may mean that she's feeling unbearable pressure to eat. Perhaps it's time to back off and let her take the initiative about eating. Allowing your child to make choices limited to the food you've already selected is fine.

Jason was born with a heart murmur. His pediatrician told Jason's parents that the murmur required no treatment and would disappear as the baby grew. "In a baby with normal growth," the doctor assured them, "a murmur of this type clears up by about 14 months of age."

Jason had few health problems. He began to eat solid foods, in addition to breast milk, at about 6 months. However, his parents worried because he was smaller than other babies they knew. They were afraid that if he didn't grow enough, the heart murmur would not go away. Each time Jason finished a meal, they urged him to swallow a few more spoonfuls. Jason turned his face away; he knew when he'd had enough and didn't want extra food forced on him. Finally, the parents stopped insisting.

At Jason's 1-year checkup, his pediatrician smiled. "Small, yes, but well proportioned," she said to his parents. "Jason is growing steadily and he's almost walking. His development is fine. Don't worry about his eating. You're right to let him decide how much he wants. This is a boy who knows his own mind!"

I'M AFRAID MY CHILD ISN'T EATING ENOUGH
When it comes to persuading children to eat, pediatricians advise parents to step back: Healthy children don't starve as long as food is available, and attempts to get them to eat more may backfire.

KEEP THE FOCUS OFF FOOD
Foster your toddler's growing independence by letting him make choices, but don't overwhelm him. In other words, limit the food selections you offer.
Let him take part in preparing the meal and the table. Given a job he can manage, no matter how small it seems to you, your toddler will focus more on his sense of accomplishment and less on the food.

A LEARNING EXPERIENCE
Your toddler is experiencing everything through her senses for the first time. She wants to explore the taste and feel of food, not just with her tongue but with her hands as well, just as she loves to squish mud between her toes and let sand run through her fingers. Let her play with the textures and finger paint with food on her tray table—it only takes a minute to rinse it off in the sink. This phase, like most others, will be over before you know it.

EATING TIME IS OVER
Toddlers have a limited attention span. This applies to eating just as it does to play. If your toddler wants to get down from the table, let her do so. But clear away the plates and don't offer cookies or crackers away from the table to make up for what she didn't eat during the meal. If she's hungry, she'll enjoy her next regularly scheduled meal.

Results of studies on children's eating habits show that children are born with the ability to instinctively regulate their food intake according to the energy they use. Parents who try to control their child's food intake or insist on a clean plate at every meal are interfering with this natural system. A typical example of misguided control is withholding dessert as a punishment for not finishing vegetables. If you're serving dessert, think of it as neither more nor less important than broccoli. All parts of the meal should have equal value. Let dessert be just another healthful part of the meal, and don't hold it out as a reward for good behavior.

One way to stop some feeding battles before they start is to let your toddler take part in meal preparation. When you set the table, let him choose between, say, the red cup and the blue. Even if he has a favorite plate or cup of his own, he might like to use a different, "special" one for a change. Put a little milk or juice in a pitcher he can lift and let him pour a drink for himself. Don't worry if most of it ends up on the high chair tray; your toddler will also enjoy helping to wipe up the mess. A child who dislikes baby bibs may feel more grown up having a cloth napkin tied under his chin.

Remember, when it comes to eating, a child's drive for independence is incredibly strong. An illustration of this is an experience Dr Dietz had with a patient with cerebral palsy so severe that he was unable to feed himself. Despite his limitations, the need to self-feed was so strong that he refused to let anyone feed him despite how hungry he was. It took weeks to figure out how to help him feed himself. Finally, it was found that by cutting food into manageable pieces, he could manually place each bite on a spoon that he then directed into his mouth.

"I Want to Do It Myself!"

As their muscular coordination steadily improves, toddlers learn to feed themselves. You'll still need to help out for a while and you shouldn't expect neatness at mealtimes for a long time yet. However, the sooner you let your toddler feed herself and get a bit messy, the earlier she'll reach the next stage of development—using utensils properly, quitting the high chair, and joining the rest of the family at the table.

Helping your child eat isn't the same thing as force-feeding with a spoon. Offer help when it's needed, but let your toddler assume increasing responsibility for getting the food from the plate to her mouth. At first, your toddler will eat mainly by finger feeding. As her

SERVING SIZES FOR TODDLERS

A toddler's energy requirements are not very large. Here's a general guide for feeding your toddler. Each day, a child between ages 1 and 3 years needs about 40 calories for every inch of height. This means, for example, that a toddler who measures 32 inches should be taking in an average of about 1,300 calories a day, but the amount varies with each child's build and activity level. The child's serving size should be approximately one-quarter of an adult's. For example, here's an average toddler-sized meal.

- One ounce of meat, or 2 to 3 tablespoons of beans
- One to 2 tablespoons of vegetable
- One to 2 tablespoons of fruit
- One-quarter slice of bread

Your toddler will get enough calories along with all the protein, vitamins, and minerals he needs from an average daily intake similar to the following:

Food Group	Servings Per Day	Number of Calories Per Day	One Serving Equals
Grains	6 servings	250 calories	Bread, ¼ to ½ slice Cereal, rice, pasta, cooked, 4 tablespoons Cereal, dry, ¼ cup Crackers, 1 to 2
Vegetables	2 to 3 servings	75 calories	Vegetables, cooked 1 tablespoon for each year of age
Fruits	2 to 3 servings	75 calories	Fruit, cooked or canned, ¼ cup Fruit, fresh, ½ piece Juice, ¼ to ½ cup (2–4 oz)
Dairy	2 to 3 servings	300 to 450 calories	Milk, ½ cup Cheese, ½ oz (1-inch cube) Yogurt, ⅓ cup

(continued on next page)

SERVING SIZES FOR TODDLERS, *CONTINUED*			
Food Group	**Servings Per Day**	**Number of Calories Per Day**	**One Serving Equals**
Protein group: meat, fish, poultry, tofu	2 servings	200 calories	1 oz (equal to two 1-inch cubes of solid meat or 2 tablespoons of ground meat) Egg, ½ any size, yolk and white
Legumes: dried beans, peas, lentils	2 servings	200 calories	Soaked and cooked, 2 tablespoons (⅛ cup)
Peanut butter (smooth only)		95 calories	1 tablespoon spread thin on bread, toast, or cracker

coordination improves, she'll enjoy learning to use cutlery, taking care to avoid sharp knives. Give her the right tools for the job—unbreakable dishware, a plate with a suction cup that won't slide around the tray table, a blunt-edge spoon with a handle little fingers can easily grasp, a stubby fork, and a 2-handled cup with a firmly fitting, spouted lid.

How Much Does My Toddler Need to Eat?

A toddler's eating habits tend to be unpredictable. One day he may devour enough breakfast for 2 people but at later meals, leave his plate almost untouched. The next day, he may eat 3 square meals plus a couple of snacks.

The amount of food a toddler needs is the amount that keeps up a good rate of growth and general health. Although the average toddler's daily intake rounds off at about 1,000 calories, he doesn't need a fixed number of calories every day, nor do you have to count every calorie he consumes. In fact, children's calorie needs vary widely according to their activity levels and their rates of growth and metabolism. If your toddler doesn't eat as much as the child next door—or seems to devour twice as much—it's because his needs are different.

Resist the urge to coax another mouthful and, by the same token, don't forbid a moderate second helping.

One of the best lessons about the need for your child to be in charge of what and how much was taught to us by a 25-month-old girl named Cassie who required repeated operations for a skeletal abnormality. Her mother brought her to us because she was small and a picky eater. Because her mother was hopeful that Cassie would regain her weight after surgery, she would urge Cassie to eat. At one meal that we observed, her mother told Cassie that if she finished the cracker that she was eating, she could have some candy. Looking directly at her mother, Cassie put the cracker down, and refused to eat any more. (See "Who's in Charge?" on page 52.)

Snacks to Stoke the Fire

With all the energy your toddler uses, his stomach can't hold enough to keep him from getting hungry between meals. Many children need a morning and afternoon snack, which should be timed so they won't interfere with lunch or dinner. Snacks should include a satisfying balance of healthful foods.

Raw vegetables are mostly too difficult for toddlers to manage, and some—carrots, whole cherry tomatoes, whole green beans, celery—are a serious choking hazard for toddlers (see "Unsafe for Toddlers" on page 68). But there's no reason that a toddler shouldn't enjoy well-cooked vegetables cut into manageable pieces. Big chunks of any food and glob-like spoonfuls of peanut butter are hazardous and should not be given to children younger than 4 years; the same advice is just as important for any types of nuts, peanuts, or popcorn because children aren't able to grind food and reduce it to a consistency safe for swallowing. Chunks of peanut butter can stick to their palate and end up choking them.

The Toddler's Diet: A Balancing Act

You don't have to include the exact number of daily servings from each food group at every meal or snack. The idea is to provide a varied diet that includes a good amount from each group when averaged out over a 2-week period. If you follow the general guide in "Serving

Sizes for Toddlers" (pages 57–58), your toddler will get a good balance of grains and cereals; vegetables and fruits; meat, fish, and eggs; and dairy products.

While many parents say that their toddler doesn't like meat, often because of its texture, they are afraid that their child will not get enough protein in a meatless diet. But bear in mind that there are plenty of other foods that contain protein, including milk, eggs, and even some vegetables (eg, rice, beans), so your toddler doesn't have to eat meat every day to consume enough protein.

Keep the Menu Simple

Young children prefer simple foods. Don't wear yourself out making elaborate recipes to tempt a picky toddler. Your child is experiencing many foods for the first time. Heavy seasonings and sauces only mask the taste and may put a toddler off the food.

Young children also tend to be more comfortable with what they know, including food. It's easy to sympathize with this conservative tendency when you consider how many things a toddler has to face for the first time and the many new activities she masters in remarkably few attempts.

There's nothing wrong with serving the same food day in, day out, if that's what your toddler prefers. It's a lot easier to achieve balanced nutrition if you vary the menu. Parents may think of their children as creatures of habit because they have a peanut butter and jelly sandwich for lunch come rain or shine. Often, it's the parents who have established the habit. Try to introduce reasonable variety with a rotating schedule of dinner dishes, different snacks, and new breakfast foods from time to time.

New Foods: A Little at a Time

When you introduce a new food, you may find that it's best to place no more than a teaspoonful on the plate alongside a favorite food until your toddler gets used to it. At every age, it's best to serve a small portion and give a second helping if the child asks for more. The sight of a plate heaped with food can overwhelm a young child.

HEALTHFUL SNACKS FOR TODDLERS	
Fresh fruits	Apples, bananas, peaches, nectarines, pears (sliced) Cherries, grapes, plums (sliced or smushed and pitted) Orange or grapefruit sections (cut into pieces) Strawberries
Dried fruits	Apples, apricots, peaches, pears (cut up) Dates, prunes (pitted, cut up) Raisins
Vegetables	Carrots, green beans (well cooked, diced) Steamed cauliflower, broccoli Yams (cooked and diced) Peas (mashed for safety; a child can inhale whole peas) Potatoes (cooked and diced)
Dairy products	Cheese (grated or diced) Cottage cheese Yogurt, fresh or frozen Milk
Breads and cereals	Whole wheat bread Bagel cut into small pieces Crackers (saltine, graham, whole grain) Dry cereal Pretzels Rice cakes
Meat/protein group	Fish (canned tuna, salmon, sardines; whitefish) Peanut butter (smooth, spread thin on bread or cracker)

FOOD FADS AND JAGS
A 2-year-old on a food jag may insist on the same food 10, 20, or 30 days in a row. On the 11th, 21st, or 31st day, however, he'll make a face at the food he used to cry for and say, "I don't eat that!" According to toddler reasoning, he's right. In his mind, he used to eat it, but he doesn't anymore.

The parents of a toddler learn to take nothing for granted, especially when it comes to eating. Toddlers are notorious for food fads and food strikes. Don't make an issue of them; instead, simply let your child choose from what's on the table. If he repeatedly refuses a particular food, give it a rest, and then reintroduce it, without comment, after a few weeks. Or serve it again when your toddler asks for it and it fits into your meal plan.

If he insists on the same food several days in a row, there's no harm in serving it, provided it's nourishing and healthful. Place a small helping of something new or different alongside the favorite; sooner or later he'll try it.

Four-year-old Nicole wasn't interested in eating when the family sat down to a hot dog lunch. Her mother wrapped Nicole's hot dog in foil and put it in the refrigerator. At snack time 2 hours later, Nicole retrieved her now-cold hot dog. She declined her mother's offer to warm it up and instead ate it with real enjoyment.

It's far better to skip a meal than to risk a standoff with bad feelings on both sides of the table. Whether you're a child or a grown-up, food is always more appealing when you're really hungry.

Fear of Trying

As if children eating less, being picky, and having food jags weren't enough to deal with, many parents find themselves across the table from a person with conservative views about food. You make something new and serve it up to your 2-year-old, certain that the color and aroma will pique her appetite. But with arms crossed and teeth clenched, she stares straight ahead like a face on Mount Rushmore. Nothing will induce her to eat.

When it comes to food, children at the toddler stage know what they're comfortable with. They mistrust the idea of trying something new, no matter how much trouble you took to make it and how good you think it looks and tastes.

Without drawing unnecessary attention to it, let your child see you eating and enjoying the new food. Your child will learn from your example.

TRY, TRY, TRY AGAIN
One study showed that children did not accept a new food until they'd been served it an average of 10 times. (By that time, it was an old food.) Some accepted it earlier, but many had to see it even more than 10 times. So if at first you don't succeed, don't give up; keep offering small servings without making an issue of it. Sooner or later, your young child will try and perhaps work the food into his routine.

SOFT-SELL APPROACH
You can't force a new food on a toddler. Instead, try a soft-sell approach by serving a very small portion alongside an established favorite when the child is hungry.

Food Strikes and Mealtime Wars

Refusing food brings a fast, emotional response from parents that the toddler interprets as caring attention. Toddlers enjoy extra time and focus from their parents.

Toddlers often choose mealtimes to put on a show of independence. This is extremely trying for a parent who has put time and effort—not to mention imagination—into preparing a meal. To make it worse, these wildcat actions often take place at the end of a tiring work day or when you're caught up with the needs of others in the family. Quick to pick up new habits, toddlers soon learn that refusing food is an effective way to get attention. So maintain a relaxed conversation, focused on the family's events and activities of the day, and not about what your toddler is or isn't putting into her mouth. (See "Managing Mealtimes" on page 64.)

No Liquid Lunches

Some toddlers drink so much milk and juice that they have no appetite when it's time for more nourishing meals and snacks. Excessive milk intake, beyond what your child consumes as solid foods, can have serious harmful health consequences, such as severe anemia. Also, children who drink a lot of juice can develop toddler diarrhea (the fruit sugar fructose and sorbitol, a sugar that is not digested well, can cause diarrhea). With this condition, an otherwise healthy child passes numerous semiliquid bowel movements over the course of the day, usually containing fairly large amounts of undigested food. This is not a serious health prob-

---

MANAGING MEALTIMES

Here are a few tips for keeping mealtimes pleasant, reflecting on common issues raised by the parents of toddlers and young children.

- *Keep mealtimes fun.* Don't let frustration set in. Allow your toddler to feed herself with her fingers if she wants, and expect there to be a mess. Wait until she's finished eating before cleaning up.

- *Show a little creativity.* Your toddler is more likely to eat particular foods if you make them look appealing. Why not use a cookie cutter to cut sandwiches into unusual shapes? Or freeze a banana, and then encourage him to dip it in a cup of yogurt or applesauce?

- *Prepare a healthy snack together.* Make and share a fruit smoothie. Give her sliced bananas, avocado, or yogurt.

- *During meals, your toddler should eat with the rest of the family rather than separately.* The entire family should sit at the dining room table and talk with one another while eating. **Keep the television off.**

Adapted from American Academy of Pediatrics. *"I Won't Eat It!" Answers to Your Questions About Feeding Babies and Toddlers.* Birch L, Dietz W, eds. Elk Grove Village, IL: American Academy of Pediatrics; 2009

lem. In this condition, important nutrients are digested and absorbed normally and weight gain continues unaffected. The major problem is the diaper rash that might occur.

Milk is an important and inexpensive source of necessary fats, protein, calcium, and vitamins A and D. But it's OK to limit milk intake to 16 to 24 oz (2–3 average glasses) a day. Your child's appetite for meals may improve if you offer water instead of juice when she's thirsty. Water is more thirst quenching than sugary drinks such as juice. Juices do supply some vitamin C, which occurs naturally in citrus juices or may be added, as in apple juice. Also, calcium-fortified orange juice is a good source of calcium. However, giving juices can be a rather expensive way to provide these nutrients. Juices mainly provide calories that the toddler can get in a more nourishing form from solid foods.

If you tell your toddler there's no juice available and offer water instead, she'll drink it without protest. Or you may cut down gradually over a week or two by giving a slightly smaller serving each time she asks for juice and diluting it with increasing amounts of water.

AVOIDING CONFLICTS OVER FOOD

You can help keep things peaceful at the family dining table by following these simple rules.

- No foods should be totally forbidden. If children know a particular food is in the home and they can't have it, that food will become much more desirable and is much more likely to be over-eaten when it's available. The way to avoid conflict over these foods is simply to keep them out of the home. Foods that are considered unhealthy for children should not be kept in the home for adults to eat. This approach makes them unavailable, not forbidden, and reinforces what foods are healthy for the whole family.

- Toddlers should not have free access to the pantry and refrigerator. Parents are the ones who should decide what foods are available for the child to eat.

- Serve your children appropriate portions rather than letting them serve themselves. This will allow you to regulate portion sizes. (See "Serving Sizes for Toddlers" on pages 57–58.)

- As should be the case for everyone in the family, generally avoid high-calorie (high-fat content) foods to be routinely served at meals.

- Don't give in. Consistency is important. If your toddler does not want to eat what's served and you offer something else, the next time the issue arises he will be that much more stubborn because he knows you will give in. His insistence may lead to tantrums because he figures that the harder he works, the more likely you will be to give in to his wishes. But a temper tantrum never hurt anyone. Let him blow off steam, but do not give in.

PHASING OUT BOTTLES

A toddler who is still drinking from a bottle may skip meals if she knows the bottle is available. So encourage your child to drink from a cup. When you serve water, for example, always serve it in a cup. Bottles should be phased out between 12 and 24 months of age.

Sippy cups can be used as a transition between bottles and open cups—and they can minimize spills (unless your toddler unscrews the top). When you start using a sippy cup, use it for all liquids, including milk, right away, and then switch to an open cup (such as a 2-handled cup) as soon as your child can manage it, usually before age 2. But keep in mind that your toddler only needs to drink when she's thirsty or with meals. If you let her hold on to the cup most of the day like a security blanket, she may end up overdrinking (and need more frequent diaper changes). Also, frequently drinking milk, juices, or sodas can lead to tooth decay because teeth are continually being bathed in sugary liquids that help bacteria grow. Do not let your child go to bed with a bottle or sippy cup to drink from.

Don't be concerned that you're depriving your child of calcium and vitamins if you limit her milk consumption to a limit of 16 to 24 oz per day. She'll get plenty from other dairy products and foods in a balanced diet (check the sources of vitamins and minerals on pages 199–206).

Lights! Food! Action!

Some parents are so anxious about feeding that they feel driven to provide diversions such as toys and videos during meals. Food is nourishment, not entertainment, and you don't have to turn your dining area into a theme restaurant to get your child to eat. In the long run, such measures can prove counterproductive. Your child may find it difficult to eat without distractions and may not learn socially acceptable behavior.

Turn the television off when it's time to eat and clear away toys, reading materials, and other distractions. Encourage your children to express their opinions and take part in the conversation at mealtimes.

Make family mealtimes special. Sit down to eat with your toddler. Serve meals at the table, not in front of the television. Even your toddler's snacks should be served at a special place, not eaten on the run. Avoid serving snacks while children are watching television. Doing so can lead to unconscious overeating and unwanted weight gain later in life.

Food Safety

Choking on food is a serious hazard that's all too common among toddlers. Lumps of food can easily lodge in a little throat and block the airway.

Children don't learn to chew with a grinding motion until about 4 years of age. That's why firm, smooth foods such as nuts and hard candies are so dangerous for children younger than 4 years—they simply don't have the ability to chew them well. Choking often happens when a toddler tries to do everything at once, such as eating as he runs or talks. If a toddler likes the taste of something, he may try to stuff the entire portion into his mouth until his cheeks bulge like a chipmunk's and he can't move his jaw to chew and swallow properly. Especially risky are hard foods such as raw carrots and celery; foods with a resistant, rubbery texture such as large chunks of boiled waxy potatoes; round, firm foods; hot dogs and other meat; and thick lumps of firm, gloppy spreads such as peanut butter. Foods can generally be considered safe if they dissolve in the saliva (eg, graham crackers, cereal, pasta). Take other preventive steps as follows:

- Chop food to a texture that's easy for a young child to manage.
- Don't let your toddler eat while running or playing.
- Make sure that older children don't give unsuitable foods to a toddler.
- Never leave your toddler alone while eating.
- Teach your toddler to finish a mouthful before speaking.
- Keep an eye on your toddler whether or not you're eating with him. A choking child may be unable to make any sound at all.

Pouching

David, at 18 months, ate a relatively limited range of foods and disliked meat but was growing well and had plenty of energy. His parents weren't concerned; they were confident he'd eventually enjoy a wider variety, just as his elder brother did.

When David was served a hamburger at a barbecue lunch hosted by family friends, the toddler took a large bite and chewed it for a long time. Unwilling to swallow the detested meat but anxious to be a well-mannered guest, David pouched the hamburger in his cheeks and resisted all suggestions that he swallow or spit it out. At bedtime that evening, his mother, worried that the toddler could choke, coaxed him and pleaded to no avail. Finally, she gently pinched David's nostrils and he immediately sprayed her with a stream of chewed-up hamburger, to his brother's delight.

Although David's mother hadn't actually forced food on him, she recalled that she had warned him several times to "be a good boy at the barbecue." David interpreted this as an order to eat. Despite his mother's good intentions, David felt pressure and resisted in the most tactful way he could, by pouching. He would allow the food he apparently didn't like into his mouth but no farther.

It's not unusual for toddlers to leave the table with food in their mouths. Some children chew for a while, then spit out the food. Others wad it up in their cheeks for hours until they look like chipmunks. A child who pouches in this way may take more than he wants just to satisfy a parent who insists on "one more mouthful." Some children also dislike the taste or texture of certain foods or are afraid to swallow.

Where Does Fat Fit In?

Young children need calories from fat for growth and brain development. This is especially important very early in your child's life. Even as adults, we all need a moderate amount of fat to supply energy, keep our skin healthy and supple, help wounds heal, and keep our hair

---

UNSAFE FOR TODDLERS

- Hot dogs (unless cut in quarters lengthwise before being sliced)
- Hard candies, including jelly beans
- Nuts
- Chunks of peanut butter (Peanut butter may be spread thinly on bread or a cracker—but never give chunks of peanut butter to a toddler.)
- Popcorn
- Raw carrots, celery, green beans
- Seeds (such as processed pumpkin or sunflower seeds)
- Whole grapes, cherry tomatoes (Cut them in quarters.)
- Large chunks of any food such as meat, potatoes, or raw vegetables and fruits

---

FIRST AID FOR A CHOKING CHILD

Choking becomes life threatening when a child swallows or inhales an object—often food—that blocks airflow to the lungs. This is an emergency that calls for immediate first aid. If your child is CHOKING and can't breathe, have someone call emergency medical services (911) while you start emergency measures. For specific and complete choking instructions, familiarize yourself with the chart in Appendix F. But if the child is coughing, crying, or speaking, DO NOT do any of these procedures; instead call EMS (911) or your pediatrician for advice.

growing thick and shiny. Fat helps us absorb certain vitamins that are essential for health. It also adds flavor and a pleasing texture to foods.

However, too much fat can add to our risk of developing heart disease and other associated medical disorders. Heart disease is the leading cause of death in the United States and other developed countries. We can reduce the risk of heart disease by cutting down on excessive fat in the diet from childhood onward.

Nutrition experts now recommend that after age 2, children's diets should be gradually modified until they are getting about one third of their daily calories from fat. This is the same fraction advised for adults, so it's a fairly simple matter to keep the whole family on a low-fat program. It's especially important to do so if heart disease runs in the family.

After age 2, you can switch your toddler to reduced-fat (2%), low-fat (1%), or nonfat (skim) milk, like the rest of the family.

TO REDUCE FAT CALORIES	
Instead of	**Serve**
Hamburgers, hot dogs	Lean chicken, fish, vegetable "burgers"
French fries, processed potato nuggets, instant potatoes made with butter or margarine	Baked potatoes, homemade oven fries, mashed or scalloped potatoes made with low-fat yogurt or buttermilk
Fried chicken and fish, commercial breaded chicken and fish preparations	Baked or grilled chicken and fish
Doughnuts, Danish pastries, croissants, toaster cakes	Whole-grain bread, bagels, English muffins
Chocolate-chip cookies, frosted cupcakes, brownies	Graham crackers, fat-free fig bars, oatmeal-date cookies
Ice cream, milkshakes	Sherbet, ice milk, nonfat frozen yogurt, juice popsicles, fruit and yogurt shakes

Help your children develop a preference for low-fat foods. As they approach kindergarten age, start buying fat-free yogurt. Serve cheese in moderate portions and select cheeses made from skim milk. Goat's milk cheeses and yogurts are lower in saturated fats than most cow's milk products (read more about the different types of fats in Chapter 6, Is My Child Overweight?). Compare labels. Sherbets, juice popsicles without added sugar, and nonfat frozen yogurt are more healthful frozen treats than ice cream.

You can cut down on dietary fat by substituting lower-fat for higher-fat foods (such as grilled fish for a hamburger) or serving a reduced-fat version of a food (broiled fish instead of deep-fried, breaded fillets).

Treats or Tricks

A treat of potato chips, ice cream, or candy now and then for family special occasions won't do any harm, but there's no need to put temptation in your child's way. Don't keep large containers of ice cream in your freezer or giant bags of cookies and salty snacks in the pantry. Buy or make small batches only for treats on special occasions. Then, when your child asks, you can honestly reply, "There aren't any in the house," and offer fresh fruit, a vegetable snack, or whole-grain crackers instead.

Nutritional Supplements: Save Your Money

Vitamin and mineral deficiencies are rare in the United States, even among those who are eating poorly balanced diets. That's because many of our basic foods—breads, cereals, rice, milk, and margarine—are fortified with vitamins, minerals, or both.

Like many consumers, you may do a quick calculation as you scan food labels to make sure that what your child is eating will cover the recommended dietary allowances (RDAs) of vitamins and minerals. Health authorities often use the term *dietary reference intake* to assess nutrient intake. The name may have changed, but the levels are close to the old RDAs and the purpose is the same—to safeguard health.

The RDAs are set well above the amounts we actually need. A balanced diet based on the *Dietary Guidelines for Americans* (www.cnpp.usda.gov/DietaryGuidelines.htm) supplies more than enough of most vitamins and minerals for every age group. A toddler who is getting the right number of daily servings from the various food groups—even in very small portions—will always get enough of these essential nutrients.

Our bodies use vitamins to convert food into energy, and minerals, such as calcium, are necessary for building bone and muscle. We get the small amounts we need from a normal diet.

Advertisements and promotions for processed food and supplements try to plant the idea that our children's diets lack vitamins and minerals. They put pressure on families to use supplements as a kind of insurance against nutritional shortfalls. These claims are written not by health professionals but by ad writers who work to sell the products. The majority of children do not need most vitamin or mineral supplements. Healthy people retain only as much of the water-soluble vitamins (vitamin C and the B vitamins) as they need; the rest passes out in the urine. The other supplement story—which the ads don't bother to tell—is that too much of a good thing can be bad. For example, fat-soluble vitamins like vitamin A and D are stored in the tissues. When excessively high doses are taken, the tissue stores can build up to toxic levels and make people sick. High doses of iron, zinc, and other minerals taken over a prolonged period can accumulate in the body and may have adverse effects on the digestive tract, liver, heart, kidneys, and other organs. So spending money on most supplements (except possibly vitamin D) is not only costly but also wasteful for most children.

Pills and potions won't make up for a poor diet. If a young child is undernourished or has problems related to an inadequate diet, what's needed is a change in eating habits or the kind of food that's provided, not necessarily supplements. In conditions such as chronic illness in which a child can't eat enough, is unable to absorb certain nutrients, or has sensitivity to certain foods, pediatricians may prescribe supplements to meet special needs. In general, however, give your child supplements only if your pediatrician advises you to do so.

FOOD PROBLEMS THAT TODDLERS' PARENTS OFTEN WORRY ABOUT

No matter what I put on the table, my toddler says, "No!"

This resistance is just a normal sign of growing independence. Continue providing regular, healthful meals and snacks and let your toddler choose what to eat and how much at a time. (See page 61.)

How much does my toddler need to eat?

Most young children do well with 3 small meals and 2 snacks daily. The guideline is about 40 calories a day for every inch of height, or about 1,000 calories a day for the average toddler, but appetites vary among children and in the same child from day to day. (See pages 57–58 for recommended servings.)

Does each meal have to include every food group?

Base your toddler's meals on the US Department of Agriculture dietary guidelines so that the overall intake balances out over the course of 2 weeks or so. (See Chapter 6, Is My Child Overweight?)

How much milk does my toddler need?

Two or three 6- to 8-oz glasses a day is about right. Offer water when your child is thirsty and don't overdo milk and juice between meals. (Check page 63 for more about toddlers and liquids.)

When is the right time to cut down on fat?

After your child turns 2, cut down gradually, until the diet supplies about one third of daily calories from fat. This is also the percentage recommended for adults. Consciously limiting fat calories at 1 year of age is only appropriate if recommended by your child's pediatrician if there's concern for obesity. (See page 69.)

My toddler never finishes a plateful of food.

Serve smaller portions. Your child is growing more slowly than in the first year of life and doesn't need to eat so much. If you put too much food on your child's plate, you may discourage him from eating appropriate proportions, and he may not eat the amounts that he would if you placed smaller portions in front of him. You can always give a second helping if your toddler asks for it. (See pages 57–58.)

Chapter 4

Nutrition During the School Years

During the middle years boys and girls grow an average of a little more than 2 inches a year. In turn, they gain about 6½ pounds a year. These numbers, however, are only averages. Heredity, nutrition, and general health are a few of the many factors that influence your child's growth rate.

When Lauren Maier found herself juggling pots and pans to cook an alternative main course for the umpteenth time, a light finally went on: "This is my house, my family. I cook the dinner and I call the shots. Let's make ourselves happy."

She stopped asking the children what they wanted to eat. Instead, she prepared food and served it without comment. To Lauren's surprise, her 4- and 6-year-olds quickly adjusted to the new system. When they objected to the food they found on their plates, they could always fill up on the whole-grain bread and raw vegetable sticks she usually served as part of the meal. Lauren stopped wheedling, pleading, and begging if the children didn't seem to eat much. She remembered what her pediatrician had said: "It may not seem like much to you, but it's enough for a 4- or 6-year-old. You wouldn't want to be force-fed, would you?" As tension around eating decreased, Lauren began to look forward to meals as a relaxing, stimulating time of the day, instead of a test of wills that ended in tears and time-outs.

Choosing Food: A Job for Grown-ups

The family kitchen is no place for short-order cooking or bargaining over food. As in a restaurant kitchen, one person has to be the chef and make the decisions. In overwhelming numbers, parents buy the food and decide what's available in their home. Thus, although children may choose what to eat at various times, they can only select from the food that's offered. Parents decide what to buy, and parents, therefore, determine what children eat.

Mealtimes are social occasions that provide important opportunities for families to talk and share the events of the day. Even if your child doesn't like the food that's served, you should still expect her to join the rest of the family at the table. Let her help herself to bread, salad, and whatever else is on the table, but don't offer an alternative food in place of the dish she has turned down. If she's hungry later, offer to reheat the leftovers or suggest another healthy choice. The one food you shouldn't offer is the alternative she originally demanded.

Children as Educated Consumers

During the school years children are bombarded with television advertising. About half the ads that children see on television are for processed foods, and most of the foods are high in fat and simple sugars but low in fiber and protein. Explain to your children that an ad is designed to get them to buy the product, even though it may not be a healthy choice. Help them learn to be thoughtful, critical consumers, not swayed by promotional pitches. Explain how a food budget works. Finally, keep in mind that there's one fail-safe defense against television: you can turn it off and organize other activities.

Supermarket shelves are stacked on purpose with heavily advertised, high-profit items at children's eye level. That's why it's a good idea to write out a shopping list at home and keep to it. If you find yourself giving in to demands for "this" cereal or "those" cookies just for the sake of peace and quiet, have someone else mind your children so you can shop without being distracted. For example, you could trade shopping time and child care with a neighbor to help both of you cope. Older children may enjoy helping out in the supermarket. Equip them with a list of items and challenge them to compare brands for nutrient content and unit price, then pick the best values.

Too Many Children Are Not Eating Well

While Americans may enjoy the most abundant and economical food supply in the world, a survey by government health experts revealed worrisome eating patterns in children and adolescents ranging in age from 2 to 19 years. Few children and adolescents consume the recommended daily servings of fruits and vegetables. Children 2 to 5 years old have better diets than children 12 to 17 years old when it comes to total fruits, whole grains, and milk. Among school-aged children and adolescents, almost half consumed less than a cup of fruit daily, and more than a quarter failed to consume more than a cup of vegetables daily. No matter which group they were in, all the young people surveyed were eating too much fat and too much added sugar.

Make sure your children are offered a healthful, balanced diet. To keep fat consumption low,

- Trim all fat from meat before cooking.
- Use cooking methods that require little or no fat, such as broiling, steaming, and roasting.
- Switch to skim or low-fat milk and dairy foods for children older than 2 years. Children aged 12 to 24 months can be given low-fat milk, especially if their body mass index (see Chapter 7, Is My Child Too Thin? Too Small? Too Tall?) is greater than the 85th percentile, there is a concern about developing obesity, or there is a family history of heart disease.

Promote your family's fiber intake and vitamins by providing plenty of vegetables and fruits. If your children balk at unadorned vegetables and fruits, try incorporating more of these foods into favorite recipes. For example, you can mix applesauce in waffle batter or mix blueberries or sliced bananas into pancakes. Replace the ground meat in spaghetti sauce or taco filling with a mixture of minced and chopped vegetables, such as onion, carrot, celery, mushrooms, zucchini, squash, and eggplant. For a change from the usual snacks, let your children make their own colorful kebabs with raw fruit chunks and diced cheese, or serve raw vegetable sticks with low-fat dips.

When in Rome...

While you're doing your best to keep the healthy food flag flying, there'll be times during playdates and sleepovers when your child has foods you'd never serve at home. What's more, he'll probably enjoy them and tell you so. Relax. An occasional lapse isn't going to wreck the healthy foundation you've laid. Besides, the emotional benefit your child gains from spending time with a friend counts for much more than any potential harm done by a few fatty or nutrient-poor meals.

Compliment your child for having the good manners to eat what he was offered even though it wasn't the kind of food he's used to—and continue to serve healthful meals at home.

Bigger, Not Better

As you stroll through any mall or amusement park, you may notice that many young people look as if their diets are based on quantity rather than quality. There is no mystery here—children are getting heavier because they're eating too much and exercising too little.

To meet a surge in the demand for fashionable clothing for overweight children, several major retail chains have added new extra-large sizes to their children's wear lines and are making some of their regular sizes fuller than they used to. Besides pressing retailers for larger clothes, however, parents who recognize that their children are overweight should develop ways to help them control their weight. Paying attention to food choices and becoming more active is a proven way to control weight. One approach to help your family stay slim and cut the risk of many illnesses in later life is by following the principles of the *Dietary Guidelines for Americans* (www.cnpp.usda.gov/DietaryGuidelines.htm).

Main dishes should emphasize complex carbohydrates such as brown rice, beans, and whole-grain pasta. Properly prepared and served in moderate portions, these foods are good,

---

WHAT YOU SEE IS WHAT YOU EAT

While it's true that children have an inborn ability to regulate their calorie intake according to their needs for growth and energy, they may not always get their calories from the most healthful and nutritious foods. Researchers who studied children's food choices many years ago claimed that children instinctively balanced their diets. But the children were allowed to choose only from an array of fresh, unprocessed foods without added seasonings, sugars, flavor enhancers, or artificial dyes. These young children were not given cookies, candy, potato chips, or other nutrient-poor foods.

In today's world, children are exposed to many commercial foods that try to cover up their poor nutritional quality with advertisements claiming they're "fun to eat." That's why you should get into the habit of comparing the nutritional value of foods served at home and at school with the recommendations of the *Dietary Guidelines for Americans*. Food labels are also an essential source of information. To keep healthy nutrition in focus, educate your children to choose healthful foods for themselves when you aren't around.

low-fat sources of protein and other nutrients. The body has to work hard to digest them so children feel fuller longer, and they are less likely to promote weight gain than high-fat foods. Switch to skim milk and other low-fat dairy products. For treats, serve sherbets, frozen juice popsicles without added sugar, and nonfat frozen yogurts instead of ice cream. Join your child in regular, moderate exercise such as walking, bicycling, or swimming. Discourage snacking while watching television, which can lead to a habit of overeating.

The key factor in regulating weight is balancing total daily calories with energy expended. Although 10 years ago it was thought that the amount of fat consumed was an important determinant of weight gain, more recent data emphasize that the source of calories is not as important as the number of calories that are eaten. The type of fat that is eaten is still a very important concern for the development of heart disease. Trans fat and saturated fat require attention. Current recommendations are that children and adolescents should avoid trans fat and limit the calories from saturated fat to less than 10% of total calories. (For more information about overweight in children, including how to tell if your child is overweight, see Chapter 6, Is My Child Overweight?)

Karen remained an unwavering size 6 by means of constant dieting. She was also determined to protect her daughter Alison from the taunts that had made Karen miserable throughout a chubby childhood and adolescence. Karen never cooked from scratch. With just 2 in the family, she found it simpler to let Alison choose from frozen dinners at the supermarket and managed her own weight with frozen, calorie-controlled diet entrees. She and Alison also ate out several times a week. After a long day at work, Karen often complained, "I'm too tired to zap anything!" and chose greens from the salad bar while Alison ordered pizza or a double cheeseburger.

Alarmed at Alison's noticeable weight gain as puberty approached, Karen redoubled her efforts and replaced the sweet snacks Alison preferred with fat-free cookies, low-fat ice cream and frozen yogurt, fat-free toppings, and other reduced-fat substitutes. At Alison's next checkup, Karen expressed her concerns: "I keep her on fat-free everything and still she doesn't lose weight."

Their pediatrician explained that fat free does not mean low in calories; many reduced-fat foods, for example, are high in sugar and calories. Although you may be attracted to

100-calorie snack packages on supermarket shelves, remember that even an extra 100 calories over what your child requires can contribute to weight gain.

Also keep in mind that 100 calories in an apple is more filling than 100 calories of cookies. So it's important to choose foods that make children feel full with the least amount of calories. In humans, fullness after a meal is determined by the bulk of food that is eaten rather than the number of calories. Because fruits and vegetables have a high water and fiber content, they contain few calories, occupy a lot of space in the stomach, and help children feel full after eating. This effect is just another reason to encourage your child to eat fruits and vegetables. Conversely, because fast foods and many processed foods have low water content, they tend to have more calories per unit of volume, and more of these foods tend to be eaten before children feel full. In addition, a fruit, like an orange or apple, is more filling than the juice of that fruit, like orange or apple juice.

What else will make your child feel full? Put lean protein on the table, such as lean meat, poultry, and fish (although even with protein, you can overdo it; see "Protein: How Much Do Children Need?" on the next page). Protein is much more important in creating a sense of fullness than fat or carbohydrates.

By the way, Alison's moderate weight gain was not unusual in an adolescent. The best way for mother and daughter to keep trim was to eat a balanced diet with plenty of fresh vegetables

---

DO OVERWEIGHT CHILDREN GROW UP OVERWEIGHT?

Most chubby children younger than 3 years whose parents are not overweight are likely to trim down as they grow, without further action. However, at any stage of childhood, having an obese parent increases the risk that a child will become an overweight adult. Furthermore, some children with rapid weight gain in the first several years of life will go on to become obese teenagers or adults. Cutting calories is not the right approach for children, who need a balance of nutrients for growth. All children can benefit from limiting sugar-sweetened beverages, juices, and fast foods. Never restrict a young child's diet except under your pediatrician's close guidance. Your pediatrician can suggest measures to prevent or control overweight that are aimed at altering the family lifestyle. Such measures will emphasize a sensible diet and regular physical activity.

Any child who has a drastic weight change, whether upward or downward, should be seen by a pediatrician.

and fruits as well as lean protein. By choosing meals containing foods like these, Karen found them easier to regulate because they contained fewer carbohydrates that children are likely to overconsume.

Karen's pediatrician suggested that she try making more meals from basic ingredients and involve Alison in the preparation. He pointed out that a dinner of fresh pasta with vegetable sauce from the refrigerated section was hardly more trouble than juggling different frozen entrees. Premixed greens from the produce display could make a quick salad. Finally, he suggested that Karen and Alison restrict their television viewing time and instead keep up a program of regular, moderate exercise to use up calories.

Starches to Center Stage

After infancy, children should get about half of their daily calories from carbohydrates, especially starchy foods like whole-grain breads and cereals, beans and rice, potatoes, and pasta. Less emphasis should be placed on sugars, which are simple carbohydrates.

If less than 50% of children's calories come from carbohydrates, their plates may be overloaded with meat, cheese, and other foods high in protein and fat. Too much fat in childhood adds to the risk of heart disease and other disorders later on.

Protein: How Much Do Children Need?

Protein is needed for growth as well as to maintain muscle, bone and cartilage, teeth, and every system in the body (also see Chapter 8, Nutrition Basics). As a primary constituent of muscle and bone, protein provides structural support. However, protein is so abundant in the foods Americans eat that most of us, children and adults alike, consume more than we need. Protein overload may be a more serious problem than protein deficiency. While it's important to eat enough protein, researchers believe that eating *too much* protein over many years may contribute to kidney disease and osteoporosis. What's more, our main sources of high-quality (complete) protein are animal products, such as meat and dairy foods, which have relatively high saturated-fat content. Thus, a diet that includes more protein than necessary may also be too high in saturated fat.

PROTEIN RECOMMENDED DIETARY ALLOWANCES WITH SOURCES AND SERVINGS BASED ON AGE AND WEIGHT				
Age (years)	Child's Weight (lb)	RDA Protein (g/day)	Protein Sources	Protein Content (g)
1–3	29	16	Milk (1 cup)	8
			Bread, whole wheat (1 slice)	3
4–6	44	22	Egg, boiled (1 large)	6.25
			Cheese, cheddar (1 oz)	7
7–10	61	28	Macaroni and cheese (1 cup)	17
			Corn muffin (1 medium)	21
			Bagel (1 medium)	7
11–14 (boys)	99	45	Tuna salad (½ cup)	16
			Peanut butter (1 tablespoon)	5
			Baked beans (½ cup)	9
11–14 (girls)	101	46	Chicken breast, roasted, skinless (half)	27
			English muffin (1 medium)	5

RDA, recommended dietary allowance.

Children require more protein per pound than adults because young people need it for growth as well as tissue repair. (As the Table above shows, there are other good foods besides lean meat that contain protein and that can help meet your child's protein requirements.)

Vitamins and Minerals

Surveys indicate that about a quarter of all school-aged American children are given vitamin and mineral supplements. These products are seldom necessary. A healthy child eating a balanced diet should meet the recommended dietary allowances (RDAs) for all essential vitamins and minerals. (See Chapter 8, Nutrition Basics, for where we get vitamins and what they do.) There's no evidence that levels higher than the RDAs are beneficial for healthy children; on the contrary, excessive doses of minerals and high doses, or megadoses, of vitamins A, D, and C can be harmful.

If a child's diet isn't healthy to start with, vitamin and mineral supplements won't make it right. These supplements can't help a child who is regularly consuming too many calories, too much fat, too much sugar, and not enough fiber.

In some cases, pediatricians may prescribe supplements. For example, children in homes where a strict vegetarian diet is followed, or children with medical conditions such as cystic fibrosis or malabsorption due to liver or gastrointestinal disease, may require supplements. However, these products should not be used except on your pediatrician's advice. For example, pediatricians now recommend vitamin D supplements for breastfeeding infants, beginning shortly after birth and sometimes continuing through childhood.

EXCHANGING VITAMIN AND MINERAL SOURCES	
Vitamins For children who don't like vegetables	Vitamin A: apricots, cantaloupe, mango, peaches, plums, prunes; milk; eggs Vitamin C: grapefruit, oranges, cantaloupe and other melons, strawberries
Calcium For children who don't drink milk	Part-skim and low-fat cheeses, yogurt; broccoli, dark-green leafy vegetables; chickpeas, lentils; canned sardines, salmon, and other fish with bones; calcium-fortified orange juice. Some pediatricians recommend an over-the-counter antacid containing calcium carbonate.
Protein For children who don't eat meat	Lentils, tofu; beans and other legumes in combination with grains; peanut butter; eggs; fish; nuts; dairy foods

THE CASE OF THE MISSING NUTRIENTS		
Studies in large numbers of school-aged children have shown that the nutrients most often lacking in their diets are calcium, iron, zinc, vitamin A, vitamin C (ascorbic acid), folic acid, and vitamin B_6 (also called pyridoxine). However, these essential nutrients are so plentiful in foods that a child only needs to consume the minimum number of recommended servings to get the right amount each day. The missing nutrients can be obtained from the following sources and servings:		
Whole grains, fortified cereals, and breads	6 servings	Iron, zinc, vitamin B_6, folic acid
Fruits	2 servings	Vitamins A, B_6, C; folic acid
Milk, cheese, yogurt group	3 servings	Calcium, zinc, vitamins A, B_6
Meat, fish, poultry group	2 servings	Iron, zinc, vitamin B_6
Vegetables (dark yellow; leafy greens; potatoes)	2 servings	Vitamins A, B_6, C; folic acid

If you have a picky eater in your family, you may have to juggle the food groups slightly to ensure adequate vitamin and mineral intakes, but this is a simple matter of adjusting portions. It's not necessary to spend money on expensive commercial products. (Read more in "Feeding Difficulties and Picky Eaters" on page 93.)

How Children Act and Eat at School Age

A child of early school age can be a pretty reasonable person; toddler tantrums are forgotten and adolescent turbulence is still a long way off. Most children at this age are prepared to sample a variety of foods. Their appetites vary according to their growth and activity levels. The pattern children establish as toddlers—3 full meals and a couple of snacks daily—should continue as they move into the school years.

Growth keeps up steadily, maintaining the trend that began around the first birthday and without the dramatic surges seen in infants and adolescents. Nevertheless, surges do occur. Many parents claim that their school-aged children go through phases of "stretching" and "consolidating"—looking alternately lanky and squat. Their appetites may vary in the same way—they may devour everything in sight for a month or so, then cut back as if to make up for it.

As puberty approaches, growth picks up and weight gain may increase to 9 or 10 pounds a year. The normal ranges for girls and boys from 2 to 18 years are shown in the standard growth charts in Appendix C. As the ranges indicate, it's not unusual for preadolescent young people of the same age to differ by as many as 5 inches in height.

Does Breakfast Really Matter?

Breakfast is the meal that's most likely to get lost in the daily shuffle. Time is short in the morning, even in the best-run households, and many children—especially the owls who tend to fall asleep later and make up for it by being harder to rouse in the morning—don't feel like eating during the short time available between getting up and leaving for school. Nevertheless, breakfast is important for a good start. Studies have shown that children who don't eat breakfast have trouble staying alert and concentrating during the first hours of the school day. Studies also have shown that eating breakfast improves performance on standardized tests.

WHERE CHILDREN ARE CONCERNED, YOU CAN'T HAVE TOO MANY COOKS

As their sense of independence grows, school-aged children gain a sense of self-worth from doing worthwhile jobs. The problem is, it's sometimes difficult to find jobs that aren't too hazardous or complicated for the age level.

The kitchen is a great place for children to perform tasks that show real results. Cooking is important; girls and boys should be taught how to plan and prepare healthful meals. Best of all, cooking jobs start with simple skills that a preschooler can manage and go right up the scale to high professional levels. Toddlers love to tear salad leaves, stir mixtures, and roll dough. Many little ones learn numbers as their parents count off the eggs, spoonfuls, and cupfuls in recipes. Preschoolers and older children enjoy assembling ingredients, measuring, mixing, and cutting under supervision.

While preschoolers and kindergartners are eager to work and learn, they're also easily distracted. Children in this age group usually need a lot of help to break jobs down into manageable parts. By age 7 or 8, however, children can harness their enthusiasm and focus on quite complicated tasks. Increasingly independent and cooperative, they like to be told that you appreciate their contribution to the family.

If breakfast is your family's stumbling block, you may have to work on scheduling and delivery. Move as many morning chores as you can to the evening before and push bedtime up 20 minutes earlier. At night, check that homework is finished and packed, ready for school. Lay out clothes for the morning. Get the table ready for breakfast so all you have to add is food.

Not only did Paige find it hard to wake up in the morning, but the thought of food right away made her queasy. She felt ready to eat only after she had washed, dressed, fed the cat, and spent her first 10 minutes on the school bus catching up with developments in her friends' lives since the afternoon before. Her mother stopped trying to force the family breakfast on Paige. Instead, she packed a box of chilled milk or calcium-fortified orange juice and a granola bar in Paige's backpack. Sometimes she added a piece of fruit or cheese as well. That way, Paige could eat her breakfast on the bus and be ready for school by the end of the ride.

Some children really can't face eating first thing in the morning. If your child is one of them, try offering her a small glass of 100% fruit juice as soon as she wakes up. By the time she's dressed, she may be ready for breakfast.

It's not the end of the world if your child skips breakfast. Above all, it's not worth nagging your child or worrying unnecessarily and thus setting the scene for confrontations and upsets first thing in the morning. If your morning routine runs like clockwork but your child still doesn't eat, pack a breakfast to eat on the bus or at snack time. She'll eat when she feels hungry. Emphasize cereals, low-fat dairy foods, and proteins, and keep the sugar and fat content moderate. Check the suggestions on the next page for breakfast ideas.

School Menus: News From the Lunchroom

The big change with the school years is that many meals are eaten away from home. Most students have lunch at school, whether they eat cafeteria food or bring a bag lunch. Some children also have breakfast at school.

Many schools teach the principles of good nutrition starting at the kindergarten level. Cafeterias usually provide sandwich or salad makings for those who don't want the dish of the day.

MENU SUGGESTIONS: BREAKFASTS TO GO
Dry cereal and yogurt with berries or sliced fruit
Bagel or toasted English muffin with peanut butter
Ham and low-fat cheese sandwich on whole wheat bread
Low-fat granola bar
Low-fat raisin-bran or fruit-oatmeal muffin
Warm cereal in an insulated container
Whole wheat waffle spread with lite cream cheese and strawberries
Whole wheat banana-nut bread
Low-fat milk or 100% fruit juice; insulated container of warm cocoa on winter mornings

To stretch limited budgets, many schools contract with fast-food chains for lunches. School administrators can request changes in the standard dishes, however, to keep the fat content moderate. Chicken nuggets and fish sticks, for example, can be baked instead of fried; the salad bar should offer a selection of raw vegetables and low-fat dressings.

Most schools regularly send schedules of cafeteria menus home. With this advance information, you can plan on packing lunch on the days when the main course is less healthful or is one your child prefers not to eat.

School Lunches: You Can Make a Difference

Meal planning for schools is a complicated process. Menus have to allow for a wide range of tastes and restrictions. Budgets are limited. Foods that are available at lowest cost and require the least preparation are often high in fat, sugar, and salt. According to the School Meals Initiative for Healthy Children set up in 1996, school lunch menus backed by federal subsidies must conform to the current guidelines for health. When it comes to fat, this means that meals may contain no more than 30% of total calories from fat and no more than

10% from saturated fat (for more about the various types of fat, see Chapter 6, Is My Child Overweight?). It also means that schools taking part in the National School Lunch Program have been required to take the following practical steps to improve menus:

- Adding more fruits, vegetables, and grains to menus
- Balancing menus by using foods from each of the 5 groups
- Reducing overall fat content by serving more vegetarian main courses, less beef and pork, and fewer fried foods
- Varying menus by serving more ethnic dishes, such as pasta and tacos

To back up efforts at the lunchroom level, the US Department of Agriculture set up Team Nutrition, a program to improve children's eating habits and raise their awareness about the links between food and health. Team Nutrition's goal is to improve children's lifelong eating and physical activity habits by using the principles of the *Dietary Guidelines for Americans.* This plan involves schools, parents, and the community in efforts to continuously improve school meals, and to promote the health and education of 50 million schoolchildren in more than 96,000 schools nationwide.

There's also a push at the state and local levels to help children eat better. In many communities, children at grade-school level are learning not only how to cook food but also how to grow a variety of produce. Courses combine food production and preparation with valuable lessons about history, economics, social science, and math.

If you're not satisfied with the choices available in your child's school cafeteria, get involved in your school's parent-teacher organization and brainstorm some healthful alternatives, as parents and teachers all over the country are doing. In a small town in upstate New York, for example, children at the only elementary school expanded their social studies project on India to include making vegetable curry with a spice mixture they had ground themselves. They learned to cook and enjoy many of the healthful grains and legumes—lentils, chickpeas, bulgur wheat, brown rice, and beans—that are staples of Indian cooking but not often seen in school lunches. As a change of pace, the children celebrated Martin Luther King, Jr, Day by combining black-eyed peas, corn, and collards in a soul-food stew. Their enthusiasm led the local supermarket to stock grains and greens that brought about a mini-revolution in the community's diet.

In West Virginia, a state-sponsored booklet shows teachers how to introduce children to foods from around the world in social studies classes. The booklet includes recipes that can be adapted to classroom and school cafeteria use. Oregon schoolchildren as young as 5 were consulted on what should be served in school lunches. The result was a surge in children eating fruits and vegetables.

Even if you haven't the time or resources to revamp the school cafeteria, you may be able to see that the salad bar offers a good selection of raw vegetables and low-fat dressings. Vending machine choices can also be modified to eliminate high-fat and empty-calorie munchies and provide healthy snacks that include more fresh fruit and low-fat dairy products, as well as water and 100% fruit juice instead of sodas.

Try to get your child's school to stock healthy choices in the vending machines. Although school administrators fear that they will lose money if they make these changes, schools that have provided healthier options have not lost money or have seen their revenue increase.

HEALTHY CHOICES FOR VENDING MACHINES	
Instead of	**Suggest**
Potato chips	Baked tortilla chips
Artificially flavored and colored corn and cheese snacks	Popcorn
Candy bars	Granola bars, trail mix
Sweetened, fruit-flavored roll-ups	Fruits, dried or fresh
Fruit-flavored drinks with added sugar, soda pop	Water, unsweetened 100% fruit juices
Whole milk; full-fat yogurt	Skim or low-fat milk, yogurt
Ice cream	Sherbet, Italian ice, pure fruit popsicles, frozen yogurt
Crème-filled sandwich cookies, chocolate-chip cookies	Fig bar cookies, graham crackers

"But All the Other Kids Have Candy!"

Packing bag lunches gives you lots of opportunities to develop your own creative ideas. It's also a good time to get children actively involved in nutrition by planning a balanced meal and helping to prepare it. When children help prepare food, they'll often eat dishes their parents wouldn't dream they'd like.

Many schools forbid lunch-box trading, which cuts the risk that your child will trade his fresh fruit dessert for someone else's candy. Sooner or later, however, you're going to hear, *"All* the other kids get candy in their lunch boxes!" or "It's not fair! Why do I always get carrots and fruit when everybody else gets potato chips and cookies?"

You can repeat the message, "Candy, chips, and other high-calorie treats are 'sometimes' foods." And there are other ways. Children at the elementary school level love to show off their learning. Ask your child to teach you what he's learned at school about proper nutrition, then pool what you know and come up with some joint guidelines for healthful choices. Even kindergartners are old enough to understand why fresh fruits and vegetables are better than chips and cookies, or why candy and soda are OK as occasional treats but not as lunch-box staples. So that your child won't feel deprived, you could let him mark the calendar with a weekly "treat day." On other days, his lunch box might include nonfat oatmeal-raisin or fig bar cookies for dessert, or a bag of baked tortilla chips with salsa for dipping.

TAKE LESSONS FROM HOME TO SCHOOL

At home, give children the job of preparing salads for family meals. Even children too young to handle a sharp knife can tear up lettuce and other greens, then toss them with just enough dressing to make the ingredients shiny without leaving a puddle in the bottom of the bowl. Suggest that your child prepare his own salads at the salad bar in the school cafeteria.

Clean Hands, Healthy Eating

When you pack a bag lunch, thoroughly wash and dry all reusable containers, and wash your hands just as you do before preparing any other meal (also see Chapter 13, Food Safety). Remember that the lunch is going to sit unrefrigerated in a backpack or locker for several hours. Choose sandwich fillings that don't need to be refrigerated and avoid meats or salads that may spoil. Pack crushable foods in plastic containers. Wash fruit well. Peel and wash vegetables such as carrots and wrap them in plastic or wax paper. Always discard partly consumed drinks and foods such as yogurt.

It's a good idea to invest in an insulated soft pack and an unbreakable insulated drink bottle. If you haven't got a cold pack, get into the routine of freezing juice boxes and plastic bottles of water. Tucked into the bag, the drink is thawed by lunchtime and helps to keep other foods cool.

After-School Snacks

Keep your kitchen stocked with healthy snack foods such as fresh fruits, raw vegetables with dips, baked tortillas and salsa, whole-grain crackers, pretzels, and low-fat yogurt to fill in after-school gaps. This is especially important when both parents work outside the home and children are in charge of their own after-school snacks and sometimes dinner as well. Avoid having a supply of cookies, cakes, ice cream, and fatty, salty snack foods on hand. Children

---

H_2O + SUGAR + FOOD DYE + BOTTLE = $$$

Sports drinks children see advertised aren't necessary and add extra calories. Water, however, is a much less expensive way to keep tissues hydrated and systems working. For extra zing, add a few slices of lemon or lime.

CHOOSING DESSERTS WISELY

The editors of this book typically ask parents of overweight children about their diets, including what the family has for dessert. Some respond by saying, "Ice cream." When we ask whether they eat ice cream every night, the response is often, "Well, not every night, but most nights."

But there are much healthier choices than ice cream. Ice cream, cake, and cookies are *treats* and "sometimes" foods; they shouldn't be consumed daily. Desserts can be fruit, yogurt, or some other healthful "sweets."

Also, never make desserts contingent on what and how well your child eats; don't coax him with statements like, "If you eat your broccoli, you can have cookies."

who have unsupervised access to such foods can gain unwanted weight. However, served as occasional treats, these foods do no harm and provide variety.

There's another important point to keep in mind—if you've been prone to keeping high-calorie, high-fat snack foods and sweets in the house, are you keeping them at home as much for yourself as for your child? If you're reluctant to banish them from your pantry, examine your motives for doing so.

School-aged Children and Sports

Children at grade-school level should be getting plenty of exercise and taking part in organized sports where there are opportunities to do so. School-aged athletes can get all the nutrition they need from recommended servings, although you may have to increase portion sizes or add a snack or two for very active children. A young athlete will feel most comfortable when performing if she eats a low-fat, high-carbohydrate meal, such as pasta with tomato-vegetable sauce, several hours before an event. High-performance supplements and weight-training programs to reduce body fat or increase muscle mass have no place in school athletics. They won't improve athletic performance and may be harmful.

Keep the Water Flowing

Apart from a balanced diet with enough calories for energy and growth, active children need plenty of water. School-aged athletes are especially vulnerable to dehydration when playing in hot, humid weather. Parents and coaches should keep a close watch to make sure that children drink plenty of water before and during practices and games, even though they may not feel thirsty. Thirst lags behind water losses; by the time children feel thirsty, they may already be dehydrated. Water is always a better choice than sports drinks, which supply calories in addition to the water they contain. A school-aged child should drink more during exercise or in hot weather. Remember, young children have a harder time coping with extremes of temperature than adolescents and adults.

Children and Constipation

Constipation is one of childhood's most overreported and least understood symptoms. Many people have the idea that constipation means not having a daily bowel movement. They think children will get sick if they don't have a movement every day, and that "toxins" will be absorbed from the bowel. Not so. Many children (and adults) have several bowel movements every day, while others go 2 or 3 days or even longer, then pass a stool of normal consistency.

Constipation consists of hard stools large in diameter that may be associated with significant pain, rectal bleeding, stool retention, and soiling. Constipation may occur when the diet lacks fiber or fluid. It's also fairly common after a viral illness, when children may not drink enough and are less active than usual.

To keep your child's bowel movements normal, make sure he eats high-fiber foods such as fruits, vegetables, and whole-grain breads and cereals. Nutrition experts recommend as a general rule that a person's daily intake of fiber should equal her age plus 5 g (thus, for a 7-year-old, 7 + 5 = 12 g a day) up to a maximum of 35 g a day. Oat bran cereal and popcorn are good sources of fiber that many young people like to eat. A couple of prunes or a small glass of prune juice can help stimulate bowel function. Prunes contain a natural laxative, called isatin, as well as lots of soluble fiber and sorbitol—a naturally occurring, nonabsorbable sugar alcohol—both of which have laxative effects. Apple juice and pear juice are also good sources of sorbitol; however, cooked apples, such as in applesauce, may contribute to constipation and are often given to help children with diarrhea. Plenty of water is needed to augment water in the stool and help keep bowel movements regular. (Also see Chapter 9, Spitting Up, Gagging, Vomiting, Diarrhea, and Constipation.)

"He Doesn't Eat, No Matter What I Say!"

There are school-aged children who seem to eat next to nothing. They have little appetite or may not enjoy eating. To their parents' amazement, these children keep on growing, which shows that they're getting enough to eat. Some of these children feel uncomfortable if they try to conform to the usual daily pattern of 3 relatively large meals. They are happier nibbling on several small meals over the course of the day.

SHOULD YOU DISGUISE FOOD?

Some books have coached parents to hide foods that they want their children to eat but the children refuse. You can help maintain balance in your child's diet by grinding up food so it's not recognizable in the pasta sauce or pureeing soup so the green bits are not visible. You can also serve mashed cauliflower (as though it were mashed potatoes), or mix the cauliflower in with mashed potatoes. If your child likes sushi, have him try it with vegetables inside as another way to slip vegetables into his diet.

At the same time, however, hiding food does not teach your child how to make healthy food selections. So try to be honest about what you're giving him to eat. Find a way that he will enjoy vegetables (dipping them in low-fat ranch dressing, for example), or put just a small amount of the refused food on his plate over and over (which may eventually get him to try it). One recent study showed that if a refused vegetable were offered along with a sweet fruit, the child was more likely to eat the vegetable.

Also, your child may have a particular sensitivity to certain tastes. For instance, vegetables such as broccoli and cauliflower may taste bitter to some children. Like all of us, they simply may not like some foods. One parent recently said that her children had asked her, "Can we please have peas once in a while?" She realized that because she herself did not like peas, she never served them. So allow for individual tastes, but only up to a point.

Coaxing a nibbler to eat larger, less frequent meals isn't helpful. In fact, studies show that children consume less when parents try to persuade them to eat. Some nibblers are also put off when parents praise them for eating. To these children, attention to eating makes them feel as if they're being forced to eat. On the other hand, leaving food out for unrestricted snacking leads to bad habits of constant picking, and the food may spoil.

Let your nibbler eat as much as he wants at the 3 meals and additional snacks you serve each day. He may eat less at mealtimes and more at snack times than other members of the family. At least you'll be sure that he's getting the amount and variety he needs while the family meal schedule is maintained.

Feeding Difficulties and Picky Eaters

Children's food preferences veer all over the menu—today they want third helpings of spinach, tomorrow they *never* eat anything green. Trying as it can be to keep up with the whims of an easygoing child, the picky eater presents a challenge of a different order. Some picky eaters are difficult feeders from the beginning. For them, picky eating and faddishness are part of a progression from fussiness and colic to extreme resistance to new foods. Some children are picky because they are unusually sensitive to certain tastes and textures, while others use food as a tool to manipulate their parents and gain attention.

Appetite and hunger are 2 different things. Hunger is the body's signal that it needs fuel. By contrast, appetite is a learned behavior involving pleasure and other emotions associated with eating. Hunger is present from birth; appetite develops over time.

Children learn positive and negative attitudes about eating from observing what goes on around them. For example, a child who takes part in relaxed family meals from her early months is more likely to look forward to eating than one who's never allowed to leave the table until she has finished everything on her plate. When parents use food as a bribe or reward ("You'll get double dessert if you clean your plate!"), children quickly learn that they can use food in a similar way and may try to manipulate their parents by eating or refusing meals. Parents worried by their daughter's refusal to eat may be surprised to learn that the child is only following her mother's example of nonstop dieting.

Many problems related to picky eating gradually disappear after a child begins eating regularly away from parental supervision. For example, children in group child care tend to copy the way their friends eat. A picky older child may eat school lunches without a fuss, although he continues his picky behavior at meals he shares with his parents. Finally, many faddish eaters get more pleasure from attention seeking than they do from feeding. Therefore, while it's acceptable to compliment satisfactory behavior at the end of the meal, food refusals and demands for attention should be ignored or managed by promptly terminating the meal. If you've come to expect your child being picky as part of your family's mealtime routine, it may be advisable to seek outside help, starting with your pediatrician. (For problems related to eating disorders, see Chapter 10.)

Some children fail to develop pleasure in eating because medical problems or treatments interfere with the normal feeding process. For example, a child who had to be fed by tube for a long period because she was premature or sick as a newborn may dislike the sensation of food in her mouth. Children with persistent nasal congestion, a frequent complication of tube feeding or allergies, have a reduced sense of taste and smell and therefore take little pleasure in eating. Nowadays, children who require special feeding techniques, such as tubes, are given appropriate oral stimulation—so-called *sham feeding*—to help them adapt to feeding by mouth. If your child has feeding difficulties related to medical problems or treatments, your pediatrician will advise you about where to find appropriate resources for help and support.

In studying how children respond to efforts to get them to eat, researchers have agreed on a few universal truths.

First, it is the parents' responsibility to provide the food, and it is the child's decision to eat it.

Second, bribes or orders are not useful. They make children resistant to foods they feel neutral about and actively dislike foods to which they're indifferent. The child may well reason, "If they have to bribe me to eat this stuff, it must be bad."

Third, mealtimes are for eating and socializing, not for playing games. Make meals a time for enjoyable family interaction in which children want to take part.

Fourth, meals should be kept to a reasonable time limit in keeping with the child's attention span.

FOOD CHALLENGES DURING THE SCHOOL YEARS

When my child stays over at friends' houses, he eats all kinds of junk foods that I never serve at home. Should I be concerned?

An occasional meal or snack including junk foods isn't going to harm your child if his normal diet at home is healthy. (See page 88.)

My child is much smaller than all her classmates. She's growing steadily but very slowly. Should she eat more?

Each child grows at her own rate, depending on thousands of inherited and environmental influ-ences. There aren't any hard-and-fast rules about how many calories a school-aged child needs to eat. As long as your child is eating a variety of foods and is growing normally, there's no cause for concern. In fact, trying to make her eat more may have the opposite effect from what you intend. (See pages 74 and 91.)

My child doesn't feel like eating right after he gets up. Is breakfast such a big deal at this age?

Breakfast is important. Children who don't eat breakfast may have trouble staying alert. Revise your child's morning schedule to allow more time. Waking him with a glass of 100% fruit juice may be helpful. Or try packing a brown-bag breakfast to eat on the way to school. (See page 83.)

My child refuses to eat in the school cafeteria, and when I look at the menus, I can see why. Aren't there any guidelines for school lunches?

School lunches backed with federal funds must conform to current health standards. For example, meals may have only 30% of total calories from fat and no more than 10% from saturated fat. There are lots of exciting, healthy developments in school lunch programs. (Read about them starting on page 84.) Surprisingly, children who eat school lunches receive more key nutrients than children who bring their lunch.

My son is really into sports. He says he could improve his performance by taking vitamin and mineral supplements. Because these products are not drugs, is there any harm in let-ting him try them?

Nutritional supplements won't help performance, and some can actually be harmful. School-aged athletes get all the nutrition they need from a normal, balanced diet. (See page 90.)

Chapter 5

The Adolescent Years

At the peak of a growth spurt, an adolescent may easily grow 4 inches in a year. This increase parallels changes inside the body. The heart, for example, doubles in size, as does lung capacity. Similar changes take place in nearly all other organs. Even after the dramatic changes of puberty, the bodies of teens continue to mature.

A mother who we'll call Marilyn Davis was very proud of her 2 teenagers—but she also felt exasperated at times when it came to their nutrition. Both of them were very involved in extracurricular activities, including sports and school clubs. Because of their busy schedules, they ate very few meals at home on weekdays. At the same time, at the urging of some of her friends, her 15-year-old daughter had decided to become a vegetarian, and Marilyn was worried that she wasn't eating balanced meals. Her 17-year-old son was on the varsity football team, and his coach was pressuring him to gain weight. Marilyn felt that her children's friends and coaches had become much more influential on dietary choices than she was. And she worried that the pressures on her children were sometimes leading them to make inappropriate food choices. Her anxiety led to a lot of sleepless nights and frequent arguments with her teenagers about what they should be eating.

Sound familiar? Adolescence is a time of enormous physical and emotional growth, yet your teenagers may have a mind of their own about their diet and are listening too much to others instead of you. When you add advertising and product placement to the mix, in which food companies pay to have their products prominently featured on television and in the movies, sometimes you may feel like throwing up your hands, convinced that you're fighting a losing battle. (See "Troubling Influences on Teen Diets" on page 99.)

How They Grow

Children's growth rate picks up even before they develop the first signs of sexual matura-tion—breast buds in girls and testes growth in boys—then accelerates rapidly. Growth reaches a peak at about age 12 in girls, before menstruation begins. In boys, the peak rate occurs later, at about age 14. These numbers are just averages. Sexual maturation and increased growth may begin as much as 2 years earlier or later.

Until puberty, boys and girls the same age are similar in size. With the onset of puberty but before the first menstrual period (menarche), girls have reached their growth peak and are looking down on their male classmates with an advantage of 1½ inches. Although boys start puberty later, they soon overtake girls. By age 14, boys equal girls in height. After growth is complete, boys are 5 inches taller, on average, than girls.

Where Energy Goes

It takes measurable energy to carry out various vital functions and keep the body healthy. The energy the body uses at rest is called the *resting metabolic rate,* which is expressed in cal-ories. Adolescents also need calories to fuel their physical activity. On a daily basis, normally active teenagers use up one third to half of all the calories they consume in physical activity. Of course, the amount of energy used for physical activity by individual teenagers varies—from less than half the energy in a sedentary adolescent's diet to much more than half for a high-performing athlete. Finally, teenagers need a small number of additional calories to power the adolescent growth spurt. An adequate energy supply is essential for this process.

During adolescence, young people become increasingly independent of their families, although a good deal of this so-called independence actually consists of doing exactly what their friends are doing. A teenager would rather join a group of friends for fast food—if that's what the group is doing—than make polite conversation around the family table. Furthermore, a typical teenager's schedule—crowded with school and extracurricular activities, sports, perhaps a part-time job, staying up late, sleeping late, and communicating with and hanging out with friends—may not leave a lot of time to join the family at meals. For these and other reasons, many adolescents seem to eat most of their meals on the run.

However, even if your teenager is eating out more often than in, you can encourage her to get balanced nutrition with low-fat, healthful choices.

Learning to Deal With Outside Pressure

Because children and teenagers are exposed to many hours of media that promote food consumption, their food choices tend to be heavily influenced by advertising. A commercial may suggest, for instance, that eating certain snacks or drinking the right soda will help teenagers fit in with the group and have a good time. Clever and memorable, ads are designed to sell products, not to instruct adolescents about healthy eating. Nutrition advice in teen magazines is generally sound. In some cases, though, it may be influenced by advertisers and often focuses on dieting, building muscle, or making a teenager more appealing to the opposite sex.

As your child enters adolescence, continue to deliver the message that ads are designed for one purpose: to manipulate consumers to buy products. Urge your teenager to read between

---

TROUBLING INFLUENCES ON TEEN DIETS

While television ads are obvious efforts by food manufacturers to create interest in and sales of their products, there are other, more subtle attempts to whet the appetites of young consumers. Food companies budget large amounts of money to have their products and their logos clearly visible in scenes in motion pictures and television shows. Whether it's an actor or athlete sipping a soft drink whose label is clearly noticeable, or a kitchen table with a container of mustard in full view, these product placements don't just happen by chance. And when a teenager sees his television or sports hero consuming a particular food product on camera, like high-fat potato chips, high-sugar breakfast cereals, or an energy drink, he may spend his own allowance on it or try to convince you to add the item to the shopping cart on the next trip to the supermarket.

Advertisers are always looking for new ways to reach young consumers and their parents. Product placements may not be as "hard sell" as a 30- or 60-second television commercial, but they're advertising all the same. Research has shown that they can influence the thinking and the food choices of children and teenagers—sometimes with serious consequences. There are many reasons why childhood obesity is more common, but television ads and product placement are certainly contributors. (For more information about childhood and adolescent obesity, see Chapter 6, Is My Child Overweight?)

JACK IS THE BEANSTALK

Hands and feet get bigger first. Then legs grow longer, giving the typical gangly, coltish look of the early teenage years. Soon the jaw begins to lengthen and facial features enlarge. Because different parts of the body grow at different rates, a child may look as if he's nothing but elbows and knees one month and all ears and nose the next. Finally, the trunk and chest catch up, and all the parts of the puzzle fit into place.

EATING PATTERNS CHANGE

Eating together has been a way to strengthen family ties throughout every age and culture. Young people entering adolescence usually have fairly well-established habits and preferences based on their families' approaches to food. However, as adolescents grow older, they eat fewer meals with their families. The way their friends eat may become the dominant influence on eating patterns.

HEALTHY AND UNHEALTHY CHOICES AT FAST-FOOD RESTAURANTS

Many of the fast-food restaurants where teenagers like to gather offer not only high-fat burgers and fries but also a selection of healthy alternatives.

- A chicken fajita instead of a breaded chicken sandwich
- A lean burger instead of an outsized special with lots of fat-laden trimmings
- A baked potato instead of high-fat french fries
- A main-course salad from the salad bar with low-fat dressing
- Nonfat frozen yogurt with a fresh fruit topping instead of an ice cream sundae or a large wedge of pie
- Water or a low-fat milkshake instead of soda or a regular shake

Still, fast-food restaurants have unhealthy features as well, including

- The food is high in fat and carbohydrates.
- The portions are large, so meals may contain as many calories as adolescents need in a whole day.
- The sodium content in some meals may be more than what teens need in a day.
- A large soda may contain 17 teaspoons of sugar.

Teenagers will eat pizza even when they turn down almost any other food. Luckily, pizza can be a healthy balance of complex carbohydrates, vegetables, protein, and a little fat—if it's garnished with vegetables such as tomato sauce, mushrooms, eggplant, and peppers instead of high-fat toppings such as sausage, pepperoni, and extra cheese.

the lines of ads and commercials and to read the labels on food products to find out what the ads don't say. (More information about dealing with outside influences follows in this chapter and also in Chapter 11, What Do I Do About Outside Influences?)

What Are Adolescents Really Eating?

Schools teach children about nutrition, often starting as early as kindergarten. The healthy message continues on up through the grades, stressing the importance of fruits and vegetables as advised by the *Dietary Guidelines for Americans,* American Heart Association, National Cancer Institute, and others; complex carbohydrates such as whole grains and cereals; low-fat dairy and protein choices; and fiber. With new government guidelines, many school lunch programs have switched to more healthful and varied menus. Yet surveys show poor eating patterns that may have adverse effects on current weight, fitness, and future health.

Researchers who compared adolescents' food intakes with government recommendations (also see Chapter 6, Is My Child Overweight?) found that on the whole, teenaged boys ate a much healthier diet than girls the same age. For example, boys met at least the minimum recommendations for grains, vegetables, and meat, though their choices tended to be high in fat. By contrast, adolescent girls failed to achieve the minimum in any food group. As they grew older, boys and girls ate more vegetables and meat, although the increase in vegetables was offset by a corresponding decrease in fruit consumption. However, nearly a quarter of the vegetables the youngsters counted as daily servings were french fries, which are high in fat and have limited nutritional value. The intake of dark-green and deep-yellow vegetables was very low compared with recommended levels.

Particularly disturbing was how few dairy foods teen girls ate. Only about 1 girl in 5 was eating the recommended 4 or 5 daily servings of dairy foods, and grain and fruit group intake was not much better. They ate a healthier amount of vegetables and meat but still far below recommended levels. The researchers suggested that the low energy (calorie) intake among teenaged girls reflected the typical overriding concern with weight in this age group.

Researchers warned that adolescents who met none of the recommended intakes were getting far less than the dietary reference intakes (formerly known as recommended dietary allowances or RDAs) for essential vitamins and minerals, including vitamin B$_6$, folic acid, calcium, iron, and zinc, and their diets had far too little fiber. (See Appendix G.) Invariably, teenagers who failed to meet the minimum in any food group were eating high levels of added sugars. In all age groups, children consumed more fat than the recommended quantity (no more than 30% of calories); they obtained 40% of their energy from fats and added

---

CALORIES TO GROW ON

A child's developing body uses food energy for vital functions of muscles, the brain and heart, physical activity, growth, and sexual maturation. If the energy supply is lacking because not enough food is being eaten or because of excessive exercise, growth suffers. But even at the height of the adolescent growth spurt, a teenager uses only about 100 calories a day to grow—equivalent to the energy in 2 slices of bread.

CARBOHYDRATES AND CALORIES IN A FEW EVERYDAY FOODS

Food, serving size	Carbohydrates (g)	Calories
Breads, cereals		
White or whole wheat, 1 slice	12	65
Bagel (1 medium)	38	200
Corn flakes, sugar-frosted, ¾ cup	26	110
Cracker, graham, 2 pieces	11	60
English muffin	27	140
Taco shell	7	50
Toaster pastry, 1	35	195
Fruits, juices		
Apple, 1 medium	21	80
Banana, 1 medium	27	105

CARBOHYDRATES AND CALORIES IN A FEW EVERYDAY FOODS, *CONTINUED*		
Food, serving size	**Carbohydrates (g)**	**Calories**
Orange juice, fresh, ½ cup	13	55
Raisins, 1½-oz package	10	40
Pasta, cooked firm, drained (1 cup)		
Macaroni	39	190
Egg noodles	37	200
Spaghetti	39	190
Rice (1 cup)		
Brown or enriched white	25	115
Vegetables and legumes		
Black beans, cooked, ½ cup	20	115
Black-eyed peas, cooked, ½ cup	18	95
Carrot, raw, 1 medium	7	30
Celery, raw, 1 stalk		5
Corn, boiled, 1 ear	19	85
Kidney beans, cooked, ½ cup	20	110
Potato, baked, 1 medium	50	220
Potato, french-fried in vegetable oil, frozen (10 pieces)	20	160
Yogurt, low-fat, 8 oz		
Plain	16	145
Fruit flavored	43	230

sugars without meeting recommendations for grains, fruit, and low-fat dairy foods. Even though teenaged boys weren't eating according to guidelines, they still had healthier diets, whereas teenaged girls and children from minority and low-income households had the least healthy eating patterns.

Adolescents are often quite knowledgeable about calories, fat, and cholesterol. However, apart from school courses in nutrition, many tend to get nutritional information from television programs, talk shows, and the Internet. Such sources are prone to deliver endless, sensational stories about instant weight loss programs and diet supplements "guaranteed" to burn off fat. What's worrisome is that these young people may skip meals in favor of eating snacks or convenience food while watching television. For some teenagers, the family dinner table may be something they see only in television situation comedies. However, family dinners for conversation as well as modeling healthy eating should be encouraged whenever possible.

It's hard to convince teenagers of the importance of good nutrition for their future years, to prevent cancer, heart disease, and other serious illnesses. However, teenaged athletes may accept the importance of eating well to improve performance. All adolescents want to be physically attractive (even though their notions of what constitutes attractiveness may differ from yours) and may adapt their diets to achieve this goal. Girls and boys alike should be encouraged to develop an interest in food, healthy eating, and exercise to stay fit and strong.

How Many Calories?

As a general rule, moderately active adolescent boys should consume about 2,700 calories a day, and girls need about 2,300 calories. It's impossible to specify an exact number of calories because individual energy needs depend on size and build, growth rate, and level of physical activity. A rapidly developing boy who is involved in a challenging athletics program, for example, may burn up 5,000 calories or even more a day, whereas a girl who tends to be sedentary might need only about 2,000 calories or less. In adolescence, as in the early school years, the best guide is a satisfactory rate of growth—if the young person is still growing—along with good levels of energy and fitness.

Where Those Calories Come From

Complex carbohydrates—starchy foods such as pasta, breads, cereals, rice, beans, lentils, and other legumes—are the bedrock of a healthful diet. Adolescents, like adults, should get 55% to 60% of their daily calories from carbohydrates. This amount allows for a large proportion of complex carbohydrates and a smaller amount of simple carbohydrates, or sugars, including the naturally occurring sugars in fruits and vegetables. Only 30% of calories, at most, should come from fats, with no more than one third of this allowance (that is, 10% of total daily calories) from saturated fat—the kind that tends to stay solid at room temperature. (Most of the fat in meat and dairy products is saturated.)

Another type of fat called *trans fats* has received a lot of attention in recent years. Like saturated fats, they can raise your child's LDL ("bad") cholesterol levels, and reduce his HDL ("good") cholesterol. Trans fats are found in foods such as french fries, pizza dough, pastries, and stick margarine, and if your teenager consumes a lot of them, they can raise his risk of developing heart disease. In 2006 the Food and Drug Administration required that trans fat content be added to the Nutrition Facts panel. Since that time, trans fats in the food supply have been considerably reduced, although not completely eliminated. (For more information about trans fats, see pages 196 and 296.)

Finally, although protein is important, it should not make up more than 10% to 12% of the calories consumed.

How Big Is a Serving?

Serving sizes for teenagers are the same as for adults. (For more about recommended daily servings, check out the *Dietary Guidelines for Americans* at www.cnpp.usda.gov/DietaryGuidelines.htm.)

The Iron Age

A teenager's blood volume expands to keep up with the body's increasing need for oxygen, which is carried by iron-rich hemoglobin in red blood cells. The RDA of iron for *adolescent* girls is 15 mg a day, and some experts recommend up to 25 mg for girls who are heavily involved in athletics. The RDA for teenaged boys is 12 mg of iron a day. (Also see "What

Makes Sammy [and Samantha] Run?" on page 112.) Male and female athletes who run a lot have excess iron needs.

Lack of iron means lower levels of hemoglobin leading to anemia, tiredness, weakness, increased susceptibility to infection, and other symptoms. Most people know that iron is important in adolescent girls' diets to make up for menstrual blood loss. Our bodies retrieve iron from old blood cells. Therefore, boys and men don't need to consume as much iron as girls and women, who lose iron during their menstrual period. However, although boys generally have higher hemoglobin levels than girls, boys can develop iron deficiency; they need plenty of iron in the diet. A boy or girl may be iron deficient without actually being anemic. Iron is also critical for optimal brain functioning.

There are 2 different types of dietary iron. Heme iron is found in foods from animals, such as meat, fish and shellfish, and poultry. Nonheme iron comes from plants; good sources are dark-green leafy vegetables, soy products, and dried fruits. Iron-fortified breads and cereals are also important sources of the mineral. Iron cooking pots may make a small contribution to iron intake.

Our bodies absorb only between 5% and 20% of the iron we eat, depending on the composition of the meal. With heme iron, about 20% is absorbed no matter how it's prepared and served. Nonheme iron is less easily absorbed, but we can increase the absorption rate by eating sources of nonheme iron—such as legumes and fortified breads and grains—together with foods that contain some heme iron, or foods rich in vitamin C. These include citrus fruits and vegetables such as cauliflower, broccoli, tomatoes, and potatoes. Meat contains a substance that is also known to promote nonheme iron absorption, although it has not yet been isolated and identified. Combining a small amount of meat, therefore, with iron-rich legumes or beans can boost the amount of iron that is absorbed.

Tannins, phytates, and calcium in foods such as tea, bran, and milk, respectively, can hinder the absorption of nonheme iron eaten at the same meal by as much as 50%. If your child has been diagnosed with iron deficiency anemia, or if you're otherwise concerned about her iron intake, have her drink tea and milk only at snack times. At mealtimes, serve fruits and vegetables rich in vitamin C or a glass of citrus juice to help her absorb more iron.

SERVING SIZES FOR TEENAGERS	
Bread	1 slice
Cereal, dry	1 oz (¾ cup)[a]
Cereal, cooked	1 oz (½ cup)
Pasta, rice (cooked)	1 oz (½ cup)
Vegetables (cooked)	½ cup
Fruit	1 medium piece, eg, 1 apple or pear
Milk, yogurt	1 cup
Cheese	1.5 oz (1½" cube or 2 precut slices)
Meat, poultry, fish	2 to 3 oz (about the size of a deck of playing cards)

[a]All cup measures are a standard 8-oz measuring cup.

Lean meat, poultry, and fish are good sources of iron. Other sources include soy products such as tofu, soy milk, chickpeas (garbanzo beans), lentils, and white beans. If you cook an acidic food, such as tomato sauce or chili, in a cast-iron pot, some of the iron in the pot is leached out into the food and can supply a little dietary iron; however, some other vitamins may be lost.

Growing Bones

A good supply of calcium is essential during adolescence. Growing children build up approximately 40% to 45% of their peak adult bone mass during the teenage years, and calcium is the main building block of bone. The National Academy of Sciences recommends 1,300 mg as the RDA of calcium for adolescents (see "Recommended Daily Calcium and Vitamin D Intake" on page 109). A teenager should easily be able to reach this level with 4 daily servings from the milk, yogurt, and cheese group plus a good intake of green vegetables. Milk and dairy products made from fortified milk may be the best source because they also contain vitamin D, which helps absorb calcium.

STRONG BONES NOW, STRONG BONES LATER

Most of the calcium in the bones is laid down during adolescence and early adulthood. After that time, calcium in the bones can be turned over or lost but not added. Therefore, a good intake of calcium during adolescence is crucial for reducing the risk of osteoporosis and disabling fractures later in life.

After about age 30, bone mass declines steadily in women and men, and the rate of loss accelerates sharply in women once they reach menopause. Greater peak bone mass in early adulthood reduces the risk of osteoporosis, or weakened bones, later in life. This is especially important for those with a family history of osteoporosis.

Women are at greater risk than men for developing osteoporosis, and women of Northern European and Asian ancestry are at higher risk than those of African and Mediterranean descent. Many other factors appear to be involved, including smoking and having a slender build, fair skin, and family history of the disease. All women, regardless of their risk factors, should try to keep their bones healthy with adequate intake of calcium and vitamin D and regular, moderate, weight-bearing exercise.

Many teenagers, particularly weight-conscious girls, shun calcium-rich dairy products because they're afraid of getting fat, but low-fat and nonfat milk products are widely available. Removing fat doesn't take away calcium, and reduced-fat dairy products are just as rich in calcium as the full-fat versions. In addition, low-fat milk does not appear to increase the risk of obesity.

Girls who avoid milk are susceptible to osteoporosis. Serious effects on bone formation may appear before such women reach age 40. In fact, girls who don't take in enough calcium are more prone to fractures and stress fractures during adolescence and heal more slowly after bone injuries.

It is crucial that adolescent girls pay special attention to getting enough calcium and vitamin D. Sports coaches and dance teachers, as well as parents, have a responsibility to help female athletes and young performers eat a healthful, balanced diet. Typical teenagers find it hard to picture themselves in middle age and beyond. Thus, preaching a diet for tomorrow's health may not be persuasive. It's better to emphasize the importance of good nutrition—including plenty of calcium—to achieve the best performance today.

RECOMMENDED DAILY CALCIUM AND VITAMIN D INTAKE

A recent Institute of Medicine report has provided new recommendations for the intake of calcium and vitamin D in children and adults. In the Table that follows, calcium and vitamin D requirements are expressed in 3 different ways. Because infants have not been the subjects of clinical trials, the levels of calcium and vitamin D are expressed in terms of adequate intake, based on the composition of human milk (calcium) or the level of vitamin D intake necessary to maintain adequate levels of vitamin D in the blood. For children and adolescents 1 to 18 years of age, levels are presented based on the recommended dietary allowance, which is the level of intake that meets the requirements of 97.5% of the population. Also included is the upper level intake. These values are the safe "high end" of the scale. These, however, *should not* be used as a goal but as a cautionary note that high amounts of these nutrients have been linked to health problems like kidney stones and kidney and tissue damage.

CALCIUM			
Age	**Adequate Intake**	**Recommended Dietary Allowance**	**Upper Level Intake**
0–6 mo	200 mg	—	1,000 mg
6–12 mo	260 mg	—	1,500 mg
1–3 y	—	700 mg	2,500 mg
4–8 y	—	1,000 mg	2,500 mg
9–18 y	—	1,300 mg	3,000 mg
VITAMIN D			
Age	**Adequate Intake**	**Recommended Dietary Allowance**	**Upper Level Intake**
0–6 mo	400 IU	—	1,000 IU
6–12 mo	400 IU	—	1,500 IU
1–3 y	—	600 IU	2,500 IU
4–8 y	—	600 IU	3,000 IU
9–18 y	—	600 IU	4,000 IU

Adapted with permission from National Academies Press. http://www.iom.edu/Reports/2010/Dietary-Reference-Intakes-For-Calcium-and-Vitamin-D.aspx. Accessed June 30, 2011

Tofu is also an excellent source of calcium. Dark-green leafy vegetables such as kale and turnip greens are low in calories and have as much calcium, ounce for ounce, as some dairy foods. Calcium intake should be limited to approximately 500 mg/dose, as additional calcium may not be absorbed. Calcium-fortified orange juice is a good choice because the vitamin C in the juice promotes the absorption of calcium. Vitamin D is also needed to absorb calcium. The body can make vitamin D when skin is exposed to the sun. Dietary sources include fortified milk, cereal, eggs, and butter. Adolescent girls who won't drink milk and don't eat enough calcium should take a vitamin D supplement of 400 IU per day. Avoid taking iron with dairy foods or calcium supplements.

Folate

All teenagers should consume plenty of leafy green vegetables, fruits, and fortified cereals for folate (another form of this vitamin is called folic acid), which our bodies need to make the DNA and RNA in cells, as well as for the formation of healthy red blood cells. Low folic acid levels in pregnant women cause serious birth defects to babies' spines and nervous systems, so folic acid is particularly important for adolescent girls and young women to make sure they have adequate levels when they eventually prepare for pregnancy. Any adolescent female who is at risk of or planning a pregnancy should take prenatal vitamins with adequate folic acid levels.

Fiber

Teenagers who eat 2,000 calories per day should aim for 2 cups of fruit and 2½ cups of vegetables every day. They may need fewer or more servings depending on their individual calorie needs, which their health care professional can help determine. This will provide teens with adequate amounts of vitamins A, C, and E, and other cancer-fighting phytochemicals, as well as fiber to keep things moving in the digestive tract, preventing constipation. Good sources of fiber are beans, various fruits, and oat products. A regular fiber intake may help prevent many disorders, including cancer and heart disease, in middle age and later. Talk to your pediatrician about how much fiber your child should get. In general, add your child's age to 5 to 10 g of fiber to determine a good target amount; thus, a 15-year-old needs to consume 20 to 25 g per day.

VITAMIN D AND SUN EXPOSURE

Foods like eggs, butter, salmon, and herring are good sources of vitamin D. But unlike other vitamins, vitamin D is also made by your child's own body, with a little assistance from the sun's ultraviolet rays. When your child is exposed to sunlight, it helps his body synthesize vitamin D in the skin. And it doesn't take much time in the sun to produce adequate amounts of vitamin D.

However, not all children and adolescents get enough sunlight, particularly during certain times of the year or in northern regions of the United States. Dense cloud covers and high levels of air pollution can reduce the ultraviolet rays reaching the skin. In addition, your teenager's own skin characteristics can affect the vitamin D that his own body makes. In particular, the pigment in his skin is an important factor to consider; darker skinned people manufacture less vitamin D than those whose skin is lighter.

As important as sunscreen is to protect your teenager from skin cancer later in life, it can also interfere with sunlight's positive effects. Talk to your pediatrician about finding a balance between brief periods of sun exposure and sunscreen use.

Exercise and Healthy Bones

Physical activity—especially strength training and weight-bearing exercise—is good for bone. Combined with a balanced diet, physical activity not only strengthens bone but also stimulates hormones that protect bones and generates electrical activity within the bones that promotes growth and repair. Exercise also boosts the flow of blood and nutrients to the bones.

PHOSPHORUS

Phosphorus is another mineral needed for bone formation. The recommended dietary allowance for phosphorus is 1,200 mg a day for 9- to 18-year-olds. Phosphorus is found in most protein-rich foods, such as meat, eggs, and legumes, and also in foods that contain calcium. In fact, phosphorus is so abundant that most people routinely consume more of it than of calcium. Also, our bodies absorb phosphorus more easily than calcium   about 70% of a given quantity of phosphorus compared with 30% to 40% of calcium.

Zinc

Zinc—found in meat, fish, poultry, and dairy products, as well as shellfish, whole grains, dried beans, and nuts—is necessary for many bodily functions as well as healing wounds and sexual maturation. Zinc (with chromium) is a cofactor in insulin action. The RDA for zinc is 15 mg a day for adolescents. A high iron and calcium intake may slightly decrease zinc absorption. But when protein is present, zinc is easily absorbed. At all ages, our bodies need zinc and iron in similar amounts.

Other Essential Vitamins and Minerals

To keep enzyme systems and metabolic processes functioning properly, we need very small amounts of copper, selenium, iodine, chromium, manganese, and molybdenum. A balanced diet provides the RDA or, if the RDA is not yet known, the recognized safe level of every known vitamin and mineral. Only in unusual cases, when a child has a chronic condition or special dietary needs, do pediatricians prescribe supplements. Still, keep in mind that a multivitamin can do no harm and might be a good idea to ensure that your teenager consumes adequate amounts of vitamin D and folic acid—although pills are never a substitute for food. When taken to excess, vitamin supplements can be harmful.

What Makes Sammy (and Samantha) Run?

At age 15, Scott was only beginning to show physical changes that most of his classmates had long since experienced. Self-conscious about his smaller size and relative lack of development, Scott was tempted to start a diet and workout program he had read about in a body-building magazine. He asked a sports nutritionist to recommend a protein supplement.

"Don't waste your money," the nutritionist told Scott. "Lots of guys think supplements will help them bulk up and mature faster. Believe me, they don't help and they could hurt you. Eat a regular diet and keep exercising. That's the best way to improve your muscle mass and increase fitness."

SPORTS SUPPLEMENTS

In the competitive world of youth sports, particularly at the high school level, many teenaged athletes are looking for an edge that might help them cross the finish line a little sooner or hit the baseball a little harder. And that has led some of them to turn to dietary supplements whose manufacturers promise greater strength and endurance—but often deliver only potential health risks.

These so-called performance-enhancing pills, powders, bars, and drinks are widely available in drugstores, gyms, and health food stores. They also are sold at many gyms and are advertised in bodybuilding magazines. But because they are supplements, not drugs, the Food and Drug Administration does not require them to be tested for safety or effectiveness, nor are their claims as tightly regulated.

There are a lot of claims about these products, but very few are supported by scientific studies; in fact, almost no research has been conducted on these supplements in teenaged athletes. Manufacturers of a popular supplement called creatine, for example, claim that it can provide short bursts of high-intensity muscle activity; but these studies only show a 3% to 5% improvement in performance. This is trivial when compared with gains athletes will make with normal growth and development.

Other products are associated with serious problems like decreased height, acne, and baldness.

In addition to worries about safety, there are other concerns as well. When you read the active ingredients on the bottle, you expect them to be accurate. But when independent laboratories have evaluated these supplements, they have found that some do not deliver the ingredients that have been promised. To complicate matters, certain supplements may contain small doses of stimulants that can cause athletes to test positive for banned substances. Consumers shouldn't ignore the cost of these products. They are much more expensive than the same amounts of nutrients like protein and carbohydrates found in food.

Some of the highest risk supplements are illegal, particularly anabolic steroids, which are synthetic hormones. As you can read in "Anabolic Steroids and Other Performance Enhancers" on page 114, some boys and girls in high school and even middle school still use anabolic steroids despite their illegal status. They are associated with severe liver disease, heart disease, behavioral changes (like marked mood swings), and many other side effects. They may also interfere with sex hormones and sexual function, and may damage sexual organs. Some of these changes may not be reversible.

No wonder the American Academy of Pediatrics discourages these supplements. The best and safest approach to improve sports performance is by following a properly supervised exercise routine and good nutrition. (For information about sports drinks, see "Replacing Fluid and Electrolytes" on page 117 and Chapter 4, Nutrition During the School Years.)

ANABOLIC STEROIDS AND OTHER PERFORMANCE ENHANCERS

Athletes may be tempted to use supplements to improve athletic performance. Expensive nutritional products such as energy bars and shakes are popular but haven't been shown to enhance performance. Amino acid preparations, such as arginine and ornithine, have no proven value; one product, tryptophan, was banned by the Food and Drug Administration because of serious toxicity. (See "Sports Supplements" on page 113.) Anabolic steroids can stimulate muscle development but are dangerous to health and illegal. In boys, these synthetic male hormones can damage the testicles, cause the breasts to grow, and stunt growth. In girls, anabolic steroids cause a masculine appearance, including abnormal development of the sexual organs. Steroids alter blood cholesterol levels and may increase the risk of heart disease in boys and girls. They can have profound effects on the personality. Long-term use has been associated with severe liver disease, including cancer.

Although adverse effects are widely known, anabolic steroids are still distributed illegally among adolescents in middle school and high school. Make sure your teenagers are aware of the dangers of these and other illicit drugs. Work with your adolescent's coach to find alternative, healthy ways of building strength and gaining an edge on the competition.

MASTER OF THE UNIVERSE IN 3 EASY STAGES

Boys' growth follows a distinct 3-part sequence that's tied directly to the rate of sexual maturation, not to height. First, a boy rapidly grows taller. Then, about a year after his growth has peaked, he starts to develop muscle mass. By this time, his beard and chest hair have started to grow. Finally, he develops strength and endurance. A scrawny, late-maturing kid won't turn into a master of the universe by taking nutritional supplements.

After a boy has reached the right stage of development, he should be able to gain muscle by keeping to a well-planned and supervised strength-training program and diet. In fact, for pre-adolescents strength training can produce significant strength improvements and appears to be safe.

Teenaged athletes are prepared to work hard and train for hours at a time, but many are also susceptible to the notion that there is a magic formula for gaining a competitive edge. The formula generally involves manipulating the diet.

There's no nutritional magic trick for improving athletic prowess. A balanced intake from the 5 food groups should provide the nutrients a young athlete needs for growth and performance. At a minimum, the daily intake should include

- Six servings from the grain group
- Two servings from the meat and beans group
- Three servings from the vegetable group
- Two servings from the fruit group
- Four servings from the dairy group

Carbohydrates for Energy

About 50% to 55% of an athlete's daily energy requirement should come from carbohydrates. In practical terms, this works out in the following way: a young athlete consuming 2,500 calories a day needs on average about 1,250 carbohydrate calories daily, equivalent to about 312 g (11 oz) of carbohydrate food, or 6 to 11 servings.

TO LOAD OR NOT TO LOAD?

For short, intense bursts of activity, such as sprints or weight-lifting events, athletes get their energy from glucose stored as glycogen in the muscles and liver. Longer events requiring sustained effort draw calories first from glycogen, then from body fat. Some athletes try the technique known as *carbohydrate loading* to boost their glycogen stores just before a major competition. The idea is to consume as many carbohydrates as possible while cutting down on the time spent training on the day before the event. Carbohydrate loading also requires extra water and juices because glycogen needs extra water for storage.

Although carbohydrate loading can help athletes taking part in endurance events lasting 90 minutes or longer, it is not recommended for shorter competitions or for athletes taking part in sports at the high school level. Teenaged athletes should meet at least half of their daily energy requirements with carbohydrates.

A carbohydrate snack or a drink of juice right after a training session helps to replace the glycogen in muscles. Carbohydrates at the next meal will help to keep the muscles primed for training.

Protein

Protein is essential for growth, energy, and tissue repair. Athletic performance depends on muscle strength, and muscles are made of protein. Although athletes who are involved in strength and endurance training may need slightly more protein, it's a mistake to think you can simply build up muscles by eating lots of protein. Exercise, not dietary protein, increases muscle mass.

The amount of protein adolescents need varies at different stages of development. As a rule, boys and girls between ages 11 and 14 need half a gram per pound of body weight daily. Thus, a young teenager weighing 110 pounds needs about 50 g of protein a day. Between ages 15 and 18, the RDA drops slightly. As with all essential nutrients, common sense is the rule—you don't have to weigh every gram on a scale. Each gram of protein provides 4 calories—the same as carbohydrates—and protein should make up about 10% to 12% of each

PROTEIN AND CALORIE CONTENT OF FOODS MOST TEENAGERS LIKE TO EAT		
Food (portion size)	**Protein Content (g)**	**Calorie Average**
Bagel (1 medium)	7	200
Bread, whole wheat, 1 slice	3	60–65
Cheese, processed, American (1 oz)	6	105
Cheeseburger (4-oz meat patty)	30	525
Lean meat, fish, or poultry (3-oz serving)	22	180/120/140
Milk—reduced-fat (2%), low-fat (1%), or nonfat (skim) milk	8	120/100/85
Peanut butter (1 tablespoon)	5	95
Pizza, cheese (1 slice)	15	290
Taco	9	195
Yogurt, low-fat, coffee or vanilla (8 oz)	8	195

day's calories. As a general rule, there are approximately 22 g of protein in 3 oz of meat, fish, or poultry. An 8-oz glass of milk contains about 8 g of protein. Therefore, an average teenager who is drinking 3 glasses of milk a day does not need enormous amounts of meat to meet his daily protein requirement.

The protein in foods of animal origin is termed *complete* or *high-quality* protein because it contains all the essential amino acids (see Chapter 8, Nutrition Basics) in about the proportions humans need. Vegetable proteins are called *incomplete* because, except for soybeans, they have low levels of one or more essential amino acids. You don't have to eat animal products to obtain high-quality protein, however. People on vegetarian diets (see Chapter 15, Alternative Diets and Supplements) take care of their protein needs by pairing plant foods that balance each other's shortfalls. Pairing foods in this way is called protein complementation. Eating a grain and a legume does the trick; beans and tortillas, a peanut butter sandwich on wheat bread, and black-eyed peas and rice are good examples of protein complementation. You can also compensate for any lack in a plant-based food by adding a small amount of animal-derived protein, such as in pasta with cheese or cereal with milk.

Water

Without water, the most abundant substance in the body, many of the processes that produce energy couldn't take place. Every cell is bathed in water, which carries nutrients around the body. Water helps regulate body temperature. Finally, water flushes out waste products left over from energy metabolism.

Water is lost through sweating, urination, and evaporation from the lungs as a person breathes. During exercise, the rate of loss is faster as the athlete breathes faster and sweats

---

REPLACING FLUID AND ELECTROLYTES

If an event lasts longer than 1 hour or the weather is hot and humid, an athlete may need to replace not only water but also electrolytes—sodium, potassium, and chloride—that help regulate the body's balance of fluids. In these cases, sports drinks are appropriate. However, athletes taking part in less strenuous or shorter activities should drink cool water. Juice or commercial sports drinks are unnecessary. Never use salt pills; they can be dangerous.

HIDDEN CAFFEINE

Your anxious, wakeful teenager may not be aware of how much caffeine she's consuming in the course of a day. Obvious sources include colas, coffee, tea, and energy drinks, but there are hidden ones, such as over-the-counter headache remedies and other kinds of soda. The following chart includes common caffeinated products and the amounts of caffeine they contain:

CONTENTS OF A SAMPLING OF ENERGY DRINKS,[a] PER SERVING (240 mL [8 oz])

Product	Calories	Caffeine (mg)
Java Monster	100	Yes[b]
Java Monster Lo-Ball	50	Yes
Monster Energy	100	Yes
Monster Low Carb	10	Yes
Red Bull	106	77
Red Bull Sugarfree	9.6	77
Power Trip Original Blue	100	105
Power Trip "0"	5	105
Power Trip The Extreme	110	110
Rockstar Original	140	80
Rockstar Sugar Free	10	80
Full Throttle	110	Yes

[a]Selection of specific energy drinks for this table was based on the most commonly available products at the time this report was under development.

[b]If "Yes" rather than a milligram amount is listed, it is because milligrams were not specified on the nutritional content label.

American Academy of Pediatrics Committee on Nutrition, Council on Sports Medicine and Fitness. Sports drinks and energy drinks for children and adolescents: are they appropriate? *Pediatrics.* 2011;127(6):1182–1189

more. Even more water is lost if exercise takes place in hot weather or in a warm indoor area. An athlete who loses too much water loses the ability to regulate his body temperature and runs a risk of heat exhaustion and life-threatening shutdown of vital bodily functions. Adolescents competing in sports in which weight is a factor, such as gymnastics, weight lifting, and wrestling, may be pressured by coaches, parents, or themselves to "make weight" for an event. Wrestlers are particularly vulnerable because they frequently train at one weight level and compete at another, lower one. Common practices athletes use to meet the required weight include restrictive dieting (eg, eating only bananas or oranges for several days in a row), water deprivation, and heavy workouts while wearing heat-retaining clothing. Such practices are dangerous—they have led to deaths among college-level wrestlers.

Children with a history of eating disorders or chronic disease, such as diabetes, cystic fibrosis, or sickle cell disease, should be especially careful about fluid loss. These teenagers sometimes fail to recognize signals from the brain's thirst center or their kidneys may not respond to signals in the blood and body salts, and they can rapidly become dehydrated before they feel thirsty.

Thirst is not a reliable guide to the need for water. In fact, by the time a child feels thirsty, she already may be seriously dehydrated.

Children have a greater surface to body area, which means they get hot faster in hot weather. In addition, they do not sweat as much and do not feel thirsty, even when they are somewhat dehydrated. Common symptoms of dehydration during sports include decreased athletic performance, noticeable thirst, fatigue, nausea, headache, cramping, dizziness, and weakness. Children and teenagers who participate in vigorous activity on a regular basis should weigh themselves before and after the activity to get a sense for how much water they have lost. Young athletes taking part in games or practice should take regular breaks for water whether or not they feel thirsty. Teenaged boys typically lose more than a quart of fluid when playing soccer in the heat, while younger boys and girls may lose 1 to 2 pints. Athletes should drink 12 to 16 oz before beginning vigorous exercise, as well as 5 oz every 20 minutes for athletes weighing less than 90 pounds (9 oz for those weighing more than 90 pounds).

PMS and Sweets

Some adolescent girls crave sweet foods and candy a few days before each menstrual period. Such cravings are similar to craving carbohydrates when under stress or trying to quit smoking. Researchers found that women with severe premenstrual symptoms felt happier and calmer if their evening meals were high in carbohydrates and low in protein on the days preceding their periods. The women were less depressed, tense, and confused, and felt calmer and more alert than women who kept to their regular diet.

Researchers traced the explanation to serotonin, a brain chemical involved in mood and appetite. Serotonin is controlled by food intake; carbohydrates boost serotonin release while protein has no effect. Nicotine, like carbohydrates, increases brain serotonin, while nicotine withdrawal has the opposite effect.

If your teenager is unusually tense or tearful around the time of her periods, she may feel better if her meals and snacks include more complex carbohydrates such as pasta and grains. She should make a corresponding cut in her intake of animal protein and avoid simple sugars such as in candy and desserts, which often include hefty amounts of fat as well. In this way, she'll lift her mood and maintain balanced nutrition while avoiding extra, empty calories. Premenstrual syndrome (PMS) can be reduced by taking 400 mg of calcium 3 times daily every day. Some data also suggest that magnesium (250 mg 1–2 times per day) may decrease PMS.

Teenage Jitters and Caffeine

Hearing sobs from her daughter's room, Robin Schneider knocked, then pushed open the door to find 17-year-old Jessica curled up in a fetal position on her bed. "Something's really wrong with me, Mom," Jessica wailed. "My heart keeps racing out of control and sometimes I can't get my breath!"

To Robin—a trained nurse—the teenager looked distressed but not ill. Her temperature and color were normal and she had no chest pain. When Jessica mentioned that she had had several episodes of bringing up a sour, burning fluid and added that she couldn't get to sleep, Robin put two and two together.

Jessica had been meeting friends 3 or 4 times a week for iced caffe latte at the new coffee bar in town. She often drank a cola for an afternoon pick-me-up, despite her mother's suggestion that she drink juice instead. When she felt drowsy during morning classes, she drank a jolt of the new extra-caffeine soda that she and her classmates saw advertised on television. Also, to ease menstrual cramps, her mother had given Jessica several tablets of an over-the-counter headache remedy (and some "cramps" remedies) containing caffeine when she'd run out of her usual pain reliever.

Robin thought Jessica's problems might be caused by too much caffeine. Caffeine is a strong stimulant that can cause the heart to race, provoke stomach upsets, and—as Jessica was aware—prevent drowsiness. The effects may bring on a feeling of anxiety that makes it hard to breathe. Jessica was a slender girl, 5 feet 4 inches and 112 pounds. A rough tally of her recent intake showed that she was consuming enough caffeine each day to give a burly man the jitters.

Jessica promised to cut down on her iced caffe latte and order only the decaffeinated version. She also agreed to drink juices and bottled waters instead of sodas. Finally, she planned to try getting up a quarter-hour earlier. That way she'd have time for breakfast.

Caffeine, a stimulant that works on the central nervous system, can stop a drowsy feeling and keep you alert. Too much can cause palpitations (the feeling that your heart is racing or thumping hard), heartburn, sleeplessness, and a jittery, anxious feeling. The effect varies according to the size of the dose as well as the size of the consumer. Some people are more sensitive to caffeine, while others build up a tolerance through regular use. A jittery, anxious teen should cut back on colas and other sodas, coffee, and tea, including iced beverages, for

---

CAFFEINE-WITHDRAWAL HEADACHE

A teenager who is used to a steady intake of caffeine may develop a caffeine-withdrawal headache and a feeling of sluggishness, fatigue, drowsiness, or tired a day or two after cutting back. Some complain of a weekend headache, which appears when a person who starts every weekday with a caffeine drink sleeps late on Saturday and misses the "dose" at the regular time. Once the caffeine habit is broken, caffeine-withdrawal headaches should disappear within a week or two.

WHAT MAKES A DIET VEGETARIAN?

Vegetarians differ in degree, just as they differ in their reasons for adopting a vegetarian lifestyle. Partial or semi-vegetarians avoid some but not all animal products. They may eat chicken or fish and dairy products but no meat. Some eat fish but no poultry. Lacto-ovo vegetarians eat eggs and dairy products but avoid all flesh—they avoid "food with a face"; lactovegetarians don't eat eggs. Vegans follow a strict diet that excludes all foods derived from animals, including eggs and dairy products. Fruitarians eat only fruit, nuts and seeds, honey, whole grains, and olive oil. (For more details, see Chapter 15, Alternative Diets and Supplements.)

ACNE TRIGGERS

There is little scientific support for food effects on acne, including chocolate. However, some diet changes may be associated with the premenstrual phase in young women or other stressors, which may provoke more pimples. Some people develop acne after consuming foods with high iodine content. The amount of iodine that will trigger acne is many times the normal dietary level. There isn't enough iodine in seafood and iodized salt to cause skin problems, but acne has been linked to the high iodine levels in kelp, a seaweed extract sometimes included in sports drinks.

A few medications can cause acne. Adolescents under treatment with certain steroids, antiepilepsy medications, or lithium should talk to their pediatricians about the effects of such medications on the skin.

---

a week or so. Decaffeinated coffee and tea can deliver a substantial dose of caffeine. When a pain reliever is necessary, check the label to make sure it doesn't contain caffeine. If your teenager is still bothered by symptoms, especially heart palpitations, talk to your pediatrician.

Fads and Diets

Teenaged opinions about food may be based on concern for the environment and our role in it, a humanitarian view of animal exploitation, or the relationship between diet and health. In many cases, such opinions are well thought out and deserve respect. At times, adolescents may be pardoned for focusing on food as a symbol of everything that's wrong in their families.

Parents can safely ignore faddish notions about food as long as the teenager continues to eat a balanced diet. Vegetarian diets, which are appealing to many, are so widely accepted that few consider them faddish any more (also see Chapter 15, Alternative Diets and Supplements). Among adolescents, the most common reason for rejecting meat is the exploitation of animals. Long-term vegetarians who maintain a proper nutritional balance have lower rates of several diseases associated with the typical Western high-fat, low-fiber diet. They are less likely to have high blood pressure and high cholesterol levels and have lower rates of some cancers, and their weight is usually closer to a healthy ideal than that of meat eaters. They may also have less constipation and other functional bowel complaints. However, eliminating animal products from an otherwise unhealthy diet will not provide the health advantages of vegetarianism.

More restricted diets increase the risk of nutritional deficiencies. Partial vegetarians usually have no difficulty getting a good balance of nutrients. They should take care, however, that complex carbohydrates make up the bulk of their diet. Some rely too much on dairy products and end up with a diet that's too high in fats and calories. All vegetarians should learn how to combine 2 or more foods, like beans and corn, to ensure that they get essential amino acids, the building blocks of protein.

Those who keep to a strict vegan diet must find alternative sources of vitamin D, important for healthy bones, and vitamin B_{12}, which is needed in all cells but especially for healthy blood. Humans can get some vitamin D from sunlight but cannot absorb the B_{12} that occurs in small amounts in a few plant foods. Vegans of all ages should consume soy milk or cereals fortified with B_{12}. Without dairy foods, a vegan diet may also lack calcium. Your pediatrician or a qualified dietitian may recommend supplements to ensure that your child receives adequate amounts of vitamins, calcium, iron, and zinc.

Any adolescent planning to go on a weight-loss diet should first talk with a pediatrician, who may recommend books on nutrition or provide a referral to a nutrition counselor. When it comes to adopting a vegetarian diet, it's as much about what your teenager does eat as what he doesn't.

Image and Eating Disorders

Teenagers sometimes develop notions about food that are based on a distorted body image and an overconcern with reshaping it. Food fads and refusals are not unusual during adolescence and usually pass quickly. Eating disorders, however, are serious problems that are associated with health risks and serious emotional disturbances. These disorders usually affect girls but also occur in boys. They are not always easy to detect because adolescents with eating disorders may maintain normal weight or wear bulky clothing to disguise weight loss. The major types of eating disorder involve self-starvation, gorging, binge eating, and purging. (Also see Chapter 10, Eating Disorders.)

A teenager with an eating disorder urgently needs professional help. If your child has had unusual weight loss or gain, seems obsessed with food preparation or dieting, or is exercising compulsively for hours on end, talk to your pediatrician.

VITAMIN PILLS AND ACNE

For a teenager being treated for acne, vitamin supplements could be not only unnecessary but dangerous as well. Certain acne treatments available by prescription are derived from vitamin A. This fat-soluble vitamin is stored in the body and can build up to toxic levels if too much is consumed.

When a teenager is taking a vitamin A supplement at the same time as an oral acne treatment, you should talk to his pediatrician and make sure he's not consuming toxic amounts of vitamin A, which could cause headaches, further skin and hair problems, and—in severe cases—liver and nerve damage.

THAT'S NOT CHOCOLATE, THAT'S STRESS!

People under stress often crave chocolate and sweets. After eating candy, they have an acne outbreak, then mistakenly associate the candies with the acne outbreak and overlook the real culprit—stress.

Food and Adolescent Acne

More than 80% of teenagers have acne, so if your youngster manages to get through adolescence with no more than a couple of skin blemishes, she's one of the lucky few. Contrary to what most people believe, acne is not caused by chocolate, fried foods, candies, or anything else in a teenager's usual diet. It's not the result of constipation, nor is it a sign of sexual activity or the lack of it. Instead, it's caused by increased levels of certain hormones that stimulate the fat glands in skin to step up production of sebum, an oily secretion that lubricates and protects the skin. Sebum, together with cast-off skin cells and other debris, blocks skin follicles, which can become infected or inflamed. The increase in sebum production may occur as early as 2 years before any other signs of puberty, and boys and girls as young as age 9 may have skin bumps and coarsened pores, especially in areas where sebaceous glands are numerous, such as around the nose and the middle of the face.

Acne often runs in families. Most cases are mild, and pimples and zits don't usually leave permanent scars if the lesions are left alone. Over-the-counter lotions containing benzoyl peroxide can be helpful to prevent minor blemishes and mild to moderate acne. Your pediatrician or dermatologist can prescribe treatment for more severe or persistent acne. Occasionally some girls with severe or persistent acne have an underlying hormone imbalance with excess male hormones.

Although there's no proven link between diet and acne, it won't hurt to avoid chocolate and sugary or fatty foods if your teenager believes they trigger blemishes. Indeed, it may be better for her health. Adolescence is an inherently stressful time, and if stress triggers your child's acne, measures to help her control stress may also help cut down on acne outbreaks. Some girls get more pimples before and during their periods. This is caused by changes in hormone levels.

Oily creams and lotions can block skin follicles and promote sebum buildup. Teenagers should avoid oil-based skin and hair cosmetics and use non-perfumed, water-based products.

Alcohol and Adolescents

Many young people start using alcohol during the early adolescent years, and girls, on the whole, seem to experiment with alcohol and drugs at an earlier age than boys. If alcohol were not in the picture, many tragedies among young Americans could be prevented, including car crashes, drownings, fatal falls, homicides, and suicides. Alcohol loosens inhibitions and increases the risk of irresponsible sexual behavior that can result in unplanned pregnancies and sexually transmitted infections. Alcohol combined with caffeine is an especially dangerous mix. Drinkers do not realize how drunk they are, further setting the stage for risky behavior and overconsumption.

Many adolescents don't continue to drink after an initial experimentation. For those who persist, however, the risks are great. Adolescents, especially females, are on the whole smaller and lighter—and thus get drunk faster—than adults. Some adolescents are at higher risk than others for becoming alcoholics. In fact, family history is a major risk factor for drug and alcohol addiction in teenagers. Genetic and psychological factors such as depression and anxiety can make a susceptible teenager dependent on alcohol, and dependency can develop in much less time than with an adult. Mixed drinks and beer can also add lots of extra calories that deposit fat in the waist area.

DR STERN'S LAW OF CHOCOLATE
"Life without brussels sprouts is still worth living, but life without chocolate—that's another story!"

SMOKING AND TEENAGERS
Many adolescents continue to smoke despite overwhelming evidence that cigarettes are harmful. Girls, in particular, take up smoking as a method of weight control. What they don't know is that cigarette smoking partly suppresses the female hormone estrogen, which influences fat deposits in women. Women who smoke, therefore, tend to acquire fat on the abdomen—in the male pattern—instead of on the thighs and hips. So, although a girl smokes to keep her weight down, she's redistributing her body fat in a way that can give her a potbelly.

Parents may feel torn by 2 apparent choices. Should they gradually introduce their underaged children to alcohol by allowing beer and wine on special occasions in a controlled family environment? Or should they forbid any exposure to alcohol until the legal drinking age?

The American Academy of Pediatrics (AAP) warns that children and adolescents should not use alcohol, nicotine, or any drugs except for prescribed medications. The AAP urges parents who drink to do so safely and in moderation, and to keep alcohol out of children's reach. It discourages the practice of giving alcohol to children, although it acknowledges that some parents may accept the supervised use of wine in religious ceremonies. The AAP supports a zero-tolerance policy against alcohol, tobacco, and all drugs in schools and at school-related events. This ban should extend equally to students and staff. Driver's licenses should be automatically suspended—or not granted—for minors convicted of violating alcohol and drug laws.

Introduce controlled drinking in the family home after young people have reached the legal age.

TEEN FOOD PROBLEMS THAT MAKE PARENTS WORRY

My son wants to try carbohydrate loading for his high school field day. He's been picked for the 4-man relay and may also compete in the long jump. Is carb loading all it's cracked up to be?

While carbohydrate loading can help mature athletes taking part in endurance events lasting 90 minutes or longer, it is not recommended for shorter events or for teenagers taking part in sports at the high school level. (Read about how to feed your teenaged athlete on page 115.)

My daughter often complains of a persistent, dull headache after she sleeps late on weekends. Is it because she sleeps too much?

Your daughter may be getting a caffeine-withdrawal headache. It happens when a person who is used to starting the day with a caffeinated drink sleeps late and misses the regular "dose." If she cuts down on caffeine (eg, cola, coffee) for a week or two and doesn't oversleep, she may break her caffeine dependence and get rid of the headache. (For more about hidden caffeine and its symptoms, turn to page 120.)

TEEN FOOD PROBLEMS THAT MAKE PARENTS WORRY, *CONTINUED*

My daughter has acne. Is it because she's overweight and keeps sneaking chocolate bars and french fries?

What your daughter eats has no effect on acne, but stress and hormones do. She should talk to her pediatrician about weight control and acne treatment. Additional treatment suggestions may come from a dermatologist or adolescent medicine physician. (Read more about food and adolescent acne on page 122.) An equally important problem is that she is sneaking food. In our experience, sneaking food may precede an eating disorder—at the very least it indicates a conflict about food.

I'm afraid my teenager is heading for osteoporosis because she won't drink milk. She says it's got too many calories. How can I get her to eat more calcium?

Serve low-fat and nonfat milk, yogurt, and other dairy products. These have just as much calcium as the whole-milk versions. There are also ways to get calcium other than from dairy products. (Read about dietary calcium and healthy bones on page 107.) Watch for other rigid and excessive food or nutrient restrictions.

We keep reading about teenagers being injured while driving under the influence of alcohol. Couldn't a lot of these tragedies be prevented if parents taught teens to drink responsibly at home?

Only one factor has been found to reduce teen alcohol-related accidents, and that is abstinence. The accident rate went down after the legal drinking age was raised in all states. Don't allow your teen to drink alcohol before he reaches the legal age, and teach him never, ever to drink and drive (see page 126).

My son looks pale and washed out. Is it because he won't eat red meat?

A properly balanced vegetarian diet can provide plenty of iron without the saturated fat in red meat. (Read about increasing iron absorption on page 105 and vegetarian diets in Chapter 15, Alternative Diets and Supplements.) If you suspect your son is anemic, arrange an appointment with your pediatrician.

Chapter 6

Is My Child Overweight?

In the United States, 17% of 2- to 19-year-old children are obese, and an almost equal number are overweight. Between 1980 and 1994, the percentage of obese children and adolescents aged 6 to 17 years doubled. However, between 1999 and 2008, no further statistically significant increase occurred.

Most parents are happy if their children have outstanding talent, looks, intelligence, or athletic ability. Size, however, is a different story. They prefer that their children blend in with the crowd, neither much smaller nor much larger than others the same age.

A 2008 survey by the University of Michigan C.S. Mott Children's Hospital found that childhood obesity was the most important health concern of parents in the United States. Although the rate of the increase in childhood obesity has slowed, excess body weight in children and adolescents remains a serious problem, particularly because more than 70% of obese children have at least one additional risk factor for heart disease, such as elevated blood pressure or cholesterol, and 30% have 2 or more risk factors. Childhood obesity is also linked to type 2 diabetes and increased problems with sleep apnea, liver disease, and orthopedic issues. Also, being active is harder for overweight children and teenagers. If children are overweight before 8 years of age and are unable to lose weight as they grow, they are much more likely to become severely overweight adults. Despite how common the problem of obesity has become, children who are overweight or obese are subject to bullying, teasing, and other forms of discrimination. Preventing childhood overweight and obesity will promote health and improve socialization and quality of life.

The challenge for parents is how to prevent their children from gaining too much weight, and what to do if their children are already overweight. Many parents feel blame or guilt for their child's weight problem, but the obesity epidemic comes from many changes in the food we eat and the activities we do, such as an increase in fast-food consumption and increased television watching. As this chapter will point out, families can help prevent or treat obesity in their children by paying attention to food, physical activity, and television time.

This need for information and skills led parents like Bill and Judy to bring their 8-year-old daughter, Letitia, to the pediatrician's office for an evaluation. At 48 inches, Letitia's height was nothing out of the ordinary, but at 75 pounds, she was heavier than 95% of girls her age. Always plump, Letitia had become noticeably overweight in the past few months. Her parents were of average build and insisted that Letitia "hardly ate a thing." They were concerned that a glandular problem might be causing their daughter to gain weight.

It had been a year and a half since Letitia's last checkup, and her health—apart from a possible overweight issue—was good. The family had moved to their community 12 months earlier and they had only just gotten around to finding a pediatrician. According to Bill and Judy, the weight gain had started during this time. The medical records from Letitia's former pediatrician backed them up.

Letitia had no signs of the rare medical problems that might cause excess weight gain in a school-aged child. Careful probing by her pediatrician uncovered the source of the problem. She was unhappy about the move and slow to make friends. She wasn't involved in sports or hobbies and spent all her spare time watching television. Although she was not permitted to snack between meals, she had free access to the refrigerator and was allowed to drink juice. At meals, she ate relatively few fruits and vegetables, and her parents tried to avoid rules about food because they thought that these might make her even more unhappy. The lack of physical activity and the snacking that went with television watching also had contributed to her weight gain.

Although Letitia's parents were aware that she was having problems adjusting, they hadn't linked such problems with the excessive weight gain. They saw that she was not eating much at meals, but they weren't aware of the effect that her juice intake had on her weight gain and decreased appetite at meals. Letitia didn't have a glandular problem and she didn't need a formal weight-loss program; she simply needed to get away from the television, reduce her juice intake, and develop interests that would keep her active and help her make friends.

At their pediatrician's suggestion, Bill and Judy enrolled Letitia in after-school swimming classes at their local pool. The parents made a new rule that when Letitia was thirsty, she should drink water instead of juice. After some initial complaining, Letitia began to drink ice water, much to her parents' surprise. A new sitter, who walked Letitia to and from the club, made sure that snacks included fruit, raw vegetables, and low-fat dips and yogurt. Letitia's growth continued, but with the exercise and more healthful eating, a slimmer, fit Letitia began to emerge out of her cocoon of overweight and inactivity. She found an activity she was good at and that helped build her confidence. She also made friends among her fellow swimmers and gradually shed her loneliness.

Why Do Children Become Overweight?

Children become overweight for many reasons. In most cases, overweight is probably a combination of factors such as genetics and an environment that promotes obesity. A tendency to be overweight may run in some families. Many children don't get enough physical activity. Many young people develop unhealthy eating patterns, and these often reflect their eating patterns at home. Medical problems such as hormone imbalances are rare and account for fewer than 1 out of 100 cases of childhood obesity. Children with rare disorders such as Cushing syndrome, Prader-Willi syndrome, Turner syndrome, or other metabolic or genetic disorders are often short and may have problems with speech, hearing, vision, and development in addition to overweight. Such conditions are usually diagnosed early in life. A pediatrician will perform a physical examination and diagnostic tests in the unlikely event that a problem of this type is suspected.

Although weight problems run in families, not all children with a family history of obesity will become overweight. If parents' weights are normal, slightly overweight children between the ages of 1 and 3 years do not have an increased risk for overweight later in life. However, children whose parents, brothers, and sisters are overweight have a higher risk of becoming overweight themselves. While genetic factors play a role, a shared environment that promotes unhealthy eating and inactivity also influences body weight. For example, some children overeat because their parents habitually overeat and unwittingly encourage the children to do the same.

Lack of physical activity that comes from watching television for hours on end, as Letitia did, is an important factor in the rising tide of childhood obesity. Snacking while watching television—complete with commercials promoting snack food and soda—adds to the problem. If children are in front of the television while eating, they tend to eat more fats and salty snacks, and fewer fruits and vegetables. Children who watch more than 5 hours of television a day are 4½ times more likely to become overweight than those who watch for 2 hours or less. Children who have a television in their room also watch more television and are more likely to become overweight. If your child is spending too much time in front of the box, turn it off. Keep snacks for snack times, such as after an outdoor game—not as a companion to watching television—and when your child is thirsty, give her water rather than juice.

DR DIETZ'S FIRST LAW OF THERMODYNAMICS

Children use up more energy doing almost anything besides watching television.

THE CALORIE GAP

Parents frequently ask what has changed to contribute to the obesity epidemic. The answer is, "Almost everything!" Food is available everywhere, more food is consumed outside the home, and that food tends to be high in calories. Children spend more time in front of a screen for entertainment, fewer children walk to school, and there are fewer safe opportunities for outdoor play.

Easy access to food, of course, is a major factor. When children eat more calories than their body can use, more body fat results. One recent study showed that between national surveys in 1994–1998 and 1999–2002, the extra weight US teens gained came from consuming 110 to 165 extra calories per day (which is about the number of calories in a small order of french fries or a 12-oz can of soda).

Consider the case of 4-year-old Melissa, who was clearly overweight, in sharp contrast with her lean mother. When their pediatrician questioned them about what they ate, it took a while before her mother remembered what took place every morning as she drove Melissa to preschool. Five days a week, they drove through a fast-food drive-through so mom could get a cup of coffee and Melissa could have a hot chocolate topped with whipped cream. Those few extra calories each day were enough to put extra weight on Melissa.

OVERWEIGHT AND HAPPY? MAYBE NOT

Apart from the health problems linked to overweight in children, there are also psychological and social consequences, especially if their overweight continues into adulthood. Some studies have shown that children as young as 6 years may associate overweight with negative stereotypes. For example, when children were asked to rank drawings of other children, depictions of overweight children were described as less likable than those who had various physical handicaps. Overweight children are often less likely to be chosen for team activities and may have more difficulty making friends. Because overweight children are bigger than their peers, people tend to overestimate how old they are and expect them to reach unreasonably high standards of behavior and achievement. To avoid the teasing, some overweight children turn to younger children for friendship. Also, overweight children often have trouble finding clothes that fit in styles they like. Ultimately, some overweight adolescents may develop a distorted body image, putting them at risk for eating disorders.

Studies have shown that being overweight lowers the chance of being accepted into a high-ranking college and reduces a job applicant's attractiveness to prospective employers. Overweight can translate into lower social and economic levels and, for women, less likelihood of finding a mate. Negative perceptions about weight are directly and indirectly passed on to children; thus, the consequences of overweight are carried on to the next generation.

The Internet may also contribute, especially if children are playing food "advergames." These are advertisements for food disguised as games. These games and other Internet strategies are increasingly being used to market foods to children.

As with other issues, children's perceptions about weight are influenced by their parents and peers. When Jim and Linda brought their 11-year-old son, Evan, to see his pediatrician, it was clear that Jim, a fit runner, was extremely concerned. Asked to rate Evan's weight problem on a 10-point scale, Jim gave it a 10, but when Linda was asked to do the same, she scored it as a 2. Evan was caught in the middle. Though he hadn't been bothered by his weight before, his father's attention had made it an issue. Yet his mother's apparent lack of concern sent Evan a confusing signal. An easygoing boy, he wanted to please both his parents and wasn't sure how to do so.

Their pediatrician showed the family where Evan ranked on the weight and growth charts. He explained that it wasn't unusual for boys to gain several pounds, as Evan had, with the hormonal changes leading up to puberty. In most cases, boys lose this extra weight as they enter the adolescent growth spurt. Evan wasn't seriously overweight; however, a program begun now to promote healthy eating and fitness could prevent him from becoming overweight. The pediatrician advised the family that such a plan could succeed only if everyone agreed on a common goal and how best to reach it.

In contrast to boys, puberty is a risk period for the development of overweight in girls. In boys, muscle mass increases and body fat decreases with the growth spurt. In girls, muscle mass and body fat increase with the growth spurt. Early puberty in girls is associated with a higher risk of later obesity.

Parents do not need to negotiate with younger children before making changes in the food that is served at meals, permissible snacks, or physical activity. However, to make changes for Evan, it was important for his parents to agree on the steps to be taken. If children ask why things have changed, parents can explain that the changes have been made to make everyone healthier. In older children and particularly in adolescents, it's essential to find out how an overweight child perceives his weight and whether he wants to do something about it. A weight-management program is doomed from the start if only the parents or only the

---

BEING REALISTIC ABOUT WEIGHT

When Rohan came into Dr Stern's office for his 3-year checkup, it was immediately obvious that he was overweight. Dr Stern asked his slender mother what he ate during a typical day. She responded, "He doesn't eat anything. I have to feed him."

"You mean you are hand-feeding a 3-year-old?"

"Yes, I have to. If I didn't, he wouldn't eat."

Rohan's mother had no perception that her son was overweight. All she knew was that when she thought he should be eating (and how much he should be eating), he wasn't eating. However, when Dr Stern showed her Rohan's growth curves and measurement of his body mass index (which was above the 95th percentile), she was surprised but finally became convinced that he really was overweight. Dr Stern explained to her that his appetite should be the guide for his intake, and that if he was not hungry for a particular meal, he should only eat as much as he chose.

child perceive a problem that requires action. Without this agreement, conflicts and resentments are likely to prevail when one side advocates weight loss and the other resists.

Is My Child Overweight?

Pediatricians evaluate children's growth and build by means of standardized growth charts (see Appendix C) and body mass index (BMI) (see Appendix D). Growth charts show whether a child falls within the normal range of height and weight for her age. Children whose weight or height is above the 85th or below the fifth percentile should be examined by a doctor to determine whether further evaluation is needed. Pediatricians also will watch for fluctuations in children's weight, which may mean something has changed and put them on the path toward gaining excess weight.

Body mass index is a calculation of your child's weight relative to height. A BMI above the 85th percentile means overweight, while children above the 95th percentile are considered obese, which increases their risk of chronic diseases such as heart disease and diabetes. The BMI percentile that defines severe obesity is 120% of the 95th percentile. If your child's BMI is between the 85th and 95th percentiles, her excess weight may be fat or muscle. Growth charts and BMI tell only part of the story because neither method measures body fat. Children and adolescents who are particularly athletic with unusually muscular or lean builds may have a high BMI without having excess fat or being obese. In some obesity clinics, as many as 10% to 15% of children fall into this category. Also keep in mind that there are

---

CHOOSE TO BE HAPPY

Many adolescents, particularly girls, become deeply unhappy when they realize that they are never going to be shaped like supermodels or earn multimillion-dollar contracts as movie stars.

Help your daughter feel comfortable with who she is. Reassure her that real beauty is more than skin deep. Help her develop her skills and talents and emphasize her positive attributes. Offer her female role models who have made the most of their talents, achieving intellectual and humanitarian goals or raising healthy, balanced children, instead of trading on their looks for superficial success.

small differences between African American and white children; at the same BMI measurement, African American children and teenagers tend to have more muscle and bone mass and less body fat. However, almost all children and adolescents with a BMI above the 95th percentile have too much body fat, regardless of their ethnicity or muscularity.

Some parents wonder how it is possible for 17% of 2- to 19-year-olds to be obese when only 5% of the population should have a BMI above the 95th percentile. The BMI charts were based on children and teens studied before 1988, when not as many youth were obese. At that time, only 5% of children and teens were obese.

If your child is overweight because her frame size is increased, reassure her that her extra weight is not fat and encourage her to be physically active to maintain her muscle tone. Also, be actively involved in any discussions with your pediatrician and your child about your child's weight. To prevent worries about body size, parent and child need to accept the child's body type. Other members of the family may have a similar build. If you focus

---

INTERPRETING THE PERCENTILES

When your child is weighed and measured at the pediatrician's office, the doctor may tell you what percentile your child's height and weight are. If a child is at the 50th percentile for height, for example, that means that 50% of children his age are taller and 50% are shorter. If a child's weight is at the 10th percentile, that means that 90% of children are heavier and only 10% are lighter. Although changes in weight and height percentiles are sometimes worrisome, there are times when they may not be. For example, between 9 and 15 months of age, when children start to pull up and walk, they may decrease their weight percentile somewhat. As long as their growth in height is normal, there is no reason to be concerned.

MUSCLE VERSUS FAT

A teenaged patient of Dr Stern's is an avid volleyball player. At her 13-year checkup, her body mass index was at the 90th percentile. Between that checkup and the one that followed at age 14, she had started training vigorously and changed her diet in ways suggested by her coach. At age 14, she remained at the 90th percentile, but she had lost 2 inches from her waist and about the same from her stomach. She had put on muscle and lost fat.

THE BODY MASS INDEX FORMULA

To calculate the body mass index (BMI) of your child or adolescent, use the following formula or visit www.cdc.gov:

- Multiply your child's weight (in pounds) by 703. (We'll refer to this as A.)

- Multiply your child's height (in inches) by itself. (We'll refer to this as B.)

- Dividing A by B gives you your child's BMI.

---

inappropriately on weight alone and pester your child to lose weight, she may develop a distorted body image and risk an eating disorder (see Chapter 10, Eating Disorders). It's estimated that 70% to 80% of girls perceive themselves, whether rightly or wrongly, as too fat.

Experts warn that a misperception of body image may be partly fueling the current obesity epidemic, with inappropriate dieting followed by rebound weight gain.

The case histories on pages 138 through 143 illustrate how individual growth problems might be handled.

Making a Change for the Better

If your pediatrician recommends a weight-management plan, it's important to find the best way to help your child learn to control his weight and prevent a problem that could carry over into adulthood.

Involving the whole family in weight management encourages healthful habits without singling out the overweight child. Children are quick learners and they learn best by example. If you eat a variety of foods and are physically active, you will teach your children healthy habits they can follow for the rest of their lives. How you manage changes that need to be made depends largely on your child's age. A 6-year-old, for example, doesn't need lengthy explanations; just make the changes that are in his best interest. A 10-year-old, however, may be more cooperative if he understands the reasons for change: "We're having turkey tonight

(continued on page 144)

EXAMPLE 1: EXCESSIVE WEIGHT GAIN

Boy
Birth Weight: 8 lb
Length at Birth: 21"
Health at Birth: Excellent

Current Age: 11 years old
Current Height: 57"
Current Weight: 118 lb
Current BMI: 25.5

Parents
Mother: 5', 2"; 120 lb; BMI = 21.0
Father: 5', 8"; 175 lb; BMI = 26.5

This boy was born with normal weight and length to parents who were slightly shorter than average. Although he stayed within the normal range for height and weight for a bit, his weight began to accelerate and soon he was well outside the normal range of weight for height. His pediatrician found that he was consuming 2 sodas a day and was spending a lot of time playing video games. The family was concerned about his weight, so they agreed to stop buying sodas; to provide cool, good-tasting water for when he was thirsty; and to find physical activities that were fun to reduce his screen time.

See following pages for growth and body mass index charts.

Boys, 2 to 20 years

Name _____

STATURE FOR AGE AND WEIGHT FOR AGE PERCENTILES

Record # _____

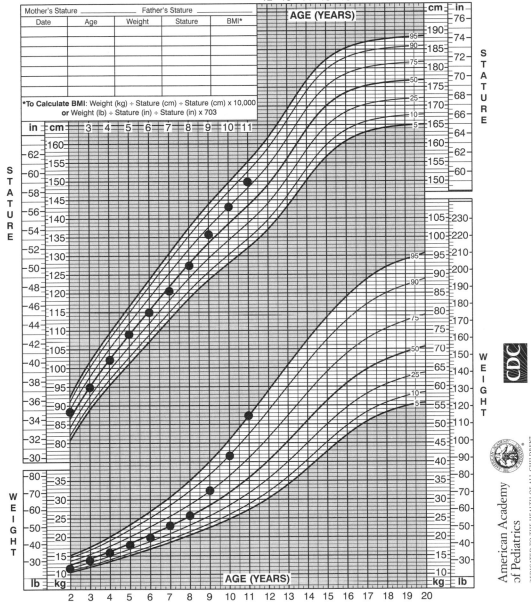

Mother's Stature _____ Father's Stature _____

Date	Age	Weight	Stature	BMI*

*To Calculate BMI: Weight (kg) ÷ Stature (cm) ÷ Stature (cm) x 10,000
or Weight (lb) ÷ Stature (in) ÷ Stature (in) x 703

AGE (YEARS)

STATURE

WEIGHT

Source: Developed by the National Center for Health Statistics in collaboration with the
National Center for Chronic Disease Prevention and Health Promotion (2000).
http://www.cdc.gov/growthcharts

Reprinted by the American Academy of Pediatrics

The recommendations in this publication do not indicate an exclusive course of treatment or serve as a
standard of medical care. Variations, taking into account individual circumstances, may be appropriate.

©2000 American Academy of Pediatrics

Additional copies are available for purchase in quantities of 100.

To order, contact:
American Academy of Pediatrics
141 Northwest Point Blvd
Elk Grove Village, IL 60007-1098
Web site — http://www.aap.org
Minimum order 100.

American Academy of Pediatrics

DEDICATED TO THE HEALTH OF ALL CHILDREN™

Boys, 2 to 20 years

Name _____

BODY MASS INDEX-FOR-AGE PERCENTILES

Record # _____

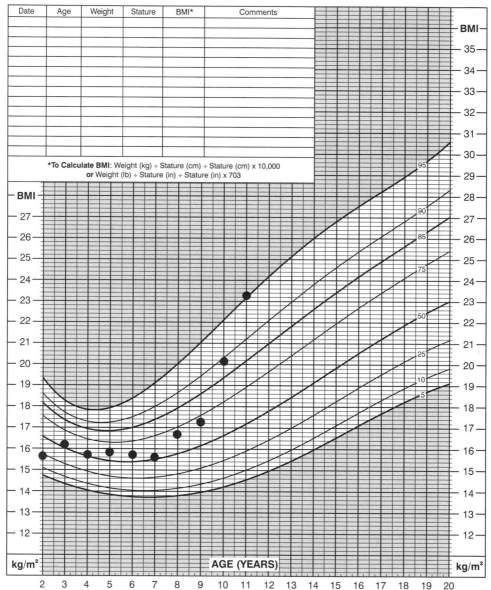

*To Calculate BMI: Weight (kg) ÷ Stature (cm) ÷ Stature (cm) x 10,000
or Weight (lb) ÷ Stature (in) ÷ Stature (in) x 703

American Academy
of Pediatrics

DEDICATED TO THE HEALTH OF ALL CHILDREN®

Source: Developed by the National Center for Health Statistics in collaboration with the
          National Center for Chronic Disease Prevention and Health Promotion (2000).
          http://www.cdc.gov/growthcharts

Reprinted by the American Academy of Pediatrics

The recommendations in this publication do not indicate an exclusive course of treatment or serve as a
standard of medical care. Variations, taking into account individual circumstances, may be appropriate.

©2000 American Academy of Pediatrics, Revised—5/01

9-8/REP1107

Additional copies are available for purchase in quantities of 100.

To order, contact:
American Academy of Pediatrics
141 Northwest Point Blvd
Elk Grove Village, IL 60007-1098
Web site — http://www.aap.org
Minimum order 100.

HE0304

EXAMPLE 2: NORMALLY LARGE

Boy

Birth Weight: 6 lb, 5 oz

Length at Birth: 17"

Health at Birth: Excellent

Current Age: 7 years old

Current Height: 51"

Current Weight: 76 lb

Current BMI: 20.5

Parents

Mother: 5', 6"; 150 lb; BMI = 24.3

Father: 6', 3"; 245 lb; BMI = 30.7

Both this boy's parents have large frames and are muscular. His father was a football player in high school and college, although he is now obese (BMI greater than 30). In reviewing the boy's growth history, it was revealed that he began to catch up to his genetic potential and developed a large frame. He was overweight for his height, but his pediatrician agreed that he was muscular and had little excess fat. There is no reason to be concerned about his size.

See following pages for growth and body mass index charts.

Boys, 2 to 20 years

Name _____

STATURE FOR AGE AND WEIGHT FOR AGE PERCENTILES

Record # _____

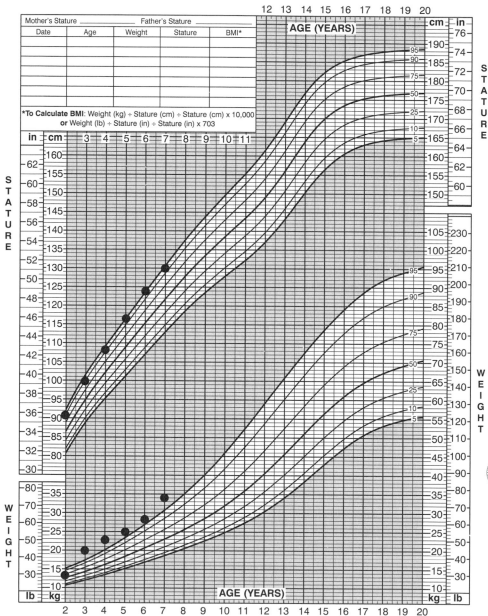

*To Calculate BMI: Weight (kg) ÷ Stature (cm) ÷ Stature (cm) x 10,000
or Weight (lb) ÷ Stature (in) ÷ Stature (in) x 703

American Academy of Pediatrics

DEDICATED TO THE HEALTH OF ALL CHILDREN™

Source: Developed by the National Center for Health Statistics in collaboration with the
National Center for Chronic Disease Prevention and Health Promotion (2000).
http://www.cdc.gov/growthcharts

Reprinted by the American Academy of Pediatrics

The recommendations in this publication do not indicate an exclusive course of treatment or serve as a
standard of medical care. Variations, taking into account individual circumstances, may be appropriate.

©2000 American Academy of Pediatrics

Additional copies are available for purchase in quantities of 100.

To order, contact:
American Academy of Pediatrics
141 Northwest Point Blvd
Elk Grove Village, IL 60007-1098
Web site — http://www.aap.org
Minimum order 100.

Boys, 2 to 20 years

Name _____

BODY MASS INDEX-FOR-AGE PERCENTILES

Record # _____

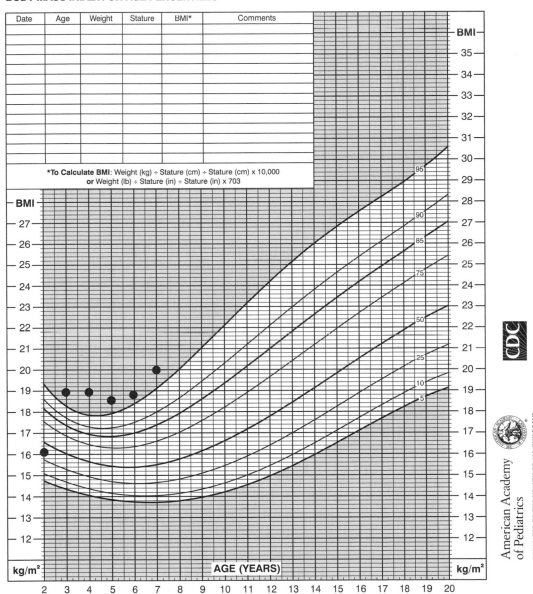

Date	Age	Weight	Stature	BMI*	Comments

*To Calculate BMI: Weight (kg) ÷ Stature (cm) ÷ Stature (cm) x 10,000
or Weight (lb) ÷ Stature (in) ÷ Stature (in) x 703

AGE (YEARS)

Source: Developed by the National Center for Health Statistics in collaboration with the
National Center for Chronic Disease Prevention and Health Promotion (2000).
http://www.cdc.gov/growthcharts

Reprinted by the American Academy of Pediatrics

The recommendations in this publication do not indicate an exclusive course of treatment or serve as a
standard of medical care. Variations, taking into account individual circumstances, may be appropriate.

©2000 American Academy of Pediatrics, Revised—5/01

9-8/REP1107

Additional copies are available for purchase in quantities of 100.

To order, contact:
American Academy of Pediatrics
141 Northwest Point Blvd
Elk Grove Village, IL 60007-1098
Web site — http://www.aap.org
Minimum order 100.

HE0304

CDC

American Academy
of Pediatrics

DEDICATED TO THE HEALTH OF ALL CHILDREN™

instead of hamburgers because it's lower in fat. And that's good for us," or, "You had cake—lots of calories—today at the birthday party, so tonight we're having fruit for dessert—no fat and plenty of fiber and vitamins."

Teenagers may resist being told what to do, even though they need direction. Giving unsolicited advice may be asking for trouble; rather, pick your moments carefully. If your teenaged daughter wails, "I'm fat!" it's your chance to ask, "Is something bothering you? Is there some way I can help?" But try not to seem overly eager or the window of opportunity may be slammed shut. To help your child or adolescent make behavioral changes and set goals for success with managing his weight, see "Making Behavioral Changes" on page 158. Here are some other helpful tips.

Be a Guide, Not a Dictator

Provide a variety of healthful foods and help your children learn to choose wisely for themselves what to eat and how much. The more you push a child to eat a particular food, the more likely she is to resist. It is also easier to say "no" if the food is not in the house. However, if a food is in the home, especially if it is where a child can see it but is not allowed to eat it, that food becomes even more desirable, and children become even more likely to eat more the next time it is available. To break this cycle, only keep enough of these foods in the house for your child to enjoy. When it is gone, it is not a forbidden fruit—it is simply not available, and your hungry child will eat something else.

Don't Limit Your Child's Calories

Your child should never be on a calorie-restricted diet unless your pediatrician prescribes and closely supervises it. Limiting what children eat can deprive them of essential nutrients and interfere with growth and development.

Remember That Simple Carbohydrates and Sugars Contribute to Excess Weight Gain Too

Even reduced-fat foods can be high in calories because of their simple sugar content and other ingredients. Although you should not be counting every calorie your child eats or restricting calories, allowing unlimited access to many "diet" foods can lead to undesirable weight gain.

Choose Foods That Make Children Feel Full Naturally

In humans, fullness after a meal is determined by the bulk of food that's in the stomach, rather than the number of calories that are eaten. Because fruits and vegetables have high water content, they contain few calories per unit of volume, occupy a lot of space in the stomach, and help children feel full after eating. This effect is just another reason to encourage your child to eat fruits and vegetables. On the other hand, because fast foods and many processed foods have low water content and are high in fat and calories, more of these foods are needed before children feel full. A piece of fruit, like an orange or apple, is more filling than orange juice or apple juice.

Let Protein Contribute to Fullness

Another strategy for making children feel full is to include good sources of lean protein in their meals, like lean meat, poultry, or fish. Protein is much more important in creating a sense of fullness than fat or carbohydrates. True, most children love carbohydrates like macaroni and cheese, potatoes, and bread. And it's easy to turn to these foods when children turn down more healthful choices. But if you offer food selections that you know are good choices, there will be enough carbohydrates in the diet to meet your child's nutritional needs.

Monitor Fat in Your Family's Diet

Reducing the fat in your family's diet may be an important step in preventing excess weight gain in children. In any case, for long-term health, children older than 2 years should take in an average of 30% of their total daily calories as fat, with one third or less (10% of calories) as saturated fat. Simple fat-cutting steps include serving low-fat or nonfat dairy products, lean meats and skinless poultry, fish or occasional vegetarian entrees, and low-fat or fat-free breads and cereals. If you plan a major dietary overhaul, you may benefit from the advice of a registered dietitian; ask your pediatrician for a referral.

Allow a Treat Once in a While

Occasional treats of ice cream, potato chips, candy, and the like do no harm. As mentioned earlier, banning these foods outright may make them seem overly desirable, and your child may crave them more. Although no food should be forbidden and any food can be part of a healthful diet, make sure that children know it is only for special occasions. If snacks and sweet foods are kept in the house, most children will want them. If and when you do have ice cream or other treats in the home, do not buy the largest sized container; it will just sit in the house, calling silently to be eaten. The readily available snacks should be fruits and vegetables.

Avoid Temptation

Free access to a supply of cookies, candy, and other treat foods will damage efforts to moderate your child's food intake. Buy or make what you need for a special event or occasion, but don't keep such foods on hand. Children should not have free reign over what they find and consume from the pantry or refrigerator. They need to ask permission before helping themselves to food in the house until they are old enough to make the right choices. However, they should have unlimited access to the faucet or water dispenser.

Limit Takeout and Fast Foods

These products tend to be high in fat and the portions are overly large. Therefore, fast-food meals contain a lot of calories but usually not much in the way of fruits or vegetables. Because people eat volumes of food rather than calories, fast-food meals can lead to overeating.

Whenever Possible, Prepare Meals at Home and Involve Children in the Preparation

It's easier to control fat content and portion sizes of foods prepared from healthful raw ingredients in your own kitchen. And children may be more likely to eat food that they help buy and prepare. But if you eat out a lot or eat on the run, rather than sitting down together as a family for more relaxed meals, your child is less likely to eat fruits and vegetables. At restaurants, portions are usually large and available choices aren't always the best. When you do eat out, consider splitting entrees, substituting a green vegetable for french fries, and ordering lower fat and lower calorie foods such as a grilled chicken sandwich rather than a hamburger. Planning ahead and freezing some healthful meals can save money and prevent relying on restaurant and takeout food in times of stress.

Offer Water for Drinks, Rather Than Juice, Soda, or Sport or Energy Drinks

Sugar-sweetened drinks, such as soda or juice drinks that contain less than 100% fruit juice, are a common source of extra calories. For example, these drinks now account on average for 7% of the total daily calories of a 2- to 5-year-old, 9% of the total for a 6- to 11-year-old, and 13% for those 12 to 19 years old. Consuming a piece of fruit is a better choice than drinking fruit juices. Also, as soft drink consumption has increased, milk consumption has decreased. This shift is double jeopardy—less calcium and vitamin D are consumed from milk, more empty calories from sugar-sweetened drinks. The solution is easy—provide water to thirsty children and low-fat or skim milk at meals. Water does not promote weight gain and is better for children's teeth than a sugary bath of juice or soft drink.

SHOULD YOU ENCOURAGE YOUR OVERWEIGHT CHILD TO DIET?

Just as it's counterproductive to try to get toddlers to eat when they don't want to (in fact, they'll probably eat less!), a recent study has shown that parental pressure may not be helpful for overweight adolescents. The study showed that parents who urged their teenager to go on a diet made it *more* likely that the adolescent would still be overweight 5 years later. In other words, the more strictly parents try to control the amount of food that children eat, the less appropriately they eat.

Children (especially toddlers) and adolescents naturally go through periods of decreased appetite and spells when they eat everything in sight. In fact, portion sizes that are right for small children are generally less than parents think, and dieting is certainly not necessary. Trying to make a child eat more because a parent thinks he should can contribute to excess calorie intake. As an alternative, parents should adopt a program for the entire family—eating more fruits and vegetables and less snack food, sharing meals together as a family, turning off the television, and increasing physical activity.

SIZING UP PORTIONS
One of the keys to managing weight is to keep an eye on portion sizes. The following information (adapted from the American Dietetic Association) will help you determine typical serving sizes: • Three oz of meat are the size of a deck of cards. • Two tablespoons of peanut butter are about the size of a ping-pong ball. • One and a half oz of cheese are equal in size to 3 dominoes. • A half cup of vegetables is about the size of a lightbulb. • One cup of pasta is the size of a tennis ball. • Half of a medium bagel is about the size of a hockey puck.

Make Sure That Your Child Consumes 24 oz (3 Large Glasses) of Reduced-fat (2%), Low-fat (1%), or Nonfat (skim) Milk, or the Equivalent in Other Dairy Foods, Per Day

Milk and dairy products are the best sources of calcium and vitamin D, which are essential for strong bones, teeth, and a healthy body. Girls, in particular, need calcium but may skimp unless persuaded that consuming good calcium sources will not lead to weight gain.

Encourage Children to Eat Slowly

Your child will be better able to judge when she has eaten enough if she eats at a moderate rate and does not rush her food.

Keep a Place for Eating and Keep Eating in its Place

Allow eating only in designated areas such as the dining room or kitchen. Keep mealtimes calm and sociable without distractions such as television. Serve meals and snacks on a regular, but not inflexible schedule.

Involve Children in Food Shopping

Grocery shopping with your child is an opportunity to pass along nutrition lessons, such as comparing the labels on sugared and nonsugared cereals for calories, sodium, and price per serving. Let your child help you plan meals, and make a shopping list together. It's all right if your child wants the same items each time you go the market together, as long as the choices are healthful. Some markets have candy-free checkout lines; when shopping with children, avoid the checkout line with a candy display.

Stay Flexible

New issues arise as a child becomes more independent and family and school schedules change. Any change that takes place after the initial treatment plan has begun will require rethinking your current weight-management techniques.

Healthful Choices

Remember that as a parent, *you* determine what food is offered and when. Your child decides whether and how much to eat. That's why the choices you offer should be healthful. Let your child choose between an apple and air-popped popcorn for a snack, not an apple or a chocolate-covered cookie. You create an atmosphere for lifelong healthy eating when children are allowed healthful choices. Above all, don't ask your child what she wants to eat unless you are prepared to serve it. For more information about balanced nutrition and age-appropriate serving sizes, check out the *Dietary Guidelines for Americans* at www.cnpp.usda.gov/DietaryGuidelines.htm.

Be consistent. You inadvertently reinforce undesirable behavior—such as demands for candy at the checkout counter—by inconsistently giving in to it. When you allow treats for parties or other special occasions, make it clear that these are exceptions.

Make any change with the idea that it's permanent and not just a temporary fix. A healthy approach to eating and physical activity should become your lifestyle, rather than a patch over a weight problem.

LET GROWTH CATCH UP

The goal for overweight children between ages 2 and 7 years is weight maintenance, not weight loss. For a heavy but otherwise healthy child, it's more important to develop habits of healthful eating and activity. If an overweight child maintains her weight as she grows, her weight and height will come back in proportion and her body mass index will drop.

Changes in diet and activity are easier to take if they are made gradually. Try only 1 or 2 changes a week and stick with them. Here are a few examples of small changes that make a big difference over time.

- For children older than 2 years, switch from whole milk to reduced-fat (2%), low-fat (1%), or nonfat (skim) milk. Also, feed them reduced-fat cheese and nonfat yogurt. While fat should not be restricted for children younger than 2, if your 12- to 24-month-old is overweight or at risk for overweight, or you have a family history of high cholesterol or heart disease, reduced-fat dietary choices may be appropriate. Check with your child's doctor before restricting fat in your child's diet.
- Go for family after-dinner walks.
- Keep unsalted pretzels on hand for snacks.
- Switch from full-fat bread spreads, such as mayonnaise and dressings, to reduced-fat or fat-free varieties. There are plenty of brands to choose from. Make sandwiches with reduced-fat spreads.
- Substitute low-fat sandwich meats such as turkey bologna and turkey ham for beef and pork products. Use ground turkey instead of beef for pasta sauces, chili and tacos, and casseroles.
- Serve frozen juice and fruit bars without fat or added sugar, instead of ice cream. Frozen yogurt, even if promoted as a low-fat or fat-free dessert, may be high in sugar and therefore high in calories.
- Serve low-fat popcorn instead of cookies for after-school snacks.
- Naturally low-fat cookies, such as vanilla wafers, graham crackers, and gingersnaps, are good choices for cookie fans, but if there is a favorite that your child just can't do without, find or make a low-fat version of it.

- Make gravies and sauces virtually fat free by reducing defatted broth or vegetable stock with seasonings.
- Experiment with child-friendly vegetarian recipes such as spaghetti or lasagna made with vegetables instead of meat, together with reduced-fat cheeses.

Getting Expert Help for Weight Management

If you find changing your family's eating habits too difficult to do alone, you could benefit from outside help. Start with your pediatrician, who may refer you to a registered dietitian who specializes in children's nutrition and can help develop a plan tailored to your family's lifestyle and preferences. However, if more intense efforts are needed or your pediatrician warns that your child's health is at risk unless she loses weight, you may need to consider a formal treatment program. A university-based medical center should be able to help you find a pediatric weight-control program suitable for your child. Contact the Weight-control Information Network for more information (877/946-4627; win@info.niddk.nih.gov; www.win.niddk.nih.gov).

Some children may need referral to a pediatric obesity center if more conservative therapies are unsuccessful. These would include a child with sleep apnea (interrupted breathing during sleep), liver disease, type 2 diabetes, or some orthopedic problems due to obesity; a child younger than 2 years whose BMI is greater than 120% of the 95th percentile; or a child older than 2 years whose BMI is above the 97th percentile.

If your older child is not ready to change or your family is not committed to helping, a weight-management program is a waste of time and may actually be harmful. A failed weight-control program can diminish a child's already low self-esteem and hinder future efforts at weight control. Also, if the child is depressed or has an eating disorder (see Chapter 10, Eating Disorders), she requires psychological evaluation and treatment in addition to weight control. A depressed, overweight child may have sleep disturbances, feelings of hopelessness and sadness, and appetite changes. A therapist may recommend counseling before or along with a weight-management program.

For older children, outside help may be essential. Take Liz, for example. Every time her mother cautiously touched on the topic of Liz's increasing weight, the 15-year-old burst into tears. Liz knew she had a problem but took her mother's unsolicited advice as a criticism of her personality. Confrontations ended with raised voices and slammed doors. Liz's mother backed off and made the wise decision to bring the girl in to see her pediatrician, with whom Liz felt comfortable. After listening to both sides, her doctor found that mother and daughter were in agreement. She referred Liz and her mother to a dietitian who specialized in working with overweight adolescents and suggested Liz call for a follow-up appointment when she had been in a weight-management program for 3 months.

Weight-Loss Programs

Commercial weight-loss programs generally are not designed with children or adolescents in mind. However, some new programs do address children's problems. As you evaluate a program, go through the following checklist:

✔ **Is it staffed with a variety of health professionals?** The best programs include one or more registered dietitians or qualified nutritionists, exercise physiologists, pediatricians or family physicians, and psychiatrists or psychologists.

✔ **Does the program focus on behavioral changes?** This includes how to select healthful foods in appropriate portions or how to exercise more while limiting sedentary behavior.

✔ **Does it include a medical evaluation?** Before your child is enrolled in a program, her weight, growth, and general health should be reviewed by a pediatrician. In addition, a health professional should monitor the child's weight, growth, and general health at regular times during the course of the program.

✔ **Does the program encompass the whole family and not just the overweight child?** The most effective programs are family based, focusing on food and activity environment, not just the affected child.

✔ **Is the program appropriate for your child's age and abilities?** A program for 8- to 12-year-olds, for example, differs from programs for 13- to 18-year-olds in terms of the responsibilities placed on the child and parents.

✔ **Does the program include a maintenance program?** Support and referral resources are essential for reinforcing behavior and dealing with the underlying issues that led to becoming overweight.

Numerous camps offer weight-control programs for young people. One advantage of such places is that all the campers are overweight so there is less fear of being teased or stigmatized. But like other marketed weight-loss programs, they have a high relapse rate. If you pick a camp program, make sure that the family environment changes so the child does not return home from a camp to the same unhealthy set of problems.

Getting Active

Children are increasingly overweight now not only because what they eat has changed but also because they are less active. One survey found that fewer than 25% of children in grades 4 through 12 take part in 20 minutes of vigorous activity or 30 minutes of any physical activity every day.

Those are unsettling statistics, particularly in light of how important exercise is to your child's well-being, now and in the future. Just like certain foods reduce the risk of specific diseases, particular types of physical activity can reduce the risk of some diseases. For example, vigorous exercise of any kind helps lower the risk of heart disease and high blood pressure, while weight-bearing activities like running or jumping reduce the risk of osteoporosis.

When weight management is a goal for your child, remember that food intake and physical activity are the 2 sides of the energy balance equation. When calories consumed are greater than calories spent on physical activity, children gain weight; when calories eaten are less than calories burned from activity, children will lose weight. However, after a child has become overweight, he may find it difficult to lose weight from physical activity alone, although exercise should remain an important component of an overall effort of weight management.

So how active should your child be? In 2008, a report by the US Department of Health and Human Services, *Physical Activity Guidelines for Americans,* answered that question. The report recommends that children aged 6 years and older do 60 minutes or more of moderate to vigorous physical activity every day. More specifically, the guidelines noted that children need the following types of physical activity as part of their 60-minutes-a-day regimen:

- **Aerobic.** Most of children's daily physical activity should be moderate or vigorous aerobic activity, meaning that they should use the body's large muscle groups through activities like swimming, hiking, dancing, bicycling, rollerblading, and walking briskly, and sports like soccer and basketball. Children should participate in vigorous activity at least 3 days a week.
- **Muscle strengthening** (or *resistance)* physical activity (eg, push-ups, climbing a tree, swinging on playground equipment, playing tug-of-war) should be done at least 3 days a week.
- **Bone-strengthening** activities, such as running, jumping rope, and hopscotch, and sports like gymnastics and tennis, should be done 2 or more times a week. Bone strengthening activities are particularly important for children and young teenagers because the largest increases in bone growth take place just prior to and during puberty; adolescents get most of their peak bone mass by the time adolescence ends.

Although 60 minutes a day is the goal, the guidelines point out that people can build up their activity time in periods of 10 minutes throughout the day. Physical activity naturally tends to be more varied in young children than in adults, but brief periods of activity add up.

Whether or not children are overweight, the challenge for parents is how to provide them with opportunities to meet the new guidelines, especially in adolescence. Budget issues have forced many schools to limit physical education, but children shouldn't depend only on organized sports for exercise. Unstructured outdoor play is a good energy outlet. However, parents in cities and suburbs are often concerned about letting young children play outside without adult supervision. If your community does not have a playground nearby, parents may have to make a special effort to find places where children can play freely and safely.

Here are some tips for becoming more active.

Be a Role Model

If your children see that you are active and enjoying it, they are more likely to be active and stay active into adulthood.

A FAMILY AFFAIR
Children younger than 10 years whose parents are overweight are more than twice as likely to become overweight adults as children the same age but with normal-weight parents.

Walk More

If you live close enough, encourage your children to walk to school with friends, or walk with them. A program called Safe Routes to School encourages children in kindergarten through eighth grade, as well as entire communities, to walk or bicycle to school, while promoting safety measures along the route. (For more information, see www.saferoutesinfo.org.) Also, recruit the whole family to take a walk through the neighborhood after dinner. When you're shopping with your child, park farther away from the store and walk up a flight or two of stairs rather than using the escalator or elevator. Even these kinds of small changes can make a difference over time, rather than trying to revolutionize your lifestyle.

Limit Sedentary Activities

The American Academy of Pediatrics recommends no more than 1 to 2 hours daily of screen time for watching television and videos or using the computer (other than for homework), sending text messages, or playing video games. (Choose only nonviolent games.)

Help Your Child Find Physical Activities

Locate activities that your child wants and likes to do. Be sensitive to his needs; overweight children often feel self-conscious about taking part in sports. Look for activities that he enjoys and that aren't embarrassing or too difficult. If your child likes a particular activity, he is more likely to stick with it for the long term.

Encourage your child to participate in age-appropriate activities. While weight lifting or a 3-mile jog may not be appropriate for a 7- or 8-year-old, there are many other activities, such as bicycle riding or swimming, that are much better choices. If your child has not been active, start slowly and make it fun. Also, make sure your child doesn't overdo it; if physical activity causes pain, he should try something less intense.

BENEFITS OF FAMILY EXERCISE

A colleague of Dr Stern's was frustrated with his inability to get his son to take walks. His son was a high school football player sidelined by a knee injury, and his orthopedist wanted him to walk not only as part of his physical therapy program but also to keep him from gaining weight while recovering. Dr Stern suggested that he go walking with his son. The next time Dr Stern ran into her colleague, he thanked her. "Not only did my son's face light up when I suggested that we walk together, but on our walks we've had some of the best conversations that we've had in a long while."

Provide Toys and Gear That Make Your Child Want to Become Active

For example, give a gift of tennis or riding lessons, along with the appropriate gear. Young children should have access to balls, jump ropes, and similar toys.

Offer Activities, Not Food, as Rewards

For example, go bowling for a treat rather than staying home to make hot-fudge sundaes.

Push Your Local School Board to Make Physical Education a Priority

While many schools reduced physical education to meet the requirements of the federal government No Child Left Behind Act, some states have more recently begun to restore it. If you live in one of those states or communities, make sure your child's school has a physical education program. If your child already has such a program, make sure it is a quality program taught by a physical education instructor who keeps children moving for most of the class time. Also push for healthy choices in lunch lines and vending machines. Get involved with your parent-teacher organization or school wellness council to ensure that school meals and snacks offer varied, healthful, and low-fat food choices.

Volunteer to Help Out With School or Community Sports Programs

If you're involved in the school's extracurricular activities, your child is more likely to take part.

Plan Activity Parties

For example, invite neighborhood children to a backyard hula hoop tournament.

Check Out Biking and Hiking Trails

Then take the family for weekend outings.

Recruit Your Children to Clean the Car

Do this instead of going to a car wash.

Go on a Mall Walk

But steer clear of the food court! Or collect a library of child-friendly exercise DVDs and exercise along with your child.

Get Your Teenager Dancing to the Music She Likes Best

Team sports such as soccer, basketball, volleyball, hockey, lacrosse, and football are excellent energy outlets. For children who dislike team sports, swimming, skating, dance classes, gymnastics, video games that include whole body physical activity, and martial arts are excellent alternatives.

Family Involvement

If parents are overweight, it's unlikely that a child's weight problem can be successfully addressed unless the family's lifestyle and eating habits are revised as well. That's another reason parents should take part in their child's weight-control program. If your child is the only family member who has to change his eating and exercise habits, he may feel resentful and is likely to relapse. In addition, slender siblings may become upset if they believe that limits are placed on their foods and activities for the sake of one family member's weight problem. Encourage children to express their feelings openly. Answer their objections truthfully and fairly. Above all, it is essential to prevent destructive sarcasm and teasing about weight by family members, and to keep others from sabotaging serious efforts at weight control.

Long-term success is more likely if all caregivers, including babysitters, child care staff, and grandparents are aware of the plan and accept responsibility to help the overweight child in her efforts while respecting her evolving independence.

The Role of Schools and Communities

The obesity epidemic did not result from conscious decisions by children to gain weight or by parents to overfeed their children or discourage them from being active. Lack of time has made us more reliant on fast or processed food. Sprawling suburban neighborhoods without sidewalks have reduced opportunities for children to walk to school. Concern about neighborhood safety has reduced opportunities for children to play outside. School cafeterias often sell attractive high-calorie foods to make the money they need for some of their expenses.

Although family rules about food and television time are essential, efforts must be made to make schools and communities healthier places for children. Some of these changes can come from active parent-teacher organizations that push schools to serve healthier options in cafeterias and vending machines, restore physical education programs, or stay open so communities can use the gyms after hours. Efforts to require new schools and parks to be located in neighborhoods where children can walk to them will encourage children to be more physically active. Walking to school with your child and other children is a twofer—it gives you and your child the health benefits of physical activity and can be a special time for talking.

Making Behavioral Changes

The Table on pages 159 through 161 provides guidelines and suggestions to help you and your child make gradual progress toward changes that can help him manage weight successfully.

STRATEGIES FOR CHANGE	EXAMPLES OF SPECIFIC BEHAVIOR CHANGES
Assess Starting Point Determine your child's starting point in the weight-control process. Identify your family and school routines, and habits and cues that may have increased your child's likelihood of consuming extra calories or remaining inactive.	Assess routines and behaviors that may make it more difficult for your child to maintain a healthy weight. For example, do you or your family • Have calorie-rich, high-fat foods in your kitchen cabinets and refrigerator? • Place too much food on your child's plate at mealtimes? • Eat away from home often? • Do little to encourage your child to be physically active? • Allow too much television viewing at home? • Expect your child to finish what is on his plate?
Determine Goals Set goals with your child to help her eat more healthfully and exercise more. Begin to formulate specific approaches to help her consume fewer calories and increase her activity level. Goals should be measurable. If the goal cannot be counted, it cannot be measured.	Set goals along with your child and make them specific, such as • Keep high-calorie snacks and sugar-sweetened beverages out of your home; for snacking, emphasize fruits and vegetables. • Limit serving sizes on your child's plate, and use smaller plates to make servings seem larger. • Limit the number of meals that your child eats outside the home, particularly at fast-food restaurants each week. Go out to dinner no more than once per week. • Help your child sign up for a program that's physically active and fun. • Do active things together as a family. • Limit the amount of time your child (and the entire family) spends in watching television, and keep a television out of her bedroom. Shut off the television during meals.

STRATEGIES FOR CHANGE	EXAMPLES OF SPECIFIC BEHAVIOR CHANGES
Monitor Behavior Monitor your child's progress in making changes, and give him feedback on how he's doing. Make adjustments as needed, and problem-solve together.	• Record the number of days your child is physically active. • Make sure he has access to fruits and vegetables in your home each day. • Keep track of how your child is doing with the other goals that you've set, and talk about how each of you can maintain or improve his progress. • Have him implement new goals 1 or 2 at a time. • Encourage him to commit to very specific behaviors ("I will have fruits and vegetables for my after-school snack"…"I will not drink any sugar-sweetened beverages"…"I will get some type of physical activity every day"). • Renew your own commitment to certain strategies ("I will walk my child to school 3 days a week"…"I will make sure the television is never on during meals"). • Work with your child to identify and resolve obstacles to success, such as eating when he's feeling stress, interference from other family members, relatives who express their love with food, high-fat meals served in the school cafeteria, and neighborhood safety concerns that keep your child from exercising outside.
Reward Changes Reward your child's successes when she makes changes. These rewards should be frequent and take place as closely as possible to her successful behaviors. Make the magnitude or value of these rewards consistent with the magnitude of your child's accomplishments.	• Praise and attention are excellent rewards. Tie this praise to specific behaviors ("I'm so proud of you for eating carrots instead of chips"). • For a reward, choose an activity that you can do together with your child, such as walking, roller-skating, bike riding, playing in the park, or buying her a new pair of athletic shoes. • Give your child an extra privilege as a reward. • Do not give expensive gifts or food as rewards.

(continued on next page)

STRATEGIES FOR CHANGE	EXAMPLES OF SPECIFIC BEHAVIOR CHANGES
Use Your Parenting Skills Work extra hard at your own parenting skills. Communicate your expectations for your child clearly, and model desirable behavior.	• Set rules for the entire family. • Set limits that support your child's good health. • All family members need to stay consistent. • Talk with your child daily about his behaviors, and express interest in the progress he's making. • Model the behaviors you want your child to copy. • Provide daily review and feedback. A sticker chart works well for young children.

Adapted from Dietz WH, Robinson TN. Clinical practice. Overweight children and adolescents. *N Engl J Med.* 2005;352:2100–2109

ISSUES PARENTS OFTEN RAISE ABOUT CHILDREN'S WEIGHT

Those really overweight children usually have glandular problems, don't they?

Medical problems linked to overweight are rare, accounting for fewer than 1 out of 100 cases of obesity in children. Many factors, such as overeating, inactivity, and parents' behavior, contribute to the rising tide of overweight among children in this country. (For more about this, turn to page 131.)

I think my 12-year-old son is getting pudgy and needs to go on a diet. His mother says I'm making a fuss about nothing.

It's not unusual for a boy to gain several pounds and look pudgy with hormonal changes leading up to puberty. In most cases, the extra weight drops off during the adolescent growth spurt. To settle the argument, ask your pediatrician to check where your son fits on the standard growth chart. This will help you plan a weight-management strategy, if one is needed. Survey his eating and activity habits. Did more screen time creep in? Has he been eating out with his friends? This is good time to join your son in healthy eating and exercise to control his weight and get fit (see pages 137 and 157). It is very important that you and his mother agree on the appropriate strategy; otherwise your child will get mixed and confusing messages about his weight.

My daughter and I agree that she needs to lose weight. I've just started a low-calorie diet, so it'll keep things simple if she does the same, won't it?

Your child should not be on a calorie-restricted diet unless your pediatrician prescribes and closely supervises it. Limiting what children eat can deprive them of important nutrients and interfere with their growth and development. However, increased physical activity, more fruits and vegetables, a good source of lean protein, and fewer desserts will benefit everyone. (For a list of suggestions on how to approach weight problems in children, turn to page 152.)

Chapter 7

Is My Child Too Thin? Too Small? Too Tall?

At regular examinations, beginning with the first one after birth, your pediatrician keeps track of your child's weight and length. During the first 2 years, her head circumference is routinely measured to track growth and development. Beginning at 2 years of age, your pediatrician will begin to measure your child's height and calculate her body mass index (BMI). Chronic illnesses can slow growth. Such illnesses sometimes occur silently, with no apparent symptoms. That's one of the reasons that regular checkups are important for your child's health.

Tracking Your Child's Growth

For you and the pediatrician tracking your child's height and weight, an unexplained major change or lack of change over time is more important than any single measurement. Dramatic growth spurts occur during the first year of life and later with the onset of puberty. A healthy infant may double her birth weight by 4 months and triple it by her first birthday. This intensive growth in the first 12 months is followed by a relative slowing of the growth rate, together with a noticeable drop in the child's appetite during the second year—a turn of events that can be disturbing to parents, at least with their first child. Because children tend to grow in spurts, a marked gain in height may be followed by a period in which height slows a bit and weight catches up, or vice versa. The appetite varies according to the rate of growth and the amount of energy the child uses. This cycle of feasting and fasting repeats itself to some degree throughout childhood, and weight gain is continuous but not always steady. Normal fluctuations in appetite do not affect your child's overall rate of growth.

In addition to these cycles, other changes in height and weight in infancy and childhood may be completely normal. For example, if a child is born large after a healthy pregnancy and her parents are small, her rate of growth in the first years of life is likely to slow until she reaches her genetic potential. Likewise, if a child is born small and her parents are large, she is likely

---

SLOWER GROWTH IN BREASTFED BABIES

Beginning at about 3 months of age, weight increases in babies who are exclusively breastfed may lag behind weight increases that occur in formula-fed infants. However, any such differences in growth between breastfed and bottle-fed babies should not concern you, as long as your child continues to grow steadily in length.

---

to grow more rapidly in the first years of life until her genetic potential is achieved. However, in an infant younger than 1 year, a marked drop-off in weight gain or growth rate can sometimes signal a feeding or developmental problem, or a medical condition such as failure to thrive (FTT). This is a potentially serious condition, the causes of which are often difficult to pinpoint. A pediatrician may suspect FTT if a baby falls below the fifth percentile for height and weight among infants her own age. Yet even in the absence of FTT, some parents worry because their child appears too thin to them (even though overweight is a more common problem in our society).

What about older children? An older child should be checked by her pediatrician if her height growth slows down but her weight gain continues. The last dramatic growth spurt occurs during adolescence, when boys may sprout up as much as 4 inches a year and girls grow and mature seemingly overnight. If your daughter has not shown signs of puberty (breast enlargement, growth of pubic hair, menarche or first period) by age 13, or your son has no corresponding signs (growth of pubic and body hair, enlargement of sexual organs) by age 14, consult your pediatrician.

WHAT DOES BMI MEAN FOR YOUR CHILD?

At the lower end, body mass index (BMI) less than the fifth percentile is considered underweight. At the other end of spectrum, children in the 95th percentile or greater are considered at higher risk for chronic health problems like diabetes or heart disease.

- BMI less than 5% = underweight
- BMI 5% to 85% = normal weight
- BMI 85% to 95% = overweight
- BMI greater than 95% = obese

WHAT IS BODY MASS INDEX? WHAT IS A PERCENTILE?

Body mass index (BMI) is a formula used to calculate a child's body weight in relation to her height. Use the following formula or go to www.cdc.gov to measure your child's BMI:

- Multiply your child's weight (in pounds) by 703. We'll call this A.
- Multiply your child's height (in inches) by itself. We'll call this B.
- Dividing A by B gives you your child's BMI score.

For example, let's say you have a 12-year-old daughter. She is 5 feet 2 inches (62") and weighs 155 pounds. Multiply her weight by 703 (108,965); multiply her height (62") by itself (3,844); then divide the first total by the second. Your daughter's BMI (108,965/3,844) is 28.3. As you can see on the following chart, this example daughter's BMI is greater than the 95th percentile for age.

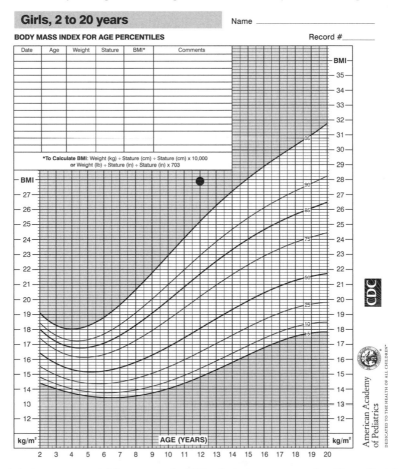

Because weight increases as children grow, the BMI calculation removes the effect of height on weight.

Now, what does the term *percentile* mean? You'll see this word mentioned several times in this chapter and others. Percentile can be applied to many things—height, weight, head circumference, blood pressure, or any other measurement. This calculation indicates where your child ranks compared with other children. If, for example, your child's height is at the 30th percentile for her age, it means that 70% of children her age are taller and 30% are smaller. As we've discussed, BMI percentiles are important for determining if someone is underweight, in the normal range, overweight, or obese. While less than the fifth percentile is considered underweight, a BMI between the fifth and 85th percentiles is a healthy weight, 85th percentile or higher is overweight, and 95th percentile or higher indicates that the child is at risk for developing chronic diseases like those mentioned previously. However, a particular child's bone structure and muscle mass may mean that even though she falls into the overweight category, she does not have too much body fat. Likewise, some children who are less than the fifth percentile, which is the cutoff percentile for underweight, have adequate body fat but reduced bone or muscle mass.

Parents concerned about their child's weight are doing the right thing by bringing him to the pediatrician's office for evaluation. In most cases, the child's weight is within the normal range and he is growing just fine. However, if he has a sudden change in the rate of growth, whether increasing or decreasing, this may signal a developing problem.

That was the case with 15-year-old Sandy. Her parents, Sharon and Bill, had noticed that their usually healthy teenager seemed fatigued and frequently complained of gas, bloating, and crampy diarrhea. One day Sharon was startled to see that Sandy's jeans and skirts suddenly looked too big for her. At first, they simply chalked the changes up to her incredibly busy schedule and irregular eating habits. But when Sandy told them she had lost 10 pounds in the last 2 months, they made an appointment with their pediatrician, who had been charting Sandy's growth and BMI for years.

At their visit, Sandy's height and weight were measured carefully. When the pediatrician's measurements confirmed that Sandy had lost weight—and that she had dropped from the 40th percentile to the fifth—Sharon and Bill were shocked. After additional tests, including a visit to a pediatric gastroenterologist, Sandy was diagnosed with Crohn disease, an inflammation of the intestinal tract. Because this chronic condition interferes with how nutrients are absorbed, it can cause weight loss in a fully grown adolescent or hinder growth and weight gain in a younger child. In severe cases, a child may become undernourished. Sandy received intensive outpatient treatment to stabilize her condition. Crohn disease is a lifelong condition that Sandy will have to manage with nutritional and medical treatments as necessary. Her parents acted wisely in consulting their pediatrician as soon as they suspected something was wrong. In this way, they may have prevented Sandy from becoming severely ill.

Growth Charts: By the Numbers

Normal children come in a dazzling variety of shapes and sizes, and their rates of growth and weight gain vary widely. A group of 8-year-olds, for example, may vary by as much as 30 pounds in weight and 8 inches in height without being considered abnormally tall, short, heavy, or thin, as long as their individual heights and weights are in proportion. Pediatricians use standardized growth charts like those in Appendix C to determine whether children fall within the normal range, and they track each child's growth rate over time. Another set of growth charts in Appendix C (for ages 0 to 2 years) has been developed by the World Health Organization, approved by the US Centers for Disease Control and Prevention, and recommended by the American Academy of Pediatrics for the first 2 years of life. Typically, pediatricians weigh and measure children at regular visits between birth and 3 years of age and then yearly after age 3. Heights and weights marked on charts provide a picture of the growth pattern.

However, weight or height alone don't tell the whole story; a child's weight *in relation to* height is what counts, as we described earlier in this chapter (see also Appendix D). As mentioned, a BMI below the fifth percentile is unusually low and needs a doctor's evaluation, just as a BMI above the 95th percentile is high. (See Chapter 6, Is My Child Overweight? for more about overweight.)

How Much Is in the Genes?

Height and weight tend to run in families. In fact, you can get a rough idea of how tall a child is likely to be by looking at the parents. Here's one way to predict a child's probable height at maturity: add together the heights of the mother and father in inches and divide by 2. For a boy, add 2½ inches; for a girl, subtract 2½ inches. Although this is just a rough estimate, it provides a guideline. Quite simply, the taller the parents, the taller the child is likely to be; on the other hand, short parents tend to have short children.

At age 11, Eric was 58 inches tall and weighed only 70 pounds. His BMI was 14.6, which was at the fifth percentile for boys of the same age. His parents, Paul and Cindy, couldn't help noticing Eric was by far the thinnest child in his class, and he seemed to look even skinnier as he grew. Paul and Cindy had no worries about Eric's eating habits and he seemed healthy and energetic, but they kept bringing up his weight at each of Eric's checkups. Their pediatrician confirmed that while Eric's height was average, he was thinner than most boys his age, falling within the fifth percentile according to the growth charts. Nevertheless, their pediatrician assured them that Eric was a healthy boy. A check of the family history revealed that in college, Paul had never weighed more than 150 pounds, although his height was 6 feet 2 inches. His BMI in college was 19.3, which is at the lower end of the range for a healthy adult. He had gained a few pounds in the intervening decades but was proud that he could still wear the suit he was married in 15 years before. Their pediatrician suggested they stop worrying about Eric's weight. Thinness, she said, was "in the genes," and Eric's build was lean and wiry, like his dad's. That perspective gave the family peace of mind, and their concerns about his "underweight" were put to rest.

As with Eric, whose lean frame resembled his father's, a child's build often reflects that of his parents. Studies with twins have confirmed this genetic connection, but environment

---

WHEN PERCENTILES CROSS

Comparing a child's growth in height, weight, and body mass index (BMI) on a growth chart provides a general summary measure of a child's health. But even though a child's rate of growth may be steady in the early years of life, the crossing of percentiles is quite common in those first several years as her body adjusts to her genetically determined percentile.

Although percentiles may change again during the adolescent growth spurt, the crossing of percentiles upward or downward after early childhood may indicate a problem. Children who are increasing their BMI percentile upward may be becoming overweight. On the other hand, those who are crossing percentiles downward may also be a cause for concern because this may be the only sign that a chronic disease is brewing.

GROWTH PROBLEMS IN ADOPTED CHILDREN

Occasionally, children adopted from other countries may have slow growth and developmental delays from inadequate care and nutrition. These children may need special help and more calories than usual to catch up to a level that fits their age. Adoption agencies can put parents in touch with support groups for those in similar situations. Your pediatrician will help with advice and referrals to specialists if they're required.

---

can play an influential role. A child may have a genetic predisposition to thinness—with thin parents, siblings, and even grandparents—but if her diet includes large amounts of high-fat, high-calorie foods and she spends most of her time watching television or playing video games, her environment may overpower her genes and she'll be at risk for becoming overweight.

When a Child Is Unusually Short or Tall

What kind of value does our society place on height? Consider the fact that once children reach school age, parents often worry if their otherwise healthy son looks considerably shorter than other boys his age, though they are generally less concerned if he is unusually tall. Girls who are short tend to elicit less attention. But in most cases, short children are simply following their genetic pattern.

It's rare that children fail to grow because they lack growth hormone, which is produced by the pituitary gland. But if a child seems significantly outside the norm, parents should raise their concerns with their pediatrician so that he can evaluate for—and most likely rule out—any medical disorders. If you have questions about growth hormone treatment, discuss it with a pediatric endocrinologist, a doctor who specializes in hormonal functions in children and who can best judge whether your child might benefit from growth hormone injections. If you are undecided or feel you don't have enough information, seek a second opinion. Growth hormone treatment has risks and side effects and costs thousands of dollars a year. Many health insurance plans do not pay for this treatment unless there is a true hormone deficiency. If your child has a proven deficiency and growth hormone is prescribed, therapy should begin as early as possible because treatment produces faster and greater growth when given to younger rather than older children.

The long-term risks of human growth hormone treatment are not yet known. However, while one purpose of giving growth hormone is to improve a child's self-image and enable him to fit in with others his age, the need for injections over a period of years may only reinforce the negative self-image that many of these children already have.

What about other causes of shorter height in a child? Some children are born small because of poor growth in the uterus, and they never catch up. They are called small for gestational age. A baby may be abnormally small for many reasons, including a decreased blood supply to the placenta, exposure to infection while in the uterus, or extreme prematurity. For these children, their small size is determined prenatally. They should not be overfed. Though growth hormone is not recommended by many and perhaps most pediatricians in such cases, this can be discussed with your pediatrician in consultation with a pediatric endocrinologist if you feel otherwise.

On the other end of the spectrum, when a child is abnormally tall, a rare cause may be a tumor of the pituitary gland that releases excessive amounts of growth hormone. This stimulates growth, particularly of the jaw and the long bones in the arms and legs. Disproportionate height cannot be reversed, but the condition can be treated with surgery, medications, or irradiation.

Although genes influence a child's growth potential, the size of a baby born after a full-term pregnancy with no medical problems has little or no relationship to that baby's size at maturity. As described earlier, most children grow and gain weight rapidly for the first 12 months. However, parents are taken by surprise when the growth rate suddenly slows at about 1 year and the child's appetite falls off to compensate for a corresponding decrease in energy requirements. This phase, which many pediatricians refer to as *catch-down growth,* is part of normal development, although parents of toddlers typically worry that their child isn't eating enough when this appetite drop-off occurs. Remember, provided the child continues to grow and gain weight steadily, even though more gradually, there is no cause for concern. Pushing her to eat will not increase her appetite or growth and may foster resistance. On pages 171 through 180 are some examples of children and their growth patterns, showing what varying growth rates can mean.

EXAMPLE 1: CATCH-DOWN GROWTH

Girl
Birth Weight: 7 lb
Length at Birth: 19"
Health at Birth: Excellent

Current Age: 2 years old
Current Height: 31½"
Current Weight: 21 lb
Current BMI: 14.9

Parents
Mother: 5', 1"; 100 lb; BMI = 18.9
Father: 5', 6"; 145 lb; BMI = 23.4

Although this girl's weight at 24 months falls below the normal range, it is in proportion to her length, which is below the fifth percentile. Because both her parents are small, this is normal growth adjustment. Her BMI at age 2 is within the normal range

---

See next page for growth chart.

Birth to 24 months: Girls
Length-for-age and Weight-for-age percentiles

NAME _____

RECORD # _____

Mother's Stature		Gestational		
Father's Stature		Age: _____ Weeks		Comment
Date	Age	Weight	Length	Head Circ.
	Birth			

Published by the Centers for Disease Control and Prevention, November 1, 2009
SOURCE: WHO Child Growth Standards (http://www.who.int/childgrowth/en)

Reprinted by the American Academy of Pediatrics

The recommendations in this publication do not indicate an exclusive course of treatment or serve as a
standard of medical care. Variations, taking into account individual circumstances, may be appropriate.
© 2011 American Academy of Pediatrics   9-284

Additional copies are available for purchase in quantities of 100.

To order, contact:
American Academy of Pediatrics
141 Northwest Point Blvd
Elk Grove Village, IL 60007-1098
Web site—http://www.aag.org. Minimum order 100.
HE0511

American Academy
of Pediatrics

DEDICATED TO THE HEALTH OF ALL CHILDREN™

EXAMPLE 2: TALL AND SLENDER

Girl
Birth Weight: 7 lb, 12 oz
Length at Birth: 22"
Health at Birth: Excellent

Current Age: 3 years old
Current Height: 39"
Current Weight: 30 lb
Current BMI: 13.9

Parents
Mother: 5', 11"; 150 lb; BMI = 21
Father: 6', 5"; 200 lb; BMI = 23.9

This girl was born tall and has remained outside the normal range for height and weight. Because her parents are tall and lean, chances are she will continue to be taller and leaner than most children her age.

See following pages for growth and body mass index charts.

Girls, 2 to 20 years

Name _____

STATURE FOR AGE AND WEIGHT FOR AGE PERCENTILES

Record # _____

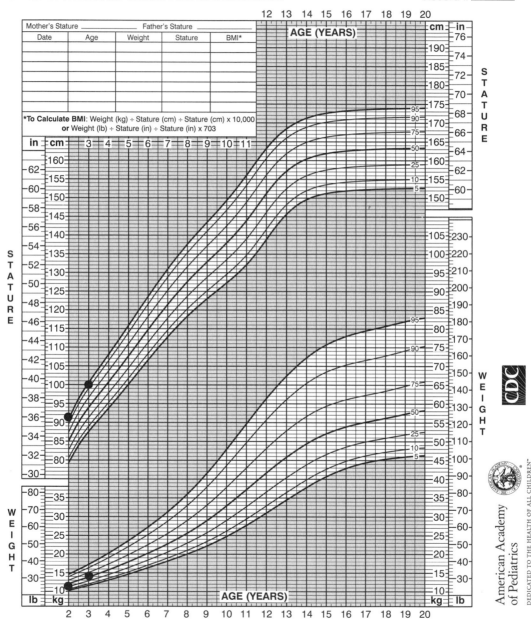

Source: Developed by the National Center for Health Statistics in collaboration with the National Center for Chronic Disease Prevention and Health Promotion (2000). http://www.cdc.gov/growthcharts

Reprinted by the American Academy of Pediatrics

The recommendations in this publication do not indicate an exclusive course of treatment or serve as a standard of medical care. Variations, taking into account individual circumstances, may be appropriate.

©2000 American Academy of Pediatrics

Additional copies are available for purchase in quantities of 100.

To order, contact
American Academy of Pediatrics
141 Northwest Point Blvd
Elk Grove Village, IL 60007-1098
Web site — http://www.aap.org
Minimum order 100.

Girls, 2 to 20 years

Name _____

BODY MASS INDEX FOR AGE PERCENTILES

Record #_____

Date	Age	Weight	Stature	BMI*	Comments

*To Calculate BMI: Weight (kg) ÷ Stature (cm) ÷ Stature (cm) x 10,000
or Weight (lb) ÷ Stature (in) ÷ Stature (in) x 703

BMI

AGE (YEARS)

kg/m²   kg/m²

2 3 4 5 6 7 8 9 10 11 12 13 14 15 16 17 18 19 20

Source: Developed by the National Center for Health Statistics in collaboration with the National Center for Chronic Disease Prevention and Health Promotion (2000).
http://www.cdc.gov/growthcharts

Reprinted by the American Academy of Pediatrics

The recommendations in this publication do not indicate an exclusive course of treatment or serve as a standard of medical care. Variations, taking into account individual circumstances, may be appropriate.

©2000 American Academy of Pediatrics, Revised—5/01

9-10/REP1107

Additional copies are available for purchase in quantities of 100.

To order, contact
American Academy of Pediatrics
141 Northwest Point Blvd
Elk Grove Village, IL 60007-1098
Web site — http://www.aap.org
Minimum order 100.

HE0306

CDC

American Academy of Pediatrics

DEDICATED TO THE HEALTH OF ALL CHILDREN™

EXAMPLE 3: UNEXPLAINED CHANGE

Boy
Birth Weight: 8 lb
Length at Birth: 20½"
Health at Birth: Excellent

Current Age: 12 years old
Current Height: 56"
Current Weight: 74 lb
Current BMI: 16.6

Parents
Mother: 5', 10"; 145 lb; BMI = 20.8
Father: 6'; 175 lb; BMI = 23.8

This tween boy has continued to grow every year, but there is a subtle drop in his rate of growth. Unfortunately, this is the time when many parents overlook the need for yearly physicals; during the first 5 to 6 years, the immunization schedule dictates frequent visits. After that, it is easy to forget how important yearly checkups really are.

There are lots of reasons for growth slowing down—hormone issues and bowel disease, to name a couple. It is important to detect growth delays early and intervene if necessary.

See following pages for growth and body mass index charts.

Boys, 2 to 20 years

Name _____

STATURE FOR AGE AND WEIGHT FOR AGE PERCENTILES

Record # _____

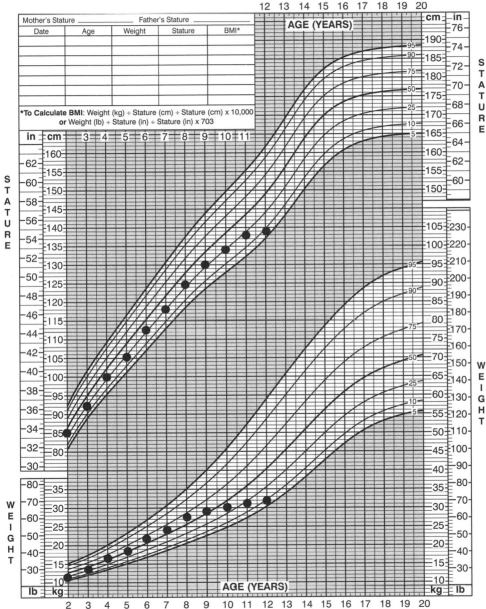

Mother's Stature _____ Father's Stature _____

Date	Age	Weight	Stature	BMI*

*To Calculate BMI: Weight (kg) ÷ Stature (cm) ÷ Stature (cm) x 10,000
or Weight (lb) ÷ Stature (in) ÷ Stature (in) x 703

AGE (YEARS)

STATURE

WEIGHT

CDC

American Academy of Pediatrics

DEDICATED TO THE HEALTH OF ALL CHILDREN®

Source: Developed by the National Center for Health Statistics in collaboration with the
National Center for Chronic Disease Prevention and Health Promotion (2000).
http://www.cdc.gov/growthcharts

Reprinted by the American Academy of Pediatrics

The recommendations in this publication do not indicate an exclusive course of treatment or serve as a
standard of medical care. Variations, taking into account individual circumstances, may be appropriate.

©2000 American Academy of Pediatrics

Additional copies are available for purchase in quantities of 100.

To order, contact:
American Academy of Pediatrics
141 Northwest Point Blvd
Elk Grove Village, IL 60007-1098
Web site — http://www.aap.org
Minimum order 100.

Boys, 2 to 20 years

Name _____

BODY MASS INDEX-FOR-AGE PERCENTILES

Record # _____

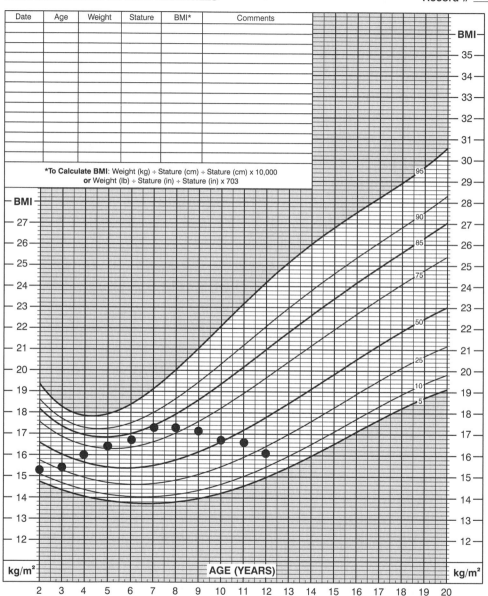

Date	Age	Weight	Stature	BMI*	Comments

*To Calculate BMI: Weight (kg) ÷ Stature (cm) ÷ Stature (cm) x 10,000
or Weight (lb) ÷ Stature (in) ÷ Stature (in) x 703

AGE (YEARS)

American Academy of Pediatrics
DEDICATED TO THE HEALTH OF ALL CHILDREN™

Source: Developed by the National Center for Health Statistics in collaboration with the
National Center for Chronic Disease Prevention and Health Promotion (2000).
http://www.cdc.gov/growthcharts

Reprinted by the American Academy of Pediatrics

The recommendations in this publication do not indicate an exclusive course of treatment or serve as a
standard of medical care. Variations, taking into account individual circumstances, may be appropriate.

©2000 American Academy of Pediatrics, Revised—5/01

9-8/REP1107

Additional copies are available for purchase in quantities of 100.

To order, contact:
American Academy of Pediatrics
141 Northwest Point Blvd
Elk Grove Village, IL 60007-1098
Web site — http://www.aap.org
Minimum order 100.

HE0304

EXAMPLE 4: PREMATURE BIRTH

Girl
Birth Weight: 4 lb, 2oz
Length at Birth: 19"
Health at Birth: Excellent

Current Age: 2 years old
Current Height: 31½"
Current Weight: 21 lb
Current BMI: 14.9

Parents
Mother: 5', 1"; 100 lb; BMI = 18.9
Father: 5', 6"; 145 lb; BMI = 23.4

Because this girl was born 8 weeks premature, she started out small but her length and weight were proportionate. If you consider that she was born early and backtrack 8 weeks on the growth chart, the adjustment puts her well within the normal range of height and weight. As with most preemies, her growth and weight gain entered normal range by her first birthday. Her BMI also is now within the normal range.

See following page for growth chart.

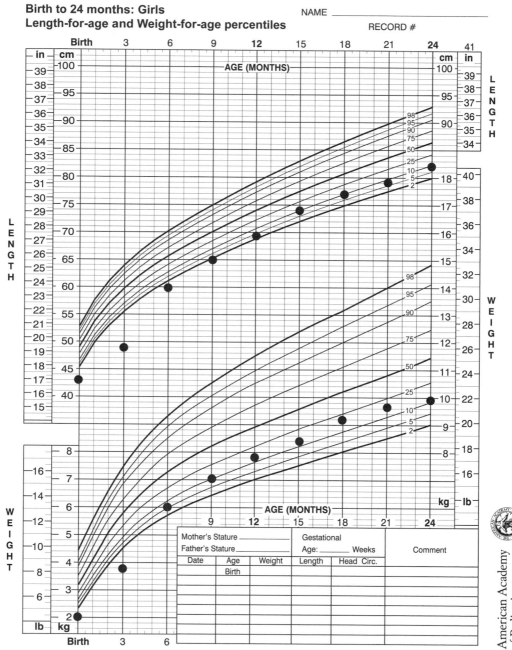

Birth to 24 months: Girls
Length-for-age and Weight-for-age percentiles

NAME _____

RECORD # _____

Published by the Centers for Disease Control and Prevention, November 1, 2009
SOURCE: WHO Child Growth Standards (http://www.who.int/childgrowth/en)

Reprinted by the American Academy of Pediatrics

The recommendations in this publication do not indicate an exclusive course of treatment or serve as a standard of medical care. Variations, taking into account individual circumstances, may be appropriate.
© 2011 American Academy of Pediatrics   9-284

Additional copies are available for purchase in quantities of 100.

To order, contact:
American Academy of Pediatrics
141 Northwest Point Blvd
Elk Grove Village, IL 60007-1098
Web site—http://www.aag/org. Minimum order 100.
HE0511

ISSUES PARENTS RAISE ABOUT SIZE AND WEIGHT

My child is noticeably taller than all the other children in his grade. Most people tell him he's lucky being very tall instead of short, but I wonder if his unusual height could be a signal that something is not quite right.

If you have any concerns at all about your child's growth, consult your pediatrician, who will examine your child and perform any necessary tests. In most cases, there's nothing to worry about. When the pediatrician assesses your child's height and weight, he'll be much more interested in an explained major change or lack of change over time. This is more important than any single measurement. (For more information, see page 169.)

My daughter was premature and although she eventually caught up in development, she has remained very small in comparison with other girls in her class. Could growth hormone treatment help her catch up in size?

For a child born very prematurely, such as your daughter, small size may be normal. Help her understand that her height is what's right for her, and help her feel comfortable with herself. Though growth hormone is generally not recommended in a case like this, this should be discussed with your pediatrician in consultation with a pediatric endocrinologist. (See page 169.)

When should my baby double her birth weight?

A healthy infant may double her birth weight by 4 months and triple it by her first birthday. However, these are only guidelines. Every child grows at her own rate, which is not necessarily identical to that of others the same age. (For more information, see page 163.)

How can I tell if my child is growing at an acceptable rate?

At every examination, beginning with the first one after birth, your pediatrician will check your child's height and weight and compare these measurements with standard growth charts. For the first 2 years, your pediatrician will also measure your baby's head circumference to track growth and development. (More information can be obtained on page 163.)

Chapter 8

Nutrition Basics

Before you eat, think about what goes on your plate or in your cup or bowl. That's one of the main messages of MyPlate, the new healthy eating food icon. It's also important to balance your calories—enjoy your food, but eat fewer high-calorie foods. When shopping with your children, look at the serving size on a product's label and determine how many servings you would actually consume. Use these messages to develop a healthy eating plan. It's also a good idea to post MyPlate on your refrigerator door as a handy guide for meal planning.

Over the years various tools have been created to provide guidance on the type and amount of food Americans should eat. MyPlate, shown on page 184, emphasizes several basic principles such as avoiding oversized portions. To build a healthy plate, make half your plate fruits and vegetables. Eat red, orange, and dark-green vegetables, such as tomatoes, sweet potatoes, and broccoli, in main and side dishes. Eat fruit, vegetables, or unsalted nuts as snacks. You should also switch to skim or low-fat (1%) milk. Vary your protein choices. Consider eating beans, which are a natural source of fiber and protein, and keep meat and poultry portions small and lean. Also, make at least half your grains whole grains by choosing 100% whole-grain cereals, breads, crackers, rice, and pasta.

Although your child may strongly dislike one or several foods within a particular group, it's important to find foods he will eat to get the nutrients the group provides. If your child absolutely refuses all foods in a group (this is so rare it almost never happens), ask your pediatrician to refer you to a dietitian who can suggest substitutes for any nutritional shortfall.

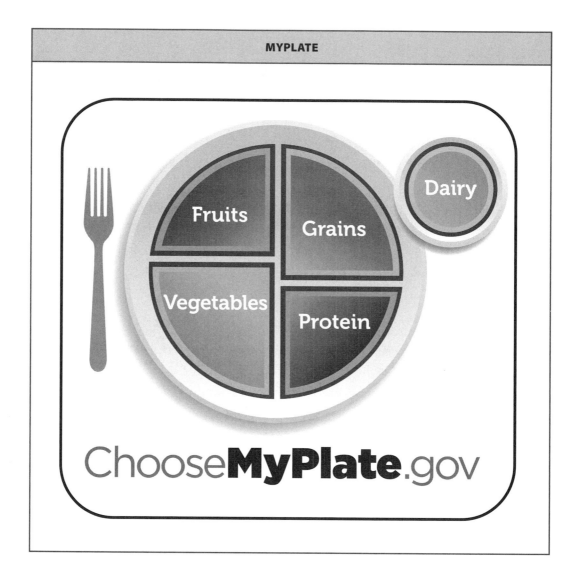

Fruit

Whole fruits provide many essential vitamins and minerals, together with a variety of disease-fighting substances like those in vegetables, and fiber. Above all, fruits are our most important source of vitamin C. We need this vitamin to produce *collagen,* the connective substance that holds cells together and helps maintain blood vessels, bones and cartilage, and teeth. Fruit juices, while containing some vitamins, do not contain the nutrients of whole fruit and should be limited in children's diets. (See pages 63, 197, and 223.)

WHEN IS VITAMIN C NOT QUITE VITAMIN C?

Fruits provide a good example of the importance of getting nutrients from foods and not from supplements. For proper nutrition, we need nutrients such as vitamins and minerals in 2 forms, oxidized and reduced, and in balance with other substances in the same food. Supplements contain only an extract of an isolated nutrient without other naturally occurring substances that promote its effects or keep them in check.

For example, to get the maximum benefit from vitamin C, we need to consume it in 2 forms, ascorbic acid (the reduced form) and dehydroascorbic acid (the oxidized form). Fruits and vegetables provide a balance of the 2 forms; supplements contain only ascorbic acid.

Vegetables

Parents worry more about their children's poor consumption of vegetables than any other food group. The recommended daily amounts of vegetables add up to only ½ to ¾ cup for ages 4 to 6 years and 1½ cups for 7- to 10-year-olds. However, surveys show that many, if not most, school-aged children do not eat 2 to 3 daily servings of vegetables.

Vegetables are the most important source of beta carotene (which our bodies convert to vitamin A for healthy skin, glands, immune system, and eye function) and many other vitamins and phytochemicals (naturally occurring plant compounds that are believed to fight cancer and other diseases). Vegetables also provide plenty of fiber.

While you should always offer vegetables to your child, keep in mind that your child's reluctance to eat brussels sprouts and many other vegetables may have more to do with genetics than fussy eating. There is a bitter chemical in dark-green, leafy vegetables and some cruciferous vegetables (eg, cauliflower, broccoli, spinach) that about 3 out of 4 children are able to taste because of a gene they inherited from one or both parents. Children who can taste this sulfur-containing chemical, called propylthiouracil (PROP), tend to eat fewer vegetables

---

COLOR ME NUTRITIOUS

Encourage your child to make colorful platefuls, with vegetables and fruits in a range of reds, yellows, and greens. The more color on the plate, the more varied and complete the nutrients are likely to be.

---

because of their distaste for them. These same "PROP tasters" also tend to prefer sweet drinks like soda rather than milk. Perhaps as a consequence of a reduced liking of vegetables and an increased preference for sweets, PROP tasters may be more prone to become overweight. Even so, many adult PROP tasters do overcome their dislikes and become adventurous eaters. Therefore, if your child is a PROP taster, she may eventually add foods like spinach and broccoli to her diet. As with any other child, she will be less likely to eat these foods if you try to force her to eat them. Just place a small amount of these foods on her plate, stay neutral, eat them yourself, and remove any uneaten vegetables without comment.

In the meantime, by using a bit of creativity, you may get even a vegetable hater to eat at least the minimum number of daily servings. A child who doesn't enjoy cooked vegetables may happily snack on carrot sticks or a selection of vegetables served with low-fat dip. Pasta can be dressed with a fresh vegetable sauce; pizza is colorful, appetizing, and healthful when topped with vegetables such as green peppers, mushrooms, asparagus, or broccoli, in addition to tomato sauce.

FOLIC ACID

Vegetables and fruits are excellent sources of folic acid, also called folate or folacin, a vitamin that is needed to make genetic material (DNA and RNA) in our cells, as well as to produce red blood cells. A good supply of folic acid is essential at every age. If women have low levels of folic acid when they conceive a child, their babies run an increased risk of serious birth defects to the nervous system and spine, as well as many other organs. Folic acid is particularly important for teenaged girls to ensure that they will be prepared when the time comes to plan their families. A child who consumes 5 fruits and vegetables a day usually gets enough folic acid. Other good sources are organ meats, eggs, chickpeas (garbanzo beans), nuts, and breads, crackers, and pasta made with whole wheat.

According to the US Department of Agriculture dietary guidelines, 4½ cups (9 servings) of fruits and vegetables are recommended for 2,000 calories a day, with higher or lower amounts depending on the caloric level. This translates into a range of 2½ to 6½ cups (5–13 servings) of fruits and vegetables each day for the 1,200- to 3,200-calorie levels.

DAILY AMOUNT OF FOOD FROM EACH GROUP (VEGETABLE SUBGROUP AMOUNTS ARE PER WEEK)ª

Calorie Level	1,000	1,200	1,400	1,600	1,800	2,000
Fruits	1 cup (2 servings)	1 cup (2 servings)	1½ cup (3 servings)	1½ cup (3 servings)	1½ cup (3 servings)	2 cup (4 servings)
Vegetables	1 cup (2 servings)	1½ cup (3 servings)	1½ cup (3 servings)	2 cup (4 servings)	2½ cup (5 servings)	2½ cup (5 servings)
Dark-green	1 cup/wk	1½ cup/wk	1½ cup/wk	2 cup/wk	3 cup/wk	3 cup/wk
Orange	½ cup/wk	1 cup/wk	1 cup/wk	1½ cup/wk	2 cup/wk	2 cup/wk
Legumes	½ cup/wk	1 cup/wk	1 cup/wk	2½ cup/wk	3 cup/wk	3 cup/wk
Starchy	1½ cup/wk	2½ cup/wk	2½ cup/wk	2½ cup/wk	3 cup/wk	3 cup/wk
Other	4 cup/wk	4½ cup/wk	4½ cup/wk	5½ cup/wk	6½ cup/wk	6½ cup/wk

Calorie Level	2,200	2,400	2,600	2,800	3,000	3,200
Fruits	2 cup (4 servings)	2 cup (4 servings)	2 cup (4 servings)	2½ cup (5 servings)	2½ cup (5 servings)	2½ cup (5 servings)
Vegetables	3 cup (6 servings)	3 cup (6 servings)	3½ cup (7 servings)	3½ cup (7 servings)	4 cup (8 servings)	4 cup (8 servings)
Dark-green	3 cup/wk	3 cup/wk	3 cup/wk	3 cup/wk	3 cup/wk	3 cup/wk
Orange	2 cup/wk	2 cup/wk	2½ cup/wk	2½ cup/wk	2½ cup/wk	2½ cup/wk
Legumes	3 cup/wk	3 cup/wk	3½ cup/wk	3½ cup/wk	3½ cup/wk	3½ cup/wk
Starchy	6 cup/wk	6 cup/wk	7 cup/wk	7 cup/wk	9 cup/wk	9 cup/wk
Other	7 cup/wk	7 cup/wk	8½ cup/wk	8½ cup/wk	10 cup/wk	10 cup/wk

ªAdapted from www.health.gov/dietaryguidelines/dga2005/document/html/appendixA.htm.

Protein

Protein foods contain 20 amino acids, building blocks that we remake into our bodies' own unique proteins and other compounds, including the compounds known as neurotransmitters that carry communications between cells. In addition, proteins play a very important role in making us feel full after eating. Nine of the amino acids (see Table on page 195) are called *essential* because we cannot manufacture them ourselves and must get them from the foods we eat. The remaining 11 are called *nonessential* because our bodies can make them even if they are not in our diet.

Body proteins and other compounds are constantly broken down and rebuilt in a process called protein turnover. The turnover rate is highest in children, who are still growing and maturing. We need a steady supply of amino acids to make and repair protein because our bodies cannot store excess amino acids from food. As a result, daily protein intake should be spaced over several meals throughout the day. This is especially important for children. However, while protein remains an essential nutrient throughout life, the need for protein decreases with age. For example, the amount of protein required for growth drops from about 56% of the amount consumed daily by a newborn to about 5% of daily consumption by age 5. At any age, the ideal protein is one that contains all the amino acids in the required amounts, without any excess. For babies up to age 1, human milk contains the ideal amino acid balance. Slightly different patterns are recommended for the changing growth rates from 1 to 6 years and again from 6 to 13 years. After age 13, the requirements are the same as for adults.

TOO MUCH OF A GOOD THING

The high amount of protein in the average American diet shows that we consume far more than we need. Too much protein in the diet may also lead to excessive loss of calcium in the urine, which increases the risk of osteoporosis, or weakening of the bones, in later life. Over the long term, too much protein may contribute to kidney disease. An extremely high protein intake can increase fluid loss, especially during activity in warm conditions, and lead to dehydration. Young athletes should eat a normal diet with moderate amounts of protein, avoid protein supplements, and drink plenty of water, especially when they exercise in warm weather

Animal foods such as milk, meat, and fish provide all the essential amino acids in the right proportions for humans. Therefore, proteins from such sources are called *complete*. Grains and legumes—plants whose seeds grow in pods, such as peas, beans, and peanuts—are also good sources of protein. Plant proteins are called *incomplete* because they have low levels of one or more essential amino acids. The only known exception is soy protein, which has a pattern of amino acids closer to animal proteins than other plant proteins.

This doesn't mean that people have to eat animal protein to be healthy. Well-informed vegetarians (also see Chapter 15, Alternative Diets and Supplements) know that it's a fairly simple matter to match up plant foods that provide complementary proteins; in other words, one food makes up for the amino acids that the other lacks. For example, cereal grains such as wheat have low levels of the amino acid lysine but plenty of methionine. By contrast, legumes such as beans, peas, and peanuts have substantial levels of lysine but little methionine. So a combination as simple as whole wheat bread with peanut butter provides a complete protein because the methionine in the wheat complements the lysine in the peanuts. In addition, eating even a small amount of animal protein, such as meat or cheese, with a plant-based food will make up for any essential amino acid lacking in the plant food. This is the system on which much healthy ethnic cooking is based; think of black beans and rice, hopping John, tortillas with beans, lentil soup with sausage, and pasta e fagioli.

The advantage of proteins from grains and vegetables is that most are naturally low in fat, in contrast with proteins in animal foods, which are packaged with substantial amounts of fat, including saturated fat. Peanuts are an exception—they contain a high proportion of fat, including saturated fat. (When opening a new jar of natural peanut butter, pour off the oil at the top.)

As far as protein is concerned, an ounce of meat, poultry, or fish is equivalent to 1 egg, ½ cup cooked beans, or 2 tablespoons peanut butter. The fat and cholesterol content varies, of course, according to the source.

ONE FAMILY'S STORY

A family who Dr Stern cared for brought their 10-year-old son in for a regular checkup. When she asked about their diet, the mother told her that they ate ground beef every night.

"Why every night?" Dr Stern asked.

"That is the only protein my son will eat—so all of us eat it."

Dr Stern did not know what to tell them first—about the problems with eating high-fat beef every night or the fact that meat is not the only source of protein that can be part of the family's diet. In fact, this family epitomizes the common misconception that many parents have about protein. It is almost impossible for children living in North America to be protein deficient. Peanut butter, nuts, dairy foods (eg, milk, yogurt [frozen or plain], ice cream, cheese), eggs, fish, bread, beans, and pizza *all* contain protein. As a nation, we eat more meat than is good for us, and we certainly don't need it every day.

A child between 1 and 3 years of age needs only 16 g of protein a day. Two cups of milk or 1 cup of macaroni and cheese meet that need.

Carbohydrates

Foods from grains, such as breads, pasta, cereal, brown rice, quinoa, and polenta, are packed with starches (complex carbohydrates), the best source of energy for active, growing bodies. Carbohydrates should make up 50% to 60% of the diet by age 5.

Foods in this group provide starch, protein, iron (a good source, though less fully absorbed than the iron in animal foods), most of the B vitamins (which are needed for the enzymes that convert food to energy, as well as for a healthy nervous system), and vitamin K (needed for normal blood clotting and bone health).

In the intestine, carbohydrates are converted to glucose, an important energy source for most tissues, especially the brain and nervous system. Glucose is stored in the liver and muscles in the form of glycogen. Our bodies contain carbohydrates in many different forms, including hormones, enzymes, and supporting structures in the connective tissues.

As we understand more about how our bodies work and the importance of avoiding unnecessary fats to prevent heart disease, cancer, and other ills, we have shed the outdated view that starches are heavy and fattening. Grain dishes are low in fat unless large amounts of fats and oils are used in preparing them. It is particularly important to choose grain dishes that are made with whole grains. Pasta, rice, and other grain-based staples can be mixed with vegetables and moderate portions from the protein and dairy groups to provide a balanced meal. When consumed together with other plant foods (a grain plus a legume, such as whole wheat bread with peanut butter, or rice and beans), grains are a good source of protein. In addition, eating a grain together with a modest serving of an animal food (such as in pizza, or rice topped with chili con carne) enhances our ability to absorb iron from the plant food. Consuming citrus or another food rich in vitamin C at the same meal increases the absorption of plant iron. As a bonus, whole grains (whole wheat bread, brown rice) include fiber. (For more, see "Whole Grains" on page 193.)

Sugars, like table sugar or the fructose and glucose in high-fructose corn syrup, are also carbohydrates and contribute significantly more calories today than they did 30 years ago. Simple sugars increase the caloric density of foods and are one of the sources of calories that may contribute to the obesity epidemic. Foods without added sugars are generally considered healthier foods. (See "Sugar" on page 197.)

Milk and Milk-Based Foods

Milk is children's best source of calcium and an important source of protein, riboflavin (vitamin B_2), and many other nutrients. Vitamin D is added to milk (including reduced-fat, low-fat, and skim milk) to prevent rickets, and vitamin A is added to skim milk to replace what's lost when fat is skimmed off. Butter and cheese provide most of the nutrients of milk and yogurt in a more concentrated form, but portions should be modest because the fat content is high. For children younger than 2 years, fats should make up about half of the total calorie intake. For that reason they should drink whole milk and eat whole-milk yogurt and cheeses. However, your child's doctor may recommend reduced-fat (2%) milk if your 12- to 24-month-old child is obese or overweight or if there is a family history of high cholesterol or heart disease. After age 2, children should drink low-fat or nonfat milk and eat low-fat or nonfat yogurt.

Adolescent girls tend to shun milk because they think it contains too many calories. They drink fruit juice and soft drinks instead. As a result, many of them have diets that are seriously lacking in calcium and vitamin D and may lead to osteoporosis once they enter the middle years. Girls should keep up their calcium intake by consuming low-fat or nonfat milk or yogurt, which provide the same nutrients as whole milk without unnecessary fat. Remind your children and their friends that nonfat milk, for example, contains fewer calories than many juices and soft drinks.

Fiber

Dietary fiber is made up of carbohydrate compounds that cannot be digested, such as cellulose and pectin. Fiber is in the cell walls of all plants but is not found in any foods from animals. Insoluble fiber, such as in wheat bran, fruit skins, and corn kernels, passes through the intestine unchanged. Soluble fiber, found in oat bran or the pectin that helps jam to jell, expands and becomes gel-like on contact with water.

Although we cannot absorb fiber, it is an essential part of a healthy diet. People who eat a lot of fiber are less likely to be obese, have heart disease, or develop problems affecting the bowel, including constipation and cancer. Fiber contributes to feeling full and makes stools larger, softer, and easier to pass. Studies show that people who consume a diet rich in soluble fiber have lower blood cholesterol levels.

Phytate compounds in fiber may reduce how some minerals are absorbed, especially zinc, which is essential for sexual maturation, and calcium, which is needed by almost every organ system but especially bones and teeth. However, phytate in whole wheat is destroyed by yeast fermentation, and most bread consumed in the United States is made with yeast. So eating yeast-risen bread blocks any harmful effect from phytates and lets the body absorb calcium. In addition, a high-fiber diet is unlikely to lead to mineral deficiencies as long as children eat a variety of foods to provide many different sources of nutrients.

Depending on your child's age, fiber intake from all sources—whole grains, vegetables, fruits—could range from 10 to 25 g a day. Recommendations that children should eat *only* low-calorie, high-fiber foods are not appropriate.

WHOLE GRAINS

Whole grains need to be part of your child's and adolescent's diet. Whole-grain foods contain all 3 elements of grains—the fibrous outer portion of the grain (known as bran), the inner part of the grain (called the endosperm), and the heart of the grain kernel (the germ). To make sure your child is getting plenty of whole grains or products made of whole grain, incorporate oatmeal, barley, whole wheat flour or bread, and wild and brown rice into her diet. (Keep in mind that wheat flour may not be the same as whole-grain flour.)

The amount of fiber in a food is not a good indicator of the amount of whole grain. That's because different grains contain different amounts of fiber. Refined grains are milled, which is a process that removes the bran and germ. These refined grains include white flour, white bread, and white rice. However, many refined grains are *enriched,* meaning that some of their vitamins that are removed during milling (eg, folic acid, niacin, thiamin, riboflavin) are put back.

So what does the term *whole grain* really mean on a food label? It indicates only that some whole grain is included. The only way to ensure that a product contains an actual serving of whole grain is if the label says so. The government's dietary guidelines recommend that Americans eat three 1-oz servings of whole grains every day.

HEALTHY READING

You can find important information for making healthy food decisions on the backs or sides of packages. This information includes the Nutrition Facts panel and the Ingredients list. The Nutrition Facts panel provides information on the number of calories per serving as well as key information about the amount of nutrients, such as total fat, saturated fat, trans fat, cholesterol, sodium, and others. The amounts of these nutrients are shown as grams and as the percentage of daily value. The percentage of daily value is based on 2,000 calories per day. The Ingredients list, which is right below the Nutrition Facts panel, lists the ingredients with the greatest amount first and the remainder in order of decreasing amounts.

Increasingly, companies are placing this information on the front of packages. Information on the front is not yet consistent, but discussions are underway to determine what nutrients the front label should contain. Such information is intended to provide a quick way to help consumers make decisions about what foods to purchase based on their nutrient content.

PORTIONS, NOT PLATEFULS			
	1–3 years 1 serving	**4–6 years** 1 serving	**7–10 years** 1 serving
Grains 6–11 servings/day	Bread, ½ slice Cereal, rice, pasta, cooked, ¼ cup Cereal, dry, ⅓ cup Crackers, 2–3	Bread, ½ slice Cereal, rice, pasta, cooked, ⅓ cup Cereal, dry, ½ cup Crackers, 3–4	Bread, 1 slice Cereal, rice, pasta, cooked, ½ cup Cereal, dry, ¾–1 cup Crackers, 4–5
Vegetables 2–3 servings/day	Vegetables, cooked, ¼ cup	Vegetables, cooked, ¼ cup Salad, ½ cup	Vegetables, cooked, ½ cup Salad, 1 cup
Fruits 2–3 servings/day	Fruit, cooked, frozen, or canned, ¼ cup Fruit, fresh, ½ piece Juice, ¼ cup	Fruit, cooked, frozen, or canned ¼ cup Fruit, fresh, ½ piece Juice, ⅓ cup	Fruit, cooked, frozen, or canned, ⅓ cup Fruit, fresh, 1 piece Juice, ½ cup
Dairy 2–3 servings/day	Milk, ½ cup Cheese, ½ oz Yogurt, ⅓ cup	Milk, ½ cup Cheese, 1 oz Yogurt, ½ cup	Milk, 1 cup Cheese, 1 oz Yogurt, ¾–1 cup
Meats and other proteins 2 servings/day	Meat, fish, poultry, tofu, 1 oz (two 1-inch cubes) Beans, dried, cooked, ¼ cup Egg, ½	Meat, fish, poultry, tofu, 1 oz (two 1-inch cubes) Beans, dried, cooked, ⅓ cup Egg, 1	Meat, fish, poultry, tofu, 2–3 oz Beans, dried, cooked, ½ cup Eggs, 1 or 2

ESSENTIAL AMINO ACIDS	NONESSENTIAL AMINO ACIDS
Histidine	Alanine
Isoleucine	Arginine[a]
Leucine	Asparagine
Lysine	Aspartic acid
Methionine	Cysteine[b]
Phenylalanine	Glutamic acid
Threonine	Glutamine
Tryptophan	Glycine
Valine	Proline
	Serine
	Tyrosine[b]

[a]May become essential if the body cannot manufacture it because of illness or prematurity.

[b]Essential for premature and healthy newborns, who cannot synthesize it.

Fats and Fatty Acids

Fats are the most misunderstood of all the food groups. They are essential to good health and add greatly to the pleasure of eating. They impart a pleasing texture and consistency to foods and because they slow down the stomach's rate of emptying, add to our feeling of fullness and satisfaction. In our bodies, fats are vital parts of cell membranes. They are a source of the fat-soluble vitamins A, D, E, and K and play a role in normal blood clotting. Fat is necessary for producing hormones that help boys and girls mature and keep adult bodies functioning properly. Above all, fat is the body's most economical way to store calories.

For children younger than 2 years, fats should make up half of their daily calories. After age 2, fat intake should be reduced until it settles at no more than one third of total daily calories.

For reasons that have not yet been fully explained, highly saturated fat interferes with removing cholesterol from the blood and so contributes to increases in blood cholesterol levels. Over a long period, high blood cholesterol can increase the risk of developing atherosclerosis—a buildup of fatty deposits on the insides of the arteries—and heart attacks. Fatty streaks come before fat deposits in arteries. Fatty streaks have been found in 7% of 10-year-olds and in more than twice as many children after age 15. These findings have led to the recommendation to reduce saturated fat to one third of the total fat intake; that is, a maximum of about 10% of the calories eaten in a day.

The terms *saturated, unsaturated, polyunsaturated,* and *monounsaturated* refer to the number and arrangement of hydrogen atoms in each molecule of fat. In general, saturated fats are those that stay firm at room temperature. Animal fats, such as butter and lard, are good examples. Some vegetable oils, including coconut and palm oils, also contain a lot of saturated fats. Monounsaturated fats, such as olive oil, are liquid at room temperature but become firmer on cooling. Polyunsaturated fats remain liquid even when refrigerated.

About half the fat in red meat is saturated; poultry fat has less. Two thirds of the fat in full-fat dairy foods is saturated. Fish fats for the most part are polyunsaturated. If they were not, the fish's body fat would harden at the low temperatures of the fish's normal habitat, preventing them from swimming. Saturation doesn't change the number of calories. All fats—butter, margarine, salad oil—contain 9 calories per gram or between 240 and 250 calories per ounce.

TRANS FATS

To create a substitute for butter, food manufacturers put vegetable oils through a process called *hydrogenation*. The addition of hydrogen makes the product firm and resistant to spoilage (also see Chapter 13, Food Safety). However, while hydrogenated or trans fats spread like butter, they also share some of the unwanted properties of saturated fats. They appear to interfere with removing LDL ("bad") cholesterol from the blood and also lower HDL ("good") cholesterol. As a result, these foods may contribute to heart disease and certain cancers.

To lower your children's consumption of saturated fats, avoid trans fats and use liquid oils and soft tub margarines instead. Since 2006, the Food and Drug Administration has required food manufacturers to list the amount of trans fats in the Nutrition Facts section of food labels, so always check labels for trans fat content. In some cities (including New York and Boston), local ordinances have been passed to eliminate trans fats in restaurant foods.

Sugar

If you look at statistics, it seems as though Americans can't get enough sugar. In 2007, the average American consumed a staggering 97 pounds of sugar. That represents an annual increase in overall sugar intake of 11% from 1977 to 2007—or about an extra 10 pounds a year.

Yet over this same 30-year period, sugar consumed as table sugar (also called sucrose) has actually decreased, while sugar consumed as high-fructose corn syrup has increased. Table sugar contains equal levels of fructose and glucose, which are the simple sugars; high-fructose corn syrup is made up of about 55% fructose and 45% glucose. Because high-fructose corn syrup is inexpensive to manufacture and can make cooking more efficient, it is now widely used in food products. While fructose is found naturally in fruits as well as some vegetables, the large majority of fructose consumed by children and adults comes from other (typically less healthy) foods. Most fructose in the American diet is found in sugar-laden soft drinks, sweetened juices, and grain products (eg, cereals, pies, cakes, breads, snacks). More than 30% of the fructose young children (aged 2 to 5 years) consume comes from sugar-sweetened drinks, while nearly half of the fructose intake of teenagers comes from sugary drinks. As a guideline, children 1 to 6 years old should drink no more than 4 to 6 oz of juice a day, and 7- to 18-year-olds should limit daily juice intake to 8 to 12 oz. Fruit juice offers no nutritional benefits over whole fruit. If your child is thirsty, replace sweetened beverages with water or reduced-fat, low-fat, or skim milk.

Also, the bar graph on page 198 shows major sources of added sugars in the American diet.

Vitamins

Vitamins are organic substances required for the body's metabolic processes to function the right way. We need only minute amounts of vitamins, but if we don't get enough, we will develop vitamin deficiency.

Thirteen vitamins are essential for human health, although there may be others still unidentified. Daily requirements have been established for 11 of them. We get most of our vitamins from food (see Table on pages 199–202) for the characteristics, effects, and sources of vitamins).

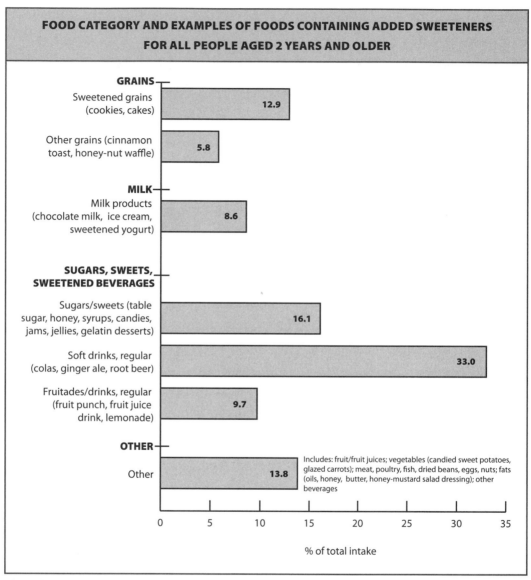

Adapted from Guthrie JF, Morton JF. Food sources of added sweeteners in the diets of Americans. *J Am Diet Assoc.* 2000;100:43–51

However, vitamin D can be made in the skin with exposure to sunlight for 10 to 30 minutes a day, and the B vitamins biotin and nicotinic acid, as well as vitamin K, are made by bacteria normally found in the intestine.

Vitamins are grouped according to how they are absorbed by the body. Vitamins A, D, E, and K are absorbed in fat or bile and are therefore known as *fat-soluble* vitamins.

(continued on page 207)

VITAMIN	EFFECT	SIGNS OF DEFICIENCY	SIGNS OF OVERDOSE	GOOD SOURCES
Fat-Soluble Vitamins				
Vitamin A	Keeps skin, hair, nails healthy. Helps maintain gums, glands, bones, teeth. Helps prevent infection. Promotes eye function; prevents night blindness.	Night blindness; dry eyes; growth delay in children; dry, rough skin; low resistance to infection	Headaches; blurred vision; fatigue; diarrhea; dry, cracked skin, rash, itch; hair loss; bone and joint pain; liver damage; irregular periods; birth defects if taken during pregnancy	Milk and dairy foods; fortified cereals; green and yellow vegetables; deep-yellow or orange fruits; organ meats
Vitamin D	Helps build and maintain bones; needed for calcium absorption.	Rickets in children; osteomalacia (bone softening) in adults; osteoporosis (thinning and weakening of bones)	Calcium deposits, mainly in heart, kidneys, blood vessels; weak bones; high blood pressure; high blood cholesterol levels; diarrhea; drowsiness; headache	Egg yolks; fish oils; fortified milk and butter; beef or chicken liver; exposure to sunlight without sunscreen
Vitamin E	Helps form red blood cells, muscles, other tissues; antioxidant; stabilizes cell membranes; preserves fatty acids.	Blood problems in premature babies; neurologic problems in older children and adults	Bleeding; changes in white blood cell function	Poultry, seafood; green, leafy vegetables; wheat germ; whole grains, seeds, nuts; butter; liver; egg yolk

(continued on next page)

VITAMIN	EFFECT	SIGNS OF DEFICIENCY	SIGNS OF OVERDOSE	GOOD SOURCES
Fat-Soluble Vitamins, continued				
Vitamin K	Needed for normal blood clotting; helps maintain healthy bones.	Excessive bleeding; liver damage	None associated with oral administration	Produced by intestinal bacteria; cow's milk; green, leafy vegetables; pork, liver; oats, wheat bran, whole grains
Water-Soluble Vitamins				
Thiamine (vitamin B_1)	Promotes carbohydrate metabolism; needed for normal appetite, digestion, nerve function; enhances energy.	Anxiety, depression; nausea; muscle cramps; appetite loss; in extreme cases, muscle-wasting disease (beriberi)	Too much of one B vitamin may cause deficiency of others (excess B_1 can interfere with B_2 and B_6).	Pork, seafood; fortified grains, cereals
Riboflavin (vitamin B_2)	Needed for all food metabolism; maintains mucous membranes; helps maintain vision; facilitates release of energy to cells.	Cracks and sores around mouth and nose; sensitivity to light; difficulty eating and swallowing	Can interfere with B_1 and B_6.	Organ meats, beef, lamb, dark meat of poultry; dairy foods; fortified cereals, grains; dark-green, leafy vegetables
Niacin nicotinic acid (vitamin B_3)	Needed in many enzymes that convert food to energy; promotes normal appetite and digestion; promotes nerve function.	Diarrhea, mouth sores; in extreme deficiency, pellagra, with skin rash, inflammation of mucous membranes, diarrhea, mental symptoms	Ulcers; liver damage; hot flushes; high blood sugar and uric acid; disturbances of heart rhythm; itchy skin	Produced by intestinal bacteria; poultry, seafood; seeds, nuts, peanuts, potatoes; fortified whole-grain breads and cereals

Water-Soluble Vitamins, continued

VITAMIN	EFFECT	SIGNS OF DEFICIENCY	SIGNS OF OVERDOSE	GOOD SOURCES
Pantothenic acid (vitamin B_5)	Needed to break down food into molecular forms required by body; involved in the manufacture of adrenal hormones and chemicals that regulate nerve function.	Unknown in humans, except when induced experimentally	May increase need for thiamine; megadoses may cause diarrhea and water retention.	Found in almost all plant and animal foods
Pyridoxine (vitamin B_6)	Required for metabolism and absorption of protein; important in carbohydrate metabolism; helps form red blood cells; promotes nerve function.	Depression, mental confusion; inflammation of mucous membranes of mouth; itchy; scaling patches on skin; convulsions in infants	Can lead to destruction of sensory nerves, with loss of feeling in limbs, fingers, and toes.	Meats, fish, poultry; grains, cereals; spinach, sweet and white potatoes; bananas, prunes, watermelon
Vitamin B_{12} (cobalamin)	Helps build genetic material (nucleic acid) required by all cells; helps form red blood cells.	Anemia and nerve damage (Deficiency is rare except in strict vegetarians who eat no foods of animal origin; B_{12} that occurs in a few plant foods cannot be absorbed by humans.)	None noted, even when intakes are well above usual levels	All foods of animal origin, including meats, poultry, eggs, seafood, dairy foods

(continued on next page)

VITAMIN	EFFECT	SIGNS OF DEFICIENCY	SIGNS OF OVERDOSE	GOOD SOURCES
Water-Soluble Vitamins, *continued*				
Biotin, a B vitamin	Required for glucose metabolism and formation of certain fatty acids; plays an essential part in many bodily processes.	Rare except in infants; scaling skin; muscle pain; fatigue; loss of appetite; sleeplessness	See vitamin B₁.	Produced by intestinal bacteria; also obtained from meats, poultry, fish, eggs; nuts, seeds, legumes; vegetables
Folic acid (folate, folacin), a B vitamin	Needed to make genetic material (DNA, RNA); needed for manufacture of red blood cells.	Anemia; gastrointestinal upsets, diarrhea, weight loss; bleeding gums; irritability; birth defects if levels are low in pregnancy	Convulsions in epileptics (can interfere with anti-convulsant medication); megadoses can interfere with zinc absorption.	Poultry, liver; dark-green, leafy vegetables; legumes; fortified whole-grain breads, cereals; oranges, grapefruit
Vitamin C (ascorbic acid)	Helps bind cells together; strengthens blood vessel walls.	Bleeding gums, loose teeth; bruising; dry, rough skin; slow healing; appetite loss; scurvy in extreme cases	Kidney stones; oxalate deposits in heart and other tissues; urinary tract irritation; diarrhea; anemia	Citrus fruits; strawberries; cantaloupe, watermelon; sweet potatoes; cabbage, cauliflower, broccoli; plantains; snow peas

MINERAL	EFFECT	SIGNS OF DEFICIENCY	SIGNS OF OVERDOSE	GOOD SOURCES
Calcium	Builds bones, teeth; promotes nerve and muscle function; helps blood to clot; helps activate enzymes that convert food into energy.	Rickets (weak, deformed bones) in children; osteomalacia and osteoporosis (softening and thinning of bones) in adults	Kidney stones and calcium deposits in tissues; mental confusion; muscle and abdominal pain; interferes with absorption of iron and other minerals.	Milk and dairy foods; canned fish (salmon, sardines) with bones; oysters; broccoli; tofu (bean curd)
Phosphorus	Works with calcium to build and maintain bones and teeth; needed by certain enzymes to convert food into energy; promotes nerve and muscle function; helps maintain body's chemical balance.	Weakness, bone pain (Deficiency is rare.)	Reduces blood calcium levels	Dairy products; egg yolks; meat, poultry, fish; legumes
Magnesium	Activates enzymes needed to release energy in body; promotes bone growth; needed to make cells and genetic material.	Muscle weakness, twitching, cramps; disturbances of heart rhythm (deficiencies rare in healthy children)	Imbalance between calcium and magnesium, leading to nervous system disorders	Green, leafy vegetables; beans; nuts; fortified whole-grain cereals and breads; shellfish

(continued on next page)

MINERAL	EFFECT	SIGNS OF DEFICIENCY	SIGNS OF OVERDOSE	GOOD SOURCES
Iron	Essential to make hemoglobin, the red oxygen-carrying pigment in blood, and myoglobin, a pigment that stores oxygen in muscles.	Anemia, with weakness, fatigue, shortness of breath	Toxic buildup in liver, pancreas, heart; diabetes; liver disease; disturbances of heart rhythm; interference with zinc absorption	Red meat, liver; fish, shellfish; legumes; fortified breads, cereals; dried apricots.
Zinc	Needed in more than 100 enzymes; instrumental in digestion and metabolism; essential for sexual maturation.	Slow wound healing; appetite loss; delayed growth and sexual development in children	Nausea, vomiting, abdominal pain, gastric bleeding	Beef, liver; oysters; yogurt; fortified cereals, wheat germ
Selenium	Interacts with vitamin E to prevent breakdown of fats and body chemicals.	Heart muscle problems; anemia	Nausea, abdominal pain, diarrhea; hair and nail damage; fatigue; irritability	Poultry, seafood; egg yolks; whole-grain breads and cereals; mushrooms, onions, garlic
Copper	Component of several enzymes, including one needed to make body's pigments; stimulates iron absorption; needed to make red blood cells, connective tissue, nerve fibers.	In infants, anemia with abnormal development of bones, nerve tissue, lungs, skin, and hair coloring	Liver disease; vomiting; diarrhea	Nuts; dried peas, beans; barley; prunes; organ meats; lobster

MINERAL	EFFECT	SIGNS OF DEFICIENCY	SIGNS OF OVERDOSE	GOOD SOURCES
Iodine	Essential for function of thyroid gland.	Goiter; delayed growth and impaired intellectual capacity (cretinism) in infants	Disturbed thyroid function; goiter	Iodized salt; seafood; vegetables grown in iodine-rich soil
Fluoride	Promotes strong teeth and bones, especially in children; enhances body's uptake of calcium.	Tooth decay	Mottling of tooth enamel	Fluoridated water; food cooked in fluoridated water; tea
Manganese	Needed for healthy tendon and bone structure; component of several enzymes involved in metabolism.	Not known in humans	Nerve damage	Tea, coffee; bran; dried peas and beans; nuts
Molybdenum	Component of enzymes essential for metabolism; helps regulate iron storage.	Not known in humans	Joint pain resembling gout	Dried peas and beans; dark-green, leafy vegetables; organ meats; whole-grain breads and cereals
Chromium	Works with insulin in glucose metabolism.	Symptoms resembling diabetes.	Not known for chromium in food; salts of chromium metal are toxic.	Whole-grain breads and cereals; brewer's yeast; peanuts

(continued on next page)

MINERAL	EFFECT	SIGNS OF DEFICIENCY	SIGNS OF OVERDOSE	GOOD SOURCES
Sulfur	Needed to make hair and nails; component of several amino acids.	Not known	Not known for sulfur in food; salts of sulfur are toxic.	Wheat germ; dried peas and beans; beef; clams; peanuts
Potassium	Works with sodium to regulate fluid balance; promotes transmission of nerve impulses and proper muscle function; essential for metabolism.	Muscle weakness; disturbances in heart rhythm; irritability	Nausea, diarrhea; disturbances in heart rhythm that may lead to cardiac arrest	Bananas; citrus fruits; dried fruits; deep-yellow vegetables; potatoes; legumes; milk; bran cereal
Sodium	Helps maintain fluid balance.	Rare, but loss of sodium can cause muscle cramps, weakness, headaches.	High blood pressure; kidney disease; heart failure	Salt; processed foods; milk; water in some areas
Chloride	Helps maintain acid-base balance of body fluids; component of hydrochloric acid in gastric juices needed for digestion.	Rare, but can upset acid-base and body fluids balance.	Upset in acid-base balance	Same as sodium

Vitamins A, D, and K are mostly stored in the liver, whereas vitamin E is probably stored in fat. The 8 B vitamins and vitamin C are water soluble and do not need fat to be absorbed. Our bodies store enough vitamins to meet general daily requirements, with a little extra in case the dietary supply should fail. The main storehouse is the liver, which absorbs and stores nutrients from the blood and then releases into the blood those nutrients that are not supplied in adequate amounts by the diet.

Contrary to what advertisements claim, most healthy children do not need multivitamin supplements to make up for nutrients lacking in their food. Nor do they need a set dose of vitamins every day. As with other trace nutrients, what's important is that the average food consumption over a week or two includes a variety of foods to provide all the essential vitamins. It is always better to get vitamins from food than in pill form. First, vitamin supplements available in pills are incomplete. Second, a pill results in a high concentration of vitamin that may interfere with the absorption of other nutrients from food. A diet based on the US Department of Agriculture guidelines provides adequate amounts of all the vitamins. However, children who are not drinking three 8-oz glasses of milk daily, and babies who are exclusively breastfed and protected from sunlight, may have inadequate vitamin D, and a supplement that provides 400 IU of vitamin D daily should be considered. Other children with intestinal malabsorption or who are taking anticonvulsant medications may also need additional vitamin D. However, vitamin supplements should not be used except on the advice of your pediatrician because excess supplement use could result in toxic levels.

Minerals

Three minerals—calcium, phosphorus, and magnesium—account for 98% of the body's mineral content by weight. Calcium and phosphorus play basic roles in countless biochemical reactions at the cellular level. They are also the main components of the skeleton, and without magnesium many metabolic functions could not take place.

Phosphorus is in almost all animal and vegetable foods and is often found in foods that contain calcium. Milk and dairy products, fish bones (such as in canned salmon and sardines), and dark-green, leafy vegetables are the best sources of calcium. Magnesium, like phosphorus, is abundant in animal and plant cells.

Healthy children do not lack phosphorus and magnesium because these minerals are easily absorbed. By contrast, low calcium intakes are very common, especially among adolescent girls who shun milk and dairy foods to avoid fat calories. These girls risk osteoporosis, or thinning of the bones, starting as early as age 30. Nonfat milk, yogurt, and other dairy foods are excellent sources of calcium and do not add unwanted fat calories to the diet.

Mineral absorption is influenced by a number of factors, including certain hormones and vitamin levels. Infants absorb calcium more easily than adults do, and the rate of absorption is increased when other nutrients are around, including the milk sugar lactose, the amino acids lysine and arginine, and vitamin C (eg, calcium-fortified orange juice). Calcium absorption may be decreased by high dietary levels of phosphate, oxalate (in rhubarb and certain leafy green vegetables), or phytate compounds in fiber. Too much protein in the diet

---

ELECTROLYTES

The minerals potassium, sodium, and chloride are known as electrolytes. In the body they conduct electrical currents and keep tissue fluids in balance, with positive sodium ions outside the cells and positive potassium ions inside.

Potassium is essential to many functions, such as those related to nerve impulses and muscle activity. A child may lose sodium and potassium through prolonged diarrhea, vomiting, or sweating, which leads to dehydration. Your pediatrician may recommend a commercial electrolyte solution to prevent serious electrolyte loss in a child with diarrhea or vomiting. For healthy children, fruits and vegetables are good sources of potassium.

A teenaged patient of Dr Stern's told her he was taking a potassium supplement. When she asked why, he said that the guy in the health food store told him it would make his muscles stronger. She told him that while a deficiency of potassium can cause weakness, too much can actually be fatal.

Sodium and chloride combine to form sodium chloride, or table salt. These minerals are so plentiful in a normal diet that even without added salt, deficiencies are rare. Even though sodium may be lost with prolonged diarrhea, vomiting, or sweating, the best way to make up for these losses is by eating normal meals and drinking plenty of fluids. Salt pills can be dangerous for children and adolescents and should never be used. (For more information about salt, see "We Don't Need to Add Salt to Food," Chapter 11, pages 251–252.)

may increase the amount of calcium excreted in the urine and decrease the amount available for building bones.

Iron

Iron is a major part of hemoglobin, the red blood pigment that carries oxygen to tissues. Lack of iron is the most common nutritional deficiency in the United States and a frequent cause of anemia.

Babies are born with enough stored iron to last about 4 to 6 months. Pediatricians usually recommend an iron-fortified cereal when babies start solid foods to prevent iron deficiency in the rapid growth phase of the first 2 years. Although cow's milk and human milk contain about the same amount of iron, a baby can absorb about 50% of the iron from human milk compared with only about 10% of that in cow's milk. In addition, sensitivity to the protein in cow's milk can cause excessive iron loss through hidden bleeding from the digestive tract in babies younger than 12 months. This is why we recommend human milk or iron-enriched formula for children up to 1 year. After age 2, the growth rate slows down, iron stores begin to build up again, and the risk of iron deficiency is lower.

Before adolescence, children normally take in adequate iron from a balanced diet that includes good iron sources such as red meat and fortified cereals. In addition, fruits rich in vitamin C promote iron absorption from plant foods. Adolescent boys may lack adequate iron around the peak growth period, the growth spurt when they seem to outgrow their clothes weekly, and iron stored in their bodies fails to meet the demands of rapid growth. Provided boys eat a balanced diet, the deficiency usually corrects itself after the growth spurt. Adolescent girls are at greater risk for developing iron deficiency anemia through loss of iron with menstrual blood. Heavy periods—a common event in young women who have not yet established a regular pattern of ovulation—increase the risk of iron deficiency. Girls who are menstruating should have a blood test for possible iron deficiency anemia at every checkup.

Meat, poultry, fish and shellfish, legumes, and fortified cereals are good sources of iron. The amount of iron absorbed depends on the source. Iron from plant foods is absorbed least well; however, the amount can be increased by consuming foods with a high vitamin C content at the same meal. Tea, bran, and milk can reduce iron absorption from plant foods. Iron absorption from dairy foods is in the middle range, and the iron in meat is well absorbed.

Other Trace Minerals

Trace elements are required only in small amounts but are involved in practically every process that takes place in the body. They are essential components of the enzyme systems that allow metabolic processes to take place. Without adequate levels, the body cannot maintain proper fluid and chemical balances or keep a steady heartbeat.

The 13 trace elements known to be nutritionally important are iron, zinc, copper, fluoride, iodine, selenium, manganese, chromium, cobalt, molybdenum, nickel, silicon, and vanadium (for mineral requirements, functions, and sources, see Table on pages 203–206.) Other minerals may also be required. Recommended dietary allowances have been established for 4 trace minerals—iron, zinc, iodine, and selenium—and "safe and adequate" amounts have been estimated for an additional 5 minerals—chromium, copper, manganese, molybdenum, and fluoride. (For more about the importance of fluoride, see Chapter 2, page 49.)

The body has a remarkable ability to regulate the balance of trace minerals. For example, if a person consumes more iron than necessary, the excess is usually excreted unchanged. However, if the body lacks iron, the rate of iron absorption from food increases to compensate. Mineral deficiencies other than iron deficiency are rare in the United States, and children do not require mineral supplements unless they have a chronic condition that limits their diet or interferes with nutrient absorption. As a result, iron, zinc, and other mineral supplements should never be given unless your pediatrician specifically recommends them.

QUESTIONS PARENTS ASK ABOUT NUTRITION BASICS

Does my child have to eat each recommended serving from the major food groups every single day?

The food guide is just that—a guide, not a prescription. It's not necessary to eat the exact number of servings from each group every day. Rather, intake should average out to the portions shown over a period of 1 to 2 weeks, to ensure a healthy intake of calories along with all the essential nutrients. (See page 194.)

Portion sizes appear small. Do they really expect a hungry teenager to survive on half a cup of cooked pasta?

Portions are standardized for easy use and reference. Obviously, a person with a moderate appetite can eat much more than half a cup of cooked pasta at a meal, and a single plateful may include several portions of one or several foods. Children's portions should be scaled according to age, appetite, and activity level (also see page 194).

With all the concerns about fats, fiber, and obesity, should I just keep my children permanently on a no-fat, low-calorie, high-fiber diet?

You should be skeptical of recommendations that children eat only low-calorie, high-fiber foods. A selection of foods from the major food groups every day ensures balanced nutrition. Children need calories for growth and activity, and some fat for health. And while fiber is good, too much of it could cause gas and other digestive problems and prevent a child from absorbing essential nutrients (see page 192 for your child's recommended daily fiber intake).

Chapter 9

Spitting Up, Gagging, Vomiting, Diarrhea, and Constipation

Most infants spit up small amounts of milk or formula during their first few months. Spitting up seldom indicates a medical problem or food sensitivity. In contrast, vomiting involves forceful muscle contractions, brings up large amounts of milk, and makes the baby uncomfortable and unhappy.

Gail Laird panicked when her newborn, Owen, started spitting up after every feeding. Responding to Gail's urgent call, her pediatrician calmed her fears. Owen wasn't really vomiting; he just opened his mouth and out came the milk. The baby was content and settling well for his naps and at night, and the amount, when Gail really examined it, was tiny. The pediatrician assured Gail that Owen was fine but asked her to call at once if the dribbling or regurgitation of milk ever changed to forceful vomiting and her baby was irritable or had other symptoms.

The tendency to spit up decreases as the baby's gastrointestinal tract matures and usually stops altogether after he begins to sit on his own.

Gastroesophageal Reflux

Spitting up is sometimes associated with gastroesophageal reflux disease (doctors often refer to this as GERD for short), which is usually a temporary mechanical hitch. If your baby's stomach is full or his position is changed abruptly, especially after a feeding, the stomach contents—food mixed with stomach acid—press against the valve at the top of the stomach called the lower esophageal sphincter. This ring of muscle normally relaxes to let food pass from the esophagus into the stomach and then tightens again to keep the food there. When it is not fully developed or it opens at the wrong time, the stomach contents move back or reflux into the esophagus. In babies, gastroesophageal reflux rarely causes symptoms or distress and usually disappears as the upper digestive tract functionally matures. Reflux is mainly a messy problem, not a serious one.

If your bottle-fed baby spits up unusually often, your pediatrician may recommend thickening his formula with a very small amount of baby cereal. Never add solids to the bottle unless your pediatrician advises it. Unless carefully supervised, this practice not only may add unnecessary calories to your baby's diet but also can interfere with the transition to solid foods (see Chapter 2, Expanding Your Baby's Diet). Be careful not to overfeed your baby. Consider smaller and more frequent feedings, but be sure her total daily intake is sufficient to keep up normal growth and development. You may find it helpful to keep your baby in an upright position in a stroller or carrier for the first hour or so after feeding.

In very rare cases, gastroesophageal reflux is severe enough to cause symptoms such as blood in vomit or stools, wheezing and hoarseness, or failure to gain weight. Such vomiting may also be caused by other medical conditions. A baby with severe reflux may refuse to feed or be irritable after feeding. An older child may complain of abdominal pain or describe the discomfort typical of heartburn, and vomit or complain of a sour taste after the food comes back up. In any such case, children with such symptoms need medical evaluation and attention.

An older child with reflux should avoid fried and fatty foods because fat slows down the rate of stomach emptying and promotes reflux. Peppermint, caffeine (an ingredient of colas and many other soft drinks), and certain asthma medications can make the lower esophageal sphincter relax and allow stomach contents to flux back into the esophagus. Some experts believe that tomato-based products have a similar effect. If any food seems to produce reflux or heartburn, keep it out of the diet for a week or two and then reintroduce it. If symptoms recur, avoid that food for a while.

Gagging

Every baby is born with the extrusion reflex, an automatic response that makes the baby push his tongue forward when an object is touched to it. As long as there is a strong extrusion response, a baby can't use his tongue to move food from the front to the back of the mouth to swallow. This is a mechanism that protects against potentially harmful material,

---

AIR SWALLOWING AND BURPING

A baby who gulps down air with her breast milk or formula is likely to spit up and burp more than others. It's usually possible to keep air swallowing (also called aerophagia) to a lower level by feeding your baby as soon as she shows signs of being ready—before she starts to cry with hunger or frustration—and holding her at an angle to prevent air from entering her mouth as she feeds (also see "Getting Started," Chapter 1, page 4).

Air swallowing and burping continue in children long past infancy. Toddlers and older children swallow air when crying or when a stuffed-up nose makes them breathe through the mouth. Help your child to clear his nose frequently when a cold makes breathing difficult.

School-aged children and adolescents gulp down air when eating or chewing gum. Carbonated drinks also lead to gas buildup. Encourage your child to take a bit more time over meals and avoid carbonated drinks if gas is bothersome. For children who deliberately swallow air to gain attention with noisy belching, the best treatment is to let them know their behavior is unacceptable. Avoid reinforcing it by paying attention. Ignore it and eventually they'll stop because they are not getting a reaction.

---

including food a baby isn't ready to chew and swallow. The extrusion reflex begins to fade when an infant is about 4 months old. (In contrast, the gag reflex continues throughout life to protect against airway blockage.) The extrusion reflex fades about the time a baby doubles his birth weight and is beginning to need more nutrition than human milk or formula (also see Chapter 2, Expanding Your Baby's Diet). Your baby will gradually learn to tolerate solids as he sucks his fingers, toys, and other objects. It's not uncommon for babies to go through a stage of repeatedly gagging themselves with their fingers and even throwing up a bit. Some make a habit of this behavior after they are rewarded by a worried reaction from their parents the first few times. Eventually, a baby learns how far he can tolerate an object in his mouth and at the same time, improves his ability to swallow. This is all part of the complex process of learning to eat. Even after the early extrusion reflex has disappeared, a child will continue to gag from time to time when he has too much in his mouth, dislikes the taste or texture of a food, or feels pressured to eat.

Pouching

It's one thing to get food as far as a toddler's mouth, but it may be quite another to persuade her to swallow it. Toddlers and preschoolers are highly sensitive to tastes and textures. In addition, until about age 4, children aren't able to chew efficiently with a grinding motion, which breaks food down to a manageable texture. A strange food or too large a mouthful may trigger a fear of choking that makes a child reluctant to swallow. In particular, meat that has been chewed for a while can have a dry, pasty texture that makes young children gag.

Perhaps this is why toddlers occasionally *pouch* their food, chewing it and wadding it in their cheeks. In some cases, pouching is a way a child resists the pressure that parents put on her to eat; the child obeys the parents by eating the food but shows resistance by pouching it rather than swallowing it. A poucher may carry food in her cheeks for hours, or leave a trail of chewed-up pellets in unexpected places. Pouching may be socially unacceptable, but it isn't a health hazard unless the wad is so large that the child could choke. It's not safe, however, to let a poucher nap or go to bed with food in her cheeks because the wad could become dislodged during sleep and choke the child. If you can't persuade your child to spit the food out, try to clear the pouches with your finger. A child who keeps her teeth tightly clenched may open her mouth in spite of herself if you make faces with her in front of a mirror. Offer a drink of water to rinse out any leftovers. (Also see "Pouching," Chapter 3, page 67)

Not only does pouching occur infrequently, but it is a phase that will eventually pass on its own. However, you may be able to help it on its way if you

- Present food in a way that your child enjoys chewing and swallowing.
- Offer alternatives if your child pouches a particular food.

RUMINATION

In rare cases, a baby repeatedly gags, mouths, and re-swallows regurgitated food to such an extent that his growth is impaired. This disorder, called rumination, is most likely to appear between 3 and 14 months, although older children may also be affected. It is more common in boys. Rumination is often associated with medical conditions such as gastroesophageal reflux disease, emotional problems, and other factors affecting development. A child who is ruminating needs the attention of a pediatrician.

For example, if meat is your child's stumbling block, make sure that the meat you offer is moist and easy to chew. Meat that's ground up and mixed with vegetables, such as in spaghetti sauce or chili con carne, is easier to manage than dry slices or grilled hamburger. In any case, meat isn't indispensable in the diet. Your child can obtain the same essential nutrients from other foods in the meat and protein group, such as fish, eggs, or dried beans and legumes, including peanut butter (thinly spread for children younger than 4 years— and serve only smooth peanut butter to this age group).

A child who continues to pouch food after early childhood may be dealing with emotional stress. Your pediatrician will evaluate the child and recommend ways to deal with the condition.

Vomiting

An isolated incident of vomiting is nothing to worry about as long as your child is not unduly distressed and has no other symptoms such as a stomachache, earache, dizziness, diarrhea, or fever. Most pediatricians consider a temperature above 100.4°F (38°C) a sign of a fever. If your baby is 2 months or younger and has a rectal temperature of 100.4°F or higher, call your pediatrician immediately. If your child is older than 1 year, is taking fluids and sleeping normally, and remains playful, you probably do not need to call your pediatrician. However, if your child vomits persistently for an hour, vomits after a fall or head injury, or has other symptoms, or if there's blood or greenish bile in the vomit, call your pediatrician immediately. If your baby is younger than 1 year, also contact your pediatrician immediately for a concern over forceful vomiting. Don't give anything to eat or drink until your pediatrician says it's safe. If your child is alert and wants to drink, let him suck on ice chips or a frozen juice-pop to moisten his mouth and lips.

If your baby's occasional vomiting or spitting up changes to forceful vomiting of fairly large amounts after every feeding, or if he is losing or failing to gain weight, call your pediatrician without delay. In a baby, these symptoms may indicate pyloric stenosis, a narrowing of the passage between the stomach and the small intestine, or another condition that requires immediate treatment.

DRINKS TO PREVENT DEHYDRATION IN A VOMITING CHILD

For vomiting children, the main risk is water loss, or dehydration, especially if fever causes them to sweat more or they are also losing fluid through diarrhea. When vomiting is severe or prolonged, a child may lose sodium, potassium, and chloride. These minerals have a crucial role in the transmission of nerve impulses and the contraction of muscles, and in regulating the body's fluid balance.

While missing a meal or two will cause no harm to an otherwise healthy child, it's important that a sick child continue to drink water to take care of normal daily needs, plus extra to make up for fluid loss and prevent dehydration. Infants and young children are especially susceptible to dehydration because they are less efficient at conserving water than older children and adults. In addition, small body size means that it takes less fluid loss to lead to dehydration.

Offer frequent sips of water or, if your child doesn't feel like drinking, ice chips to suck on. Build up to 1 oz an hour, then 2 oz an hour until the child is able to drink normally.

Your pediatrician may recommend a commercial rehydration solution to help replace lost sodium and potassium in an infant or young child. These come in liquid and Popsicle-like forms to make them more appealing to children. It also makes certain that the liquid is taken slowly. Older children may ask for commercial sports drinks, but these should be used with care. They replace salts, but they also contain large amounts of sugar, which can make diarrhea worse. A child who wants a change from plain water may enjoy sips of fruit juice diluted half-and-half with water or flat soda. If your child is too sick to drink or listless, or shows signs of progressive dehydration such as dry mouth, fewer tears, or urinates less frequently, seek urgent medical attention. Contact your pediatrician immediately.

A child may vomit as a result of intense crying, particularly during a temper tantrum. Such tantrums are especially common between the ages of 18 months and 4 years, a period marked by opposition to parents and caregivers and conflicting feelings about increasing independence. In most cases, vomiting will disappear after the cause is identified and dealt with. Toddlers generally leave tantrums behind as they gain skills and enter the preschool years. (If a child continues to have frequent emotional outbursts after age 4, you may want to ask your pediatrician for an evaluation and recommendations.)

Vomiting or retching (dry vomiting) may follow a coughing spell or may occur with persistent postnasal drip. When a child has a cold, drinking fluids is important to help thin

---

MOTION SICKNESS

A child who often feels nauseous or vomits when riding in cars, boats, or elevators suffers from motion sickness. The overwhelming nausea, vomiting, and headaches come from a difference between what the child can see and what he senses with the balance mechanism of his inner ear. If you're planning a trip by car, boat, or small plane, or know you'll be driving on winding roads, encourage your child to eat a light snack, such as a few crackers, before setting out. (He's more likely to feel sick if his stomach is empty or overly full.) Make sure that his seat in the car or boat allows a clear view to the outside, preferably forward; many people feel less nauseous if they can focus on a point in the distance.

Some motion sickness sufferers find that chewing a few pieces of candied ginger helps to control nausea, but the candy may be too spicy for a child. Over-the-counter remedies can relieve the problem, although they also may cause drowsiness. Your pediatrician can advise you about preventive medications.

---

secretions and clear mucus. When respiratory symptoms drop off, vomiting from coughing and postnasal drip may decrease.

Emotional stress from major life changes, such as starting school or family upheavals, can frequently cause vomiting. A child who vomits from stress may continue to do so when faced with stressful situations. Your pediatrician can recommend behavioral measures to help the child cope with such challenges. In all cases, no special ongoing dietary measures are necessary. Your child may resume normal meals as soon as he feels like eating again. (For the special problem of self-induced vomiting in adolescents, see Chapter 10, Eating Disorders.)

A few children have periodic vomiting that occurs irregularly, without any warning symptoms, and lasts about 24 hours. During an attack, the child may feel lethargic and ill, but she quickly recovers with no aftereffects and remains completely well and in good health until the next episode. This cyclic vomiting usually appears for the first time between 2 and 4 years. Attacks become less frequent and eventually stop as the child grows older. This is thought to be related to migraine and if frequent, may warrant treatment and medication. Migraine can also cause vomiting and abdominal pain. A child who regularly vomits with or without headaches or other symptoms should be evaluated by a pediatrician to identify possible triggers, such as food sensitivity, and to determine whether treatment is required.

POISONING PREVENTION

Post the Poison Help number (1-800-222-1222) on the emergency list next to every phone in your home and in your cell phone.

- A toddler or preschooler who vomits may have eaten or drunk something poisonous. If you suspect poisoning because of a telltale odor, unexplained stains on clothing, burns or stains around the mouth, or an open or empty container of a toxic substance, call Poison Help immediately.

  More than a million American children younger than 6 years suffer poisoning every year. Household cleaners, personal care products, and over-the-counter medications lead the list of poisons.

  Healthy preschoolers are mobile and curious enough to sample even foul-tasting substances. To complicate matters, many caustic products such as drain cleaners, which can cause devastating injuries, have no taste. A child may ingest a large amount before he stops because of a burning sensation. Vitamin pills, iron and other mineral supplements, and aspirin, while generally safe for adults, can cause serious or even life-threatening reactions in a child's small body.

- Store drugs and medications in a medicine cabinet that is locked or out of reach. Do not keep toothpaste, soap, or shampoo in the same cabinet. If you carry a purse, keep potential poisons out of your purse and keep your child away from other people's purses.

- Buy and keep medications in their own containers with child safety caps. Put the cap on completely after each use. Child resistant does not mean childproof, only that it takes longer for your child to get into it. Being alert and aware is extremely important.

- Do not take medicine in front of small children; they may try to imitate you later. Never tell a child that a medicine is candy.

- Store hazardous products in locked cabinets that are out of your child's reach. Do not keep detergents and other cleaning products under the kitchen or bathroom sink unless they are in a cabinet with a safety latch that locks every time you close the cabinet.
  - Never put poisonous or toxic products in containers that were once used for food, especially empty drink bottles, cans, or cups.
  - Empty and rinse all glasses immediately after gatherings where alcohol is served. Keep alcohol in a locked cabinet.

MEDICATIONS TO STOP VOMITING

It's not usually necessary to give a vomiting child medication (called an antiemetic) to suppress vomiting because most vomiting results from a brief, self-limited viral infection of the gastrointestinal tract, or food poisoning. However, if your child refuses liquids and you're concerned about dehydration, contact your pediatrician.

Children may have severe vomiting from an ongoing medical condition such as diabetes or cancer treatment, or following anesthesia for surgery. In these cases, pediatricians may prescribe antiemetics and other medications as necessary.

UNEXPLAINED VOMITING IN A TEENAGED GIRL

An adolescent girl who is nauseated, faint, and vomiting for several days in a row may be pregnant or fearful that she is pregnant. Parents are often unaware that their daughter is sexually active and could be pregnant. Discuss it with her calmly in a non-accusatory manner and consult your pediatrician without delay.

Diarrhea

Diarrhea is among the most common and recurrent childhood problems. Among children, diarrhea is usually a sign of a minor intestinal infection. This is when the lining of the digestive tract becomes infected by a virus—or, less often, a bacterium. In addition to loose stools, other symptoms often include nausea, vomiting, and cramping. Outbreaks of infectious diarrhea can easily occur among children in group care, especially at centers with children who aren't yet toilet trained.

While "stomach flu" is not a life-threatening infection, children with acute diarrhea can quickly lose essential fluids and salts, particularly if they are also vomiting. Children most at risk from the effects of diarrhea are those younger than 2 years, who are more susceptible to dehydration than older children and adults, and children with chronic illness, who are generally less able to ward off infection and compensate for the loss of fluids and nutrients.

Your pediatrician will advise you about giving your child drinks to make up for the fluids and electrolytes (sodium, potassium, and chloride) lost from bouts of diarrhea. Pharmacies and most supermarkets carry premixed drinks with the right balance of electrolytes. Do not use

---

TEMPORARY LACTOSE INTOLERANCE AFTER DIARRHEA

Infectious diarrhea may cause a temporary inability to digest lactose, the sugar in milk. Until bowel tissues recover, the child cannot produce enough of the enzyme lactase to break down milk sugar. Drinking milk may cause typical symptoms of lactose intolerance, including bloating, more diarrhea, cramps, and gassiness. This does not occur in most healthy children who develop a case of acute viral gastroenteritis.

If your child wants milk or milk puddings, use only reduced-lactose milk for a week or two; aged cheeses, such as cheddar and parmesan, and yogurts are usually digestible because the lactose is broken down in the manufacturing process. Breastfeeding can almost always be continued without intolerance or ill effects.

If symptoms are a result of antibiotic treatment, call your pediatrician, who may modify the prescription or recommend different therapy.

---

homemade solutions. Infants should not drink clear liquids such as juice, sport drinks, and soda to replenish ongoing fluid from vomiting or diarrhea.

Resume small servings of a normal diet as soon as your child feels up to eating. Research has shown that with a normal diet, children maintain their weight better and may have diarrhea for a shorter time than when liquids alone are given. The bananas, rice, apples, toast (BRAT) diet, once recommended while recovering from diarrhea, is no longer considered useful. Some pediatricians believe that it may actually prolong symptoms. BRAT components, however, will do no harm in a normal diet; bananas and cooked apples, in particular, have a binding effect, as do other fruits that contain high levels of the soluble fiber pectin. Oat bran is another excellent source of soluble fiber. Foods containing large amounts of insoluble fiber, such as wheat bran, promote bowel emptying and speed up bowel movements. Avoid these until bowel movements are back to normal. Breastfeeding can be continued.

Toddler Diarrhea

Ayesha's mother brought her 16-month-old in for a consultation. "Ayesha has terrible diarrhea—5 or 6 movements every day—and they're very liquid," the mother related. "Not only that, but she's losing everything she eats. I can see whole pieces of vegetables and other foods in her diapers. I'm afraid she's not getting enough nourishment."

A quick review of Ayesha's medical records showed that she was growing and gaining weight just fine. She was an active, adventurous toddler, making enthusiastic efforts to speak, and eating well, though with a toddler's typically limited attention span.

While in the pediatrician's office, Ayesha demanded, "Drink juice!" Her mother pulled a bottle of apple juice out of her bag.

"This is all she'll drink, Doctor. She practically lives on juice."

In this case, the juice was probably responsible for Ayesha's loose stools. A toddler may have several loose bowel movements every day, passing fairly large fragments of undigested food together with a lot of liquid. Parents worry that the child has something wrong with her bowels and is not absorbing her food properly. This nonspecific diarrhea is common among toddlers and is not a cause for concern provided the child is active, healthy, and gaining weight. Toddlers eventually grow out of this phase. When a cause can be found, it's often too much fruit juice in the diet. Toddlers love to drink sweet juice and parents give it to them, thinking it's nourishing.

In fact, juice has several strikes against it. First, it contains large amounts of several sugars, including fructose and sorbitol, which can lead to loose stools. Apple, pear, grape, cherry, and prune juices, among others, have high sorbitol content. Sorbitol, often used to sweeten sugarless candies and gums, cannot be digested. It's not unusual for children to develop diarrhea with gassiness and bloating if they frequently chew sugarless gum containing sorbitol. Second, toddlers tend to fill up on juice and don't have enough room left for more nourishing foods at mealtimes. Third, juice is not an important source of nutrients. It's true that citrus juices and those fortified with vitamin C are good sources of this vitamin; still, fruit juice should be limited to 4 to 6 oz a day for children 1 to 6 years old. Finally, the sugar in juice can harm developing teeth if a toddler has free access, such as in a bottle or sippy

---

OVER-THE-COUNTER MEDICATIONS

Over-the-counter antidiarrheal medications are not recommended for children 2 years and younger and should be used only on a pediatrician's advice in older children. These medications cause fluid and salt to stay in the intestine, which appears to stop the diarrhea. In fact, they may make it more difficult to recognize dehydration and can cause serious fluid and salt imbalances.

ROTAVIRUS: A COMMON CAUSE OF WINTERTIME DIARRHEA

In the United States, rotavirus accounts for about 20% of all cases of childhood gastroenteritis and is the most common reason that young children are hospitalized for dehydration. The effects can be serious—rotavirus infection has been linked to approximately 100 childhood deaths from diarrhea each year. Like the viruses for influenza and the common cold, rotavirus is most active in the winter and spring—October through May—though infection can occur at any time of the year.

Vaccines to protect against rotavirus are now available and are given between 2 and 8 months of age. They've been remarkably effective in preventing the infection and keeping children out of the hospital due to dehydration associated with this virus. In addition, simple hygiene is a good defense against the illness. Parents and others involved in children's care must not only wash their own hands but also continually teach children how important it is to wash hands before handling food and after using the toilet to curb the spread of this and other sicknesses.

---

cup that she carries about with her. When you serve juice, serve it in a cup at a scheduled snack or meal. If your toddler is thirsty, she'll find water more thirst quenching than sugary juice. Developing a preference for water may also help to eliminate a source of unnecessary calories in the future.

Diarrhea caused by bacteria (eg, *Salmonella, Shigella)* is of special concern among children of all ages, especially in schools and group child care. If your infant younger than 3 months has diarrhea and a fever, especially if there is blood or mucus in the stool, call your pediatrician right away.

If your baby is older than 3 months and has diarrhea and a mild fever for more than a day, check whether he's passing a normal amount of urine, check his temperature with a thermometer, and call your pediatrician.

If an older child has diarrhea lasting longer than 48 hours, vomiting longer than 12 hours, persistent fever, concern for dehydration, listlessness, or associated symptoms such as headache or blood in the stool, call your pediatrician.

The dietary recommendations for managing bacterial diarrhea are similar to those for viral gastroenteritis (see "Diarrhea" on page 221). An infant should continue with breastfeeding or formula; your pediatrician will advise whether additional fluids are necessary. An older child

ESCHERICHIA COLI O157:H7 AND FOOD CONTAMINATION

Serious food poisonings have been traced to *Escherichia coli* O157:H7. This microbe is a rogue strain of the bacterium *E coli,* which normally lives in human and animal digestive tracts and helps keep harmful germs from invading the body and causing illness. Strain O157:H7 produces toxins that cause severe, bloody diarrhea and may lead to fatal kidney failure (hemolytic uremic syndrome).

The most common sources of illness are leafy vegetables and undercooked ground beef from packing plants that prepare meat in bulk for fast-food chains. *E coli* O157:H7 has also been found in roast beef, raw (unpasteurized) milk, contaminated water, and vegetables contaminated with cow manure. People have become ill after drinking unpasteurized cider made from unwashed apples contaminated with cow manure. The bacteria can be passed from one person to another or through cross-contamination of foods. (Several other food-borne parasites are causing new health problems; see Chapter 13, Food Safety.) Though *E coli* O157:H7 survives freezing and can multiply at low temperatures, it is destroyed by thorough cooking.

To reduce your family's risk of food-borne illness, follow these safety rules (also see Chapter 13, Food Safety).

- Bag meats separately from other foods at the supermarket. Don't allow juices from meat to mix with other foods. Follow safe-handling labels on meat and poultry. Refrigerate meat at 40°F or freeze immediately.

- Use separate cutting boards for meat and produce.

- Wash cutting boards with hot soapy water and disinfect with a solution of 1 part bleach to 10 parts water before using again.

- Wash and disinfect knives and other utensils that have touched raw meat. Always wash your hands immediately after handling raw meat.

- Cook hamburger until brown in the center and the juices run clear. Ground beef is safely cooked when it reaches an internal temperature of at least 160°F. Reheat ground-beef leftovers to 165°F.

- Larger cuts of beef may be eaten medium to rare provided they have reached an internal temperature of at least 140°F. Use a meat thermometer if you find it hard to judge when meat is done.

- Wash fruits and vegetables.

- Don't let your children sample uncooked dough or batter made with raw eggs. Use only commercial mayonnaise, and don't use raw eggs in uncooked desserts (eg, frozen meringue made with whipped egg whites).

should drink plenty of clear fluids to keep tissues hydrated. Drinks with high sugar content, such as undiluted fruit juices and sports drinks, may worsen the diarrhea. Juices should be diluted half-and-half with water. As soon as the child feels well enough, he should resume small servings of a normal diet. If symptoms return when your child drinks milk, switch to reduced-lactose or lactose-free milk for about 2 weeks. Cheese and yogurt are usually digestible (see "Temporary Lactose Intolerance After Diarrhea" on page 222).

Intestinal Disorders

Jeffrey, at 7, had a nagging, recurrent stomachache that was making it difficult for him to go to school. He had no other symptoms like vomiting, fever, or headache, but the stomachache was severe and sometimes made him double over in pain. His parents, involved in a bitter and complicated divorce since Jeffrey was 5, at least shared concern over Jeffrey's health. They appeared at the pediatrician's office together.

The pediatrician soon saw that the parents had called only a limited truce. When the doctor asked how the pain began, Jeffrey's mother explained, "It started the day my son's dad introduced him to his new girlfriend—"

Jeffrey's father cut in. "You know it started the day I dropped Jeffrey off and you lost control. You used bad language in front of my son and called me terrible names."

Jeffrey's physical examination was normal, but the child seemed anxious and sad. The pediatrician told his parents that there was nothing physically wrong with Jeffrey's stomach. Rather, his heart and mind had too much to bear and the emotional overload was causing Jeffrey's pain. He referred the parents to a family counselor to help Jeffrey cope, and scheduled a follow-up appointment to see Jeffrey in a month.

Irritable Bowel Syndrome

Starting in the school years, many young people are troubled by a condition known as irritable bowel syndrome (IBS) or spastic colon. Typical symptoms are irregular, alternating cycles of constipation and diarrhea with pain or cramping, gas, and bloating. Although uncomfortable during the daytime, the symptoms do not awaken the child at night. Irritable bowel

---

INFLAMMATORY BOWEL DISEASE

Inflammatory bowel disease (IBD) is a term that includes ileitis (Crohn disease) and ulcerative colitis. Whatever the specific diagnosis may be, symptoms include severe diarrhea, blood or mucus in the stools, pain, weight loss, recurrent fever, mouth sores, and joint pain. When the onset is in childhood, IBD may impair growth and delay sexual maturation. In fact, in some children impaired growth becomes a problem before any bowel symptoms appear. Specific tests and consultation with a specialist are necessary to confirm the diagnosis because this is a lifelong condition and needs specific and directed treatment.

Diarrhea with bowel inflammation often leads to malnutrition because it impairs nutrient absorption. In addition to generalized malnutrition, young people with IBD suffer from specific problems depending on the site of the inflammation in the bowel. Children with IBD may need more calories than healthy children to make up for the losses due to illness. Unfortunately, children may have a poor appetite and fear that eating will make symptoms worse, so cases of childhood IBD may be associated with growth failure.

The immune system is thought to contribute to the development of IBD. No specific foods have been found to worsen symptoms. Therefore, there's no reason to restrict a child's diet unless she dislikes certain foods or they worsen symptoms. Consult your child's physician for any necessary dietary modifications.

---

syndrome symptoms don't have a consistent trigger, although anxiety plays a role and attacks may be more intense during times of stress, such as school tests or family upheaval. Food sensitivity may be a cause in some cases, bur true allergy is not a factor. The condition runs in families; often, one parent also has IBS.

Irritable bowel syndrome is not a serious disorder and it doesn't lead to more serious conditions. While symptoms are uncomfortable, they are not associated with weight loss, fever, or abnormalities in any specific laboratory test. The child is otherwise healthy in every other way. However, because all the symptoms of IBS may mimic potentially serious diseases, a child with recurrent bowel upsets should be evaluated by a pediatrician. A child with IBS should eat plenty of soluble fiber. Excellent sources are oat bran, vegetables, and fruits, which contain pectin. Your pediatrician may recommend behavioral approaches for managing stress. Occasionally, medications are prescribed.

Malabsorption

Several conditions may hinder the absorption of nutrients in the small intestine. Such malabsorption disorders may involve one or several nutrients, and the diagnosis depends on the type and number of nutrients that are lacking. No matter what the diagnosis, the general symptoms are similar—irritability, diarrhea, weight loss, bloating, and gas. The stools are often bulky and unusually foul smelling. They may also be pale and float on the water surface because of a high fat content.

Less severe malabsorption syndromes, such as lactose intolerance, can be managed by reducing or eliminating one specific nutrient and finding substitutes. Children with more severe disorders may suffer malnutrition not only because they don't absorb essential nutrients but also because they often feel too poorly to eat and they need more calories than they can consume. A child with symptoms suggesting a malabsorption disorder should be seen promptly by a pediatrician, who will perform diagnostic tests to identify the cause. Depending on the diagnosis, the child may be referred to a specialist for a consultation; a pediatric dietitian also should assist with dietary planning.

Lactose Intolerance

Primary lactose intolerance is perhaps the most widely known type of malabsorption. Passed along genetically, it is most prevalent among people of African, Asian, and Native American ancestry, and is relatively uncommon among those of Northern European descent. The symptoms of lactose intolerance can appear at about age 3 or 4 years when the child gradually stops producing lactase, the enzyme essential for the digestion of lactose, the sugar in cow's milk. Typical symptoms—cramps, gas, and diarrhea—follow consumption of dairy products. Lactose intolerance is rare in very young children except after severe gastrointestinal illness. When it occurs, typical symptoms are irritability, gas, and diarrhea.

Secondary lactose intolerance, as already discussed, can occur at any age and usually follows an acute, severe digestive illness, such as viral gastroenteritis, or is associated with a chronic digestive disease. In an otherwise healthy child, post-infectious lactose intolerance is uncommon.

Parents and children alike must become expert label readers to recognize terms that identify milk and other foods linked to intolerance. There are many children, however, who can handle milk and dairy products so long as small amounts are served as part of a meal. Breastfed infants usually continue to tolerate those feedings well. Aged cheeses and yogurts are usually acceptable because lactose is broken down in the manufacturing process. Reduced-lactose milk is widely available, as are lactase enzyme preparations that can be added to milk and dairy foods to make lactose digestible. However, in the rare cases in which milk and dairy products have to be avoided altogether, it's essential to provide alternative sources of calcium, such as calcium-fortified orange juice, canned fish with bones (eg, sardines, salmon, herring, mackerel), tofu, broccoli, and other high-calcium foods. Your pediatrician may recommend a calcium supplement. In any case of lactose intolerance, dietary modifications of your baby's formula or your child's dairy intake will have to be considered. Speak with your pediatrician about dietary counseling.

Gluten Enteropathy/Celiac Disease

People with gluten enteropathy or celiac disease cannot tolerate gliadin, a protein constituent of gluten, which is found in many grains. The symptoms of celiac disease may initially appear after a baby is first given cereal containing wheat, barley, rye, buckwheat, or millet. Affected children are irritable. They grow and gain weight poorly, and perhaps even lose weight. They often have chronic diarrhea, although some may be constipated. They may vomit or have pale or foul-smelling stools.

This food intolerance is increasingly common, affecting about 1 in 80 to 1 in 300 children, but it can be difficult to diagnose. Symptoms may appear well after infancy. It tends to run in families and is most common in those of European and Middle Eastern descent. The only treatment for celiac disease is strict, lifelong avoidance of cereals, pasta, breads, and baked goods made with grains containing gluten. Also, children with this disease need to stay away from commercially produced foods such as canned soups and stews thickened with processed grains and cereals. Even small amounts of gluten can cause symptoms in your child.

Your pediatrician will provide dietary advice and refer you to a dietitian for nutritional guidance. Many grocery stores and bakeries now sell gluten-free products (from breads to

HIRSCHSPRUNG DISEASE

If your new baby has only rare bowel movements, his stools are hard, and his abdomen appears bloated, your pediatrician will examine him to determine whether retained stool is swelling the abdomen while the rectum is empty. This group of symptoms can indicate Hirschsprung disease, a rare condition in which the baby lacks the nerves needed for having bowel movements. Hirschsprung disease is treated with surgery. Left untreated, it can lead to life-threatening complications, so be sure to bring early constipation that occurs just after birth or in early infancy to your pediatrician's attention.

DEALING WITH STOOL RETENTION AND SOILING

Stool retention is fairly common among school-aged children. What happens is that the child repeatedly ignores the urge to move her bowels. The nerve sensations in the area gradually grow weaker, and the rectal muscles and colon are not able to completely contract. The impacted stools become progressively larger, harder, and more painful to pass. This, in turn, makes the child even more reluctant to have a bowel movement. Eventually, liquid stool may leak out around the mass of impacted stool, soiling and staining the underwear and bedsheets. The child isn't aware that she's passing the liquid stool, and parents are misled into thinking she has diarrhea. When the pediatrician examines the child, however, the true problem becomes apparent.

Don't try to treat constipation or stool retention yourself with over-the-counter laxatives or enemas. Whatever the reason, your child needs a pediatrician's help to overcome it, especially because this has the potential to become a chronic problem. The goals of treatment are the following: to set regular bowel habits; to recognize and respond to the urge to defecate; to hold stool only until the time and place are right for a bowel movement; to focus the family's attention away from the child's bowels; and to eat foods and drink enough fluids that help keep bowel movements soft.

Treatment usually starts with medication to help the child pass the feces and thus let the bowel shrink back to normal size. Then the child continues taking a daily dose of a medication to ease stool passage. The pediatrician keeps a close check on the child's diet to make sure she's consuming plenty of fluids together with fiber in the form of vegetables, fruits, and whole-grain cereals and breads. Treatment may take a long time and involve the whole family. Relapses are not uncommon, but the problem usually will resolve if given the proper attention.

> **BOWEL FUNCTION IN EATING DISORDERS**
>
> Adolescents with bulimia—the binge-purge syndrome—frequently abuse laxatives to provoke diarrhea and purge unwanted calories. Constipation, by contrast, is a recognized complication of anorexia nervosa (also see Chapter 10, Eating Disorders). Apart from a diet that is woefully deficient in nutrients and bulk, an anorexic teenager has weakening of the intestinal muscles and an overall slowing of body metabolism, both of which are directly due to starvation. In addition, adolescents with this serious eating disorder typically drink very little for fear of becoming bloated. The weight of stool retained in the intestines can make it difficult to judge whether treatment is progressing. Finally, constipation may be worsened by medications used to treat anorexia.
>
> Specialists treating adolescents with anorexia manage constipation through a diet that includes adequate fiber and fluids. They also encourage moderate exercise and may recommend stool softeners and other medications if necessary.

pasta) that can be built into a healthy eating plan, and many of these products include the term *gluten free* on their packaging. Also, because celiac disease symptoms are often similar to those of other medical conditions, your doctor may recommend diagnostic tests, such as blood tests to look for high levels of particular antibodies (specialized proteins in the immune system) or a biopsy that takes a tissue sample from the small intestine through a thin tube (endoscope). Because celiac disease can be a serious disorder and is a lifelong condition, diagnostic confirmation is necessary. Because this condition tends to occur in families, the family members of a child with celiac disease may decide to be tested as well, especially if there are unexplained medical problems.

Cystic Fibrosis

Cystic fibrosis (CF) is an inherited condition that affects the function of every organ but especially the glands that produce mucus in the lungs, pancreas, liver, and intestines. Mucus blocks the ducts in the pancreas and blocks the release of enzymes and juices that are essential for digestion. Although young people with CF may eat large amounts, they often become malnourished because they cannot absorb nutrients. The stools of children with CF are pale, bulky, and fatty.

The severity of CF varies widely. Each affected child's diet must be individually prescribed and monitored to make up for specific nutrient losses as well as to make sure the child consumes enough calories. Many children with CF need supplementary digestive enzymes to offset damage to the pancreas. Children with CF lose excessive amounts of sodium and chloride when they sweat and need additional salt during hot weather, when they have a fever, or in other conditions that cause them to sweat a great deal. (In hot weather, children who do not have CF should not take salt supplements; rather, water is what they need.) Selenium supplements, once promoted as a miracle cure, have not been found to help those with CF.

Constipation

Pediatricians are often asked about constipation. People have the idea that constipation means not having a daily bowel movement. Many parents think their children will get sick if they don't have a movement every day. This isn't so. Some children (and adults) have several bowel movements every day, while others go 2 or 3 days or even longer, then pass a stool of normal consistency. A child is constipated only when the stool is hard or dry and can't be passed without straining or causing pain. Constipation may occur when the diet is lacking in fiber and fluid or when a child has been inactive and has taken fluids poorly during a viral illness.

It's quite normal for a breastfed baby to pass stools only once every 2 or 3 days, or even less frequently. This is because babies digest their mothers' milk so completely that there's not much residue. In contrast, some babies may pass stools several times a day, whether on human milk, formula, or a combination. This, too, is normal. As long as your baby is gaining weight and the stools are soft—semiliquid and seedy in a breastfed baby, no firmer than peanut butter in a formula-fed infant—the bowel movements are normal. If your baby's stools are hard and dry, like marbles; watery and filled with mucus; or whitish and claylike, talk to your pediatrician.

DON'T GIVE LAXATIVES OR ENEMAS

Never give laxatives or enemas to treat your child's constipation unless your pediatrician prescribes them. Used improperly, these products can disrupt bowel function and worsen the problem.

Occasionally, an infant becomes constipated with the introduction of solid foods between 4 and 6 months of age, or when cow's milk is introduced to the diet after about 1 year. If treatment for constipation is necessary for your child between 4 and 12 months, your pediatrician will discuss it with you and provide advice. It often helps to give the baby a small amount of diluted apple juice or prune juice, or a few teaspoons of pureed prunes. Changing from rice cereal to oatmeal to increase soluble fiber intake can help clear up the problem. Loosening foods, such as pureed apricots, also may help. In addition, a small serving (¼–⅓ cup) of prune or pear juice may have a laxative effect. Foods that tend to make stools firmer, such as bananas and applesauce, should be reduced or avoided until the problem is resolved.

A lot can be learned from vegetarians. They are rarely constipated because their diet includes a large amount of fiber. To keep your children's bowel movements regular, make sure their meals and snacks include high-fiber foods such as fruits, vegetables, and whole-grain breads and cereals. Nutrition experts recommend as a general rule that a person's daily intake of fiber should equal his age plus 5 g (thus, for a 7-year-old, 7 + 5 = 12 g a day; a safe range is age + 10 g a day) up to a maximum of 35 g a day. Oat bran cereal and popcorn are good sources of fiber that many children like to eat. A couple of prunes or a small glass of prune juice can help stimulate bowel function. Prunes contain a natural laxative, called isatin, as well as lots of soluble fiber and sorbitol—a naturally occurring, nonabsorbable sugar alcohol—both of which have laxative effects. Apple and pear juice are also good sources of sorbitol; however, cooked apples, such as in applesauce, may contribute to constipation and are often given to help children with the opposite problem—diarrhea. Plenty of water will help dietary fiber do its job. Consult your child's pediatrician about recommended fluid intake. Also, regular daily exercise helps promote regular bowel function.

There's one other approach to managing constipation that has received attention in recent years. A product called polyethylene glycol (PEG 3350) has been shown to be safe and effective for constipation in children as young as a few months old. It is not a laxative but works by drawing moisture into the stool. It is sold as a powder, is tasteless, and can be mixed in almost anything (eg, a drink, pudding, cereal). The dose varies with your child's size, and you should consult your pediatrician before using it.

When Constipation Looks Like Diarrhea

A few days before a long-planned family vacation, Carol Larson urgently called her pediatrician about her son. "We're supposed to catch a plane next weekend and Brendan has diarrhea," she told the doctor. "If I bring him over to your office, will you give him something so we can get through this?"

When the pediatrician examined 5-year-old Brendan, he found no sign of diarrhea, but he saw loose feces smeared on the child's underwear. This led the doctor to question Brendan and his mother about the child's usual bowel habits.

Brendan, it turned out, had very irregular bowel movements and was afraid to use the toilet. He often appeared to be trying to hold back a bowel movement. On the rare occasions when he couldn't hold it back, he would demand a diaper. His mother could hear him crying and straining behind the bathroom door. Finally, Brendan would emerge and give the diaper, soiled with loose stool, back to his mother, and the cycle would begin all over again.

The pediatrician explained to Carol that Brendan didn't have diarrhea. On the contrary, the child had severe constipation as a result of withholding stool. Liquid stool leaking out around an impaction—a large amount of stool in the colon—gave the appearance of diarrhea. This is called fecal soiling and is more common in boys.

The doctor outlined a treatment plan to help Brendan overcome his stool retention and fear of using the toilet. The first step was to empty the rectum of hard stool. Several enemas and continued efforts cleared enough of the impaction so that Brendan and his family could leave on their trip as planned, and he would have only a minimum amount of movements during the week's vacation. After they returned, a regular program including stool softeners and changes in toileting procedures solved the problem. It took several weeks, however, to change these habits. (Also see "Dealing With Stool Retention and Soiling" on page 230.)

ISSUES PARENTS OFTEN RAISE ABOUT DIGESTIVE PROBLEMS

My mother-in-law says my baby isn't getting enough to eat because he spits up a lot. She says if I would just add some cereal to his bottle, he wouldn't spit up.

Spitting up is normal and rarely interferes with a baby's nutrition. If your baby spits up unusually often, your pediatrician may recommend thickening his formula with a very small amount of rice cereal. Never add solids to the bottle unless your pediatrician advises it. Your baby also may do better with smaller and more frequent feedings (see page 213).

My 8-year-old has terrible gas. He embarrasses me by burping loudly when we go out.

School-aged children and adolescents gulp down air when eating or chewing gum; carbonated drinks also lead to gas buildup. Encourage your child to take a bit more time over meals and to avoid carbonated drinks if gas is bothersome. If he belches noisily to gain attention, let him know that this behavior is unacceptable, but avoid reacting with the extra notice he craves (see page 215).

My toddler wads up food in her cheeks. Is this behavior a health hazard?

Pouching isn't a health hazard unless the wad is so large that the child could choke. It's not safe, however, to let a poucher nap or go to bed with food in her cheeks. If you can't persuade your child to spit it out, try to clear the pouches with your finger and give her a drink of water to rinse her mouth (see page 216).

My daughter dreads long car trips because they make her sick to her stomach. I tried a medication from the pharmacy, but it made her sleepy.

Encourage your child to eat a few crackers or another light snack before setting out. Make sure that her seat allows a clear view to the outside; many people feel less nauseous if they can focus on a point in the distance. Avoid activities that require her to look down like video games or reading. Your pediatrician will advise you about using preventive medications (see page 219).

How long should I keep my child on a soft diet when he has diarrhea?

Resume small servings of a normal diet as soon as the child feels up to eating. Bowel movements return to normal faster with a regular diet than when only soft foods are given (see page 221). Breastfeeding should be continued.

Can irritable bowel syndrome lead to serious diseases like cancer?

Irritable bowel syndrome does not lead to more serious conditions. However, because all the symptoms of irritable bowel syndrome also may be related to potentially serious diseases, a child with recurrent bowel upsets should be evaluated by a pediatrician to rule out other conditions (see page 226).

Chapter 10

Eating Disorders

Odd behaviors and rituals with food are common in children and adolescents. In most cases, they fade away over time and have no harmful health effects. Eating disorders, on the other hand, are expressed in persistent patterns of behavior that are associated with major psychological issues that lead to serious health problems and can endanger life.

Kathleen, at 16, brought home excellent school reports, had an active social life, and was a dedicated ballet student. Her parents were understandably proud of her accomplishments.

Knowledgeable about food, Kathleen sometimes prepared elaborate dishes for special occasions. However, she was usually too busy to join the family at the table and often declined to eat with them.

When she did eat with the family, she took tiny portions, cut them into pieces, and never finished a plateful. Family meals began to turn into pitched battles, with Kathleen's mother urging her to eat and her father trying to make peace between them.

It was the ballet teacher who brought up the idea that Kathleen's behavior might be more than adolescent obstinacy. Kathleen's mother took her to see their pediatrician. Kathleen hadn't menstruated in more than 6 months, and she had covered up a dramatic weight loss by wrapping herself in oversized shirts and sweatpants.

Kathleen's pediatrician told them that Kathleen had anorexia nervosa, a serious disorder that requires the attention of a specially qualified treatment team. He referred the family to a clinic that provides nutritional, medical, and psychological support.

He also warned that treatment can be difficult and it usually takes a long time. Relapses are common, but this is a very serious physical and psychological problem, and failure to obtain treatment is very dangerous.

Who Develops Eating Disorders?

In the United States, as many as 10 million females and 1 million males are fighting a life-and-death battle with an eating disorder such as anorexia or bulimia. Millions more are struggling with binge-eating disorder. The true number is difficult to know because many people manage to hide their eating problems even from those closest to them. Once thought to be restricted to middle- and upper-income families, eating disorders are increasingly found at every social and economic level.

Eating disorders most commonly start in girls between ages 14 and 17 years but are also seen in adolescent boys and younger children. Overall, girls with eating disorders outnumber boys by about 10 to 1. The roots of the problem appear to be complex. Outside influences are one contributor to eating disorders; for example, magazines, movies, and television promote thinness. Most young people can deal with the message, but those who develop an eating disorder are more susceptible and cannot keep the media images in perspective. Young people are rarely aware of the extent to which images are altered to make models or actresses appear perfect, and they aspire to what they perceive as perfect beauty. However, there are invariably more complex and deep-seated psychological issues and genetic vulnerabilities that influence who is susceptible, including low self-esteem.

EATING DISORDER RISK FACTORS
• Family history of eating disorder or obesity
• Affective illness or alcoholism in first-degree relatives
• Ballet, gymnastics, modeling, "visual sports"
• Personality traits (eg, perfectionism)
• Parental eating behavior and weight
• Physical or sexual abuse
• Low self-esteem
• Body-image dissatisfaction
• History of excessive dieting, frequently skipped meals, compulsive exercise

Source: Rome ES, Ammerman S, Rosen DS, et al. Children and adolescents with eating disorders: the state of the art. *Pediatrics.* 2003;111:e98–e108

No age group is immune. Eating disorders in children younger than 14 years are described as *childhood onset*. Some women secretly persist in eating disorders from their teens into their 20s, 30s, and beyond. Others develop abnormal eating and exercise behaviors in response to stress long after adolescence is over. This type of eating and overconcern with body shape and image is an occupational hazard for those whose jobs or activities rely on appearance, such as fashion models, dancers and other performers, and competitive athletes like gymnasts.

Jackie, at 18, was tall and slim and a rising star in track and field. A rigorous training schedule kept her muscles toned and allowed her to eat as much as she wanted. A scout for a modeling agency tapped her at a regional track meet and invited her to audition for the agency.

Jackie had always taken pride in looking her well-groomed best. But she was first puzzled, then angry, and finally disillusioned when executives at the agency evaluated her appearance. They told her she'd have to stop running to reduce her muscle development. They also told her to follow an extremely low-calorie diet to strip 15 pounds from her already slender body.

After talking it over with her parents, Jackie decided that a modeling career was not for her. She took the next flight home to begin her college applications and resume the sports in which she excelled.

Many young women who are attracted by promises of the wealth and glamour of a modeling career are not as clear-eyed as Jackie. In their efforts to achieve the perfect form for runway or photographic modeling (far different from the average woman's shape), some adopt practices that are detrimental to health and can develop into eating disorders. Dancers and some athletes such as gymnasts, long-distance runners, synchronized swimmers, figure skaters, and wrestlers are often susceptible to similar pressures.

BEAUTY IS MORE THAN SKIN DEEP

Help your children to feel comfortable with whom they are. Encourage them to discover and develop their natural talents and activities that bring them pleasure, no matter how modest, and to look beyond appearances and media portraits in finding others to admire.

RISKS FOR ADOLESCENT ATHLETES

High school and college athletes are particularly susceptible to eating disorders. For example, some coaches encourage wrestlers to develop strength by training above their weight limits but competing at a lower weight, just under the limit. Wrestlers may be pressured to lose several pounds in the few days before a competition. Adolescent athletes are often urged to follow drastic and unbalanced weight-loss regimens (eg, eating only bananas or oranges for days). In the past, several college wrestlers died when trying to make a weight class by going without food and water and working out while wearing special clothing to promote sweating. These practices are unsafe. The American College of Sports Medicine and some states have released guidelines for weight control and monitoring high school and collegiate wrestlers (www.acsm.org). Coaches should be responsible for encouraging healthful eating and exercise. Parents who suspect that their children are subjected to dangerous or abusive practices should stop their children's involvement and bring their concerns to the attention of school or college authorities.

COMMON FORERUNNERS OF EATING DISORDERS

Be on the lookout for diet fads, especially with adolescent girls. Some, such as high-protein, very low-carbohydrate regimens, require medical supervision when used in adolescents. They've been around for decades and resurface periodically under new names. The more extreme diet routines are never intended for long-term adoption. Prescription and nonprescription over-the-counter and over-the-Internet preparations and supplements are poorly regulated and have contributed to serious and deadly problems. Ephedra-containing over-the-counter diet aids illustrate the hazards of these products. In 2004, after compounds containing ephedra or the related compound ephedrine were found to be associated with a number of deaths, they were banned by the Food and Drug Administration. Fen-phen combination prescription diet pills led to fatal heart complications in some users in the 1990s. Ipecac abuse by people with eating disorders caused permanent damage to hearts.

The principal eating disorders are *anorexia nervosa*, or self-starvation, and *bulimia nervosa*, or binge eating followed by purging through induced vomiting or laxative abuse to prevent weight gain. Another less "formal" but common eating disorder is *bulimorexia*—starvation alternating with gorging and induced purging. Whatever the specific behavior and diagnosis, those with eating disorders share a preoccupation with their food, weight, and shape;

WARNING SIGNS OF ANOREXIA

If you answer "Yes" to several of these questions, talk with your child and pediatrician.

- Does your child skip family meals and prepare her own food instead?
- Is she following her own diet?
- Are certain food groups or nutrients categorically excluded?
- Are no- or low-calorie foods and drinks a major part of daily intake?
- Has she adopted a "healthy" vegetarian diet suddenly and obsessively?
- Are diet pills or preparations in her possession?
- Is she overly concerned with losing or gaining weight?
- Have you found laxatives that you did not give her?
- Does she hide food in her room?
- Does she visit the bathroom after eating? Does she flush the toilet, run water, or turn on the shower while in the bathroom?
- Has your plumbing repeatedly and inexplicably become clogged?
- Does she have an unusual number of scratches or cuts over her knuckles?
- Does she have swollen cheeks or lymph nodes around her face, or broken blood vessels in the whites of her eyes?
- Has she lost a lot of weight in a short time?
- Does she look gaunt?
- Does she get dizzy or is she easily fatigued?
- Does she have frequent headaches, heartburn, or constipation?
- Have her periods stopped?
- Does she play with her food without actually eating it?
- Has she developed downy hair on her face, arms, and back?
- Can you see the bones of her back and collarbones clearly outlined? Does she have bruises along her backbone?
- Does she wear loose, bulky clothing?
- Does she exercise for hours on end with a routine that can't be interrupted or changed?
- Has she become withdrawn from her friends or family? Does she seem more secretive?

have a severely erratic or inadequate food intake; and can't regulate their eating and related emotions. They often have other symptoms of anxiety, depression, and obsessive-compulsive thoughts and symptoms. Some develop substance use problems over time.

Girls who start menstruating earlier than their peers tend to have more problems with body image and a somewhat higher risk of eating disorders. Children from families with eating disorders and obsessive-compulsive disorders are also more vulnerable.

Anorexia Nervosa

Anorexia nervosa affects 0.5% to 1% of women in the United States during their lifetime. Apart from drastic weight loss, the effects of anorexia include failure to menstruate, a slow-down of the body's metabolism, and other physical and psychological changes described in starvation victims. Body temperature drops and skin is cool to the touch. Hands and feet look purple from changes in circulation; the face and body may have an orange tinge from changes in the way the liver handles vitamin A and related compounds found in yellow and orange foods. Despite a woefully inadequate intake of calories, those with anorexia are often remarkably animated and energetic. They may exercise for hours on end to burn off the calories from something they've eaten. Many have trouble sleeping. Most are severely constipated because the body's metabolism slows down and the intake of food, fluid, and fiber is not enough to keep the bowel moving. Some people with anorexia drink large amounts of water or find ways to add weight with hidden metal objects under clothing before medical examinations to try to hide weight loss.

Without treatment, a person with anorexia develops severe nutritional deficiencies. In extreme cases (up to 5 out of every 100) the final result is death due to abnormal heart rhythm causing a massive heart attack or other effects of starvation.

Like many girls with anorexia nervosa, Kathleen was a high achiever who pushed herself to perform. Also like many others, Kathleen was preoccupied with food—thinking about it, planning meals, cooking it, serving it to others, playing with it, and analyzing every last calorie, fat gram, and nutrient. The only thing she didn't do with food was eat normal amounts. When she ate at all, she tried to work off the calories with punishing exercise. Although on one level Kathleen persisted in the delusion that she was fat or not thin enough, on another she recognized that she looked abnormal because she took pains to conceal her increasing emaciation under layers of bulky clothing. This had the further advantage, as she saw it, of promoting weight loss through perspiration.

If you suspect that your child is starving herself, or if someone brings it to your attention, quickly seek professional help. You might be wrong or overly worried, but you might be right, and early identification and treatment improve outcomes. Anorexia is a life-threatening condition, and one of its signs is the inability to acknowledge the problem and its seriousness. Anorexia hinders a person's ability to make rational decisions concerning her own health. One of the most promising approaches to treatment is a method that puts parents in charge of refeeding their child, with education, therapy, and support provided by a specially trained team. Inpatient therapy may be required for more severe cases. However, outpatient behavioral management that focuses on nutritional rehabilitation and normalizing eating behavior with the help of a multidisciplinary team is generally regarded as the best approach after the patient is medically and nutritionally stable. Other psychiatric problems may be identified and should be evaluated and treated by an experienced mental health professional.

A person under treatment for anorexia nervosa often passes through 3 phases. First, the eating disorder itself is the focus of attention. Second, an improvement in dietary intake is offset by a shift in attitude; the anorexic becomes hostile and sullen. Finally, the anorexic begins to eat more normally and is more pleasant and cooperative. A successful transition from the second to third phase indicates the best chance of long-term recovery; in other words, eating normally and maintaining an appropriate weight. At this stage there is restoration of physical

---

WHEN PARENTS HAVE EATING DISORDERS

Adults, most frequently women, are not immune to eating disorders. When mothers have or have had an eating disorder, they often send mixed messages to their children about body size and the foods they eat. For example, they may be less consistent or more rigid about family rules related to what children can or cannot eat. This kind of inconsistency can lead to repeated requests by their children for certain foods because children are never sure what the rules are. If mothers are overly rigid, children may consider certain foods to be forbidden fruit, which only makes them more desirable. The children of parents with eating disorders may carry a genetic vulnerability to eating disorders so the parent's behaviors may be especially difficult for them to handle.

and psychological health. About one third of anorexics have long-term problems coping with food and accepting a normal weight. The younger the child is when anorexia develops, the poorer the chances of recovery. Early intervention has a better prognosis. The disease and treatment are relatively long lasting and long term, but most individuals will get better.

Bulimia Nervosa

Stacy, at age 14, was already a veteran of the diet wars. Her figure-conscious mother waged a continual battle, counting calories, serving commercial diet meals, and pinning her hopes on "miracle" diet supplements and formulas. In her mother's presence, Stacy dutifully nibbled on calorie-controlled portions and salads without dressing. Her weight stayed the same, however, and truth to tell, Stacy wasn't fat. She had simply inherited the stocky build of her father's side of the family.

What nobody else knew, however, was that at least once or twice a week, Stacy went on an eating binge. Her allowance and earnings from a part-time job easily covered a couple of quarts of ice cream or packages of chocolate chip cookies, a whole pizza with sausage and extra cheese, party-sized bags of potato chips and cheese snacks, quarts of soda, or sometimes an entire cheesecake from the frozen-foods section of the supermarket. Occasionally she stole candy bars when she did not have the money to pay for them. Many or most of these and more went down at the same time, depending on how tense and upset she felt. The tension she felt beforehand was nothing, of course, compared with the shame she felt when the binge was over. But she found a way to fix that. As soon as the urge to binge began to wear off, Stacy would stick her fingers down her throat and bring it all up. She felt bad for a while because her stomach and throat hurt. "It's just my period," Stacy replied when her mother once asked what was going on in the bathroom. She was always careful to throw out empty food packages away from her house.

Stacy was ashamed of the bingeing and purging but told herself it wasn't wrecking her calorie intake. After all, she got rid of most of the calories before her body could absorb them.

As Stacy approached college age, she wanted to be as slender as the more popular girls in her class. Reasoning that what worked for bingeing would work even better every day, Stacy began to finish off every dinner by secretly vomiting. She knew she needed a certain amount

EATING DISORDER EMERGENCY
If your child has an eating disorder and develops a rapid or irregular heartbeat, chest pain, or fainting, or if her weight loss continues, call your pediatrician and get emergency care at once. She may have a life-threatening complication.

of food, so she kept her purging for the major meal of the day. Besides, the mornings were too rushed and school lunchtimes were difficult.

When a dental checkup revealed erosion of the enamel on her rear teeth, the dentist called Stacy's mother. "I think you'd better talk to Stacy and call your pediatrician. Her teeth look as if they've been in an acid bath. This is the sort of problem we see in young people with eating disorders. They throw up so much that the stomach acid actually erodes the teeth." Another telltale sign may be scratches on the knuckles or back of the hand, caused by the teeth when fingers are pushed down the throat.

After examining Stacy, her pediatrician recommended evaluation at a clinic that offered a team approach to the management of eating disorders.

For some people with bulimia, vomiting is a way to release built-up emotional tension in addition to ridding the body of calories. Many people practice vomiting even without bingeing as a misguided method of weight control. Some hide their disorder and may binge and purge for years undiscovered. Because of their poor self-image and impulsivity, others are vulnerable to adopting other problem behaviors such as alcohol and other drug use, a pattern of controlling and exploitative relationships.

These conditions are difficult to diagnose because people with bulimia or mixed eating disorders are often of normal weight or, in the case of bulimia, even a little overweight. In contrast to girls with anorexia, girls with bulimia usually do not completely lose their periods because their weight and body fat rarely fall below critical levels. However, they may have irregular menstrual cycles and other reproductive health problems. They also may have mood swings, swollen glands in the neck and face, stomach pain, and sore throats. Repeated vomiting creates an acid bath that burns the mucous membrane lining the esophagus and erodes the tooth enamel. Chronic heartburn and dental problems are among the consequences of long-standing bulimia. In severe cases, a patient may hemorrhage from the esophagus and develop a dangerous imbalance of potassium and other salts, which can lead to disturbances in the heart rhythm.

Once vomiting is established as a means of coping, bulimia can be difficult to treat. The person has to be willing to accept help. If you suspect bulimia in your child, talk to her and consult your pediatrician, who may provide a referral to an eating disorders clinic or recommend a psychotherapist experienced in treating adolescents with such problems. Medications may also be helpful in decreasing binging and purging behaviors.

Binge-Eating Disorder

Binge eaters repeatedly gorge on large quantities of food, sometimes equal to several days' worth of calories at once, and feel out of control. Binges are typically followed by intense feelings of guilt and shame. Unlike bulimics, however, binge eaters do not purge themselves with vomiting or laxatives. As a result, they are usually (but not always) overweight. It's estimated that about 2 out of every 100 adolescents and adults are binge eaters. They seldom have outward physical symptoms other than weight gain, but they are at risk for problems associated with obesity, including high blood pressure, elevated blood cholesterol levels, gall bladder disease, sleep apnea, fatigue, chronic headaches, asthma, diabetes, and other psychological problems.

As with bulimia, binge eating can be difficult to diagnose, although it may emerge in the course of consultations for a weight problem as a result of trust and thoughtful nonjudgmental questioning. Sometimes, parents get their first clue that a young person is binge eating when food inexplicably disappears from the kitchen. If you are concerned about your child's weight or eating, talk to her and discuss it with your pediatrician.

Recovery

The team approach for treating eating disorders involves psychotherapy, medical intervention, and nutritional counseling. Anorexia nervosa treatment is usually in 2 phases. During the recovery phase, medical problems are treated and eating is gradually reintroduced until

---

ISSUES PARENTS RAISE ABOUT EATING DISORDERS

We've been advised to see a doctor because the school nurse thinks our daughter may have an eating disorder. Her weight is normal and she's very energetic, so how could this be?

First, find out what led the nurse to make this suggestion. Often friends and school staff notice weight loss and changes in eating and attitude. It is awkward and uncomfortable for peers and adults to know what to do with their observations and worries. They may mention their concerns to a school nurse, coach, or counselor, or a parent. It is common for that adult to call a teen's parent. Such calls should be taken seriously because someone who cares is worried. Eating disorders sometimes remain undetected because the victims are of normal weight or even overweight and they can hide their behaviors from the family. Treatment is necessary to prevent serious effects on health (see page 237). Talk with your pediatrician and follow any recommendations for further consultations and treatment.

Do children with eating disorders start out as picky eaters?

Picky eaters may remain picky eaters (see page 240), but they do not necessarily develop eating disorders. Children who have anxiety problems or obsessive-compulsive behaviors are more at risk. Eating disorders most commonly appear in girls between ages 14 and 17 years, but they are also seen in adolescent boys and younger children. In fact, they can occur at any age (see page 238).

The high school wrestling coach told my son to eat very little for the next 4 days so he can make weight for a competition. Is this a safe way to lose weight?

This is a dangerous practice and it is banned by school and college athletics authorities. For more information on sports medicine and exercise science, check out the American College of Sports Medicine Web site, www.acsm.org. Keep your son on a balanced diet with plenty of fluids when he exercises, and report the coach's irresponsible advice to the high school. (Also see page 240.)

---

weight returns to close to normal. In the maintenance phase, efforts focus on normal eating patterns and preventing a relapse.

Because many people with anorexia are averse to food and cannot eat much at a time, calories are spread out through the day by way of snacks and mini-meals. Someone with or recovering from anorexia will almost always feel too full to finish their allotted food prescription. A healthy goal weight is generally higher than the level that feels comfortable, so ongoing weight gain is an uphill battle. Relapses are common.

Treating bulimia and binge eating involves teaching the young person to eat in response to hunger rather than to inappropriate cues such as loneliness or boredom. In contrast with anorexia nervosa, the goal is not weight gain if weight is within normal range or higher. Instead, the aim of treatment is to maintain weight while learning new patterns of eating. Those who are overweight must learn how to eat and exercise normally to achieve and maintain a healthy weight.

With all eating disorders, the various ways in which family members express themselves, relate to one another, and handle stress can feed into the child's feelings of lack of control and make the situation worse. Treatment that involves the whole family can change the dynamics for the better and help the person with the eating disorder.

Chapter 11

What Do I Do About Outside Influences?

You will soon find out—if you don't know it already—that your child's eating habits are affected by a lot more than your good advice. Friends, grandparents, child care providers, and last but certainly not least, the media have a great influence over children's food likes and dislikes.

When 7-year-old Greg demanded salt to shake over his meal, his mother refused. The food was well seasoned, she explained, and it isn't good for our bodies to eat too much salt.

"Dad always puts a lot of salt on his food, so is he going to get sick?" Greg countered.

Startled by the first grader's awareness, Greg's father agreed that he often added salt from force of habit, even before tasting his food. Greg's parents stopped putting the saltshaker out on the table and Greg was pleased that his watchfulness might help Dad stay healthy.

An Influential Role

As a parent, you have the first and possibly the most lasting influence on your child. That is true of many things, including food. You may not realize it, but every time you eat you're setting an example for your child. He is likely to be influenced by what, how, where, when, and with whom you eat. By watching you, your child begins to form his own ideas of the "right" way to eat. This is especially true from birth through his preschool years, and you continue to have an effect even through the stormy teenage years—although that may be difficult to believe when you watch adolescents' behavior.

While your influence is great, you don't have to be a dictator. Rather, try to take a matter-of-fact approach. Simply keep your kitchen stocked with healthful foods and prepare appealing meals on a regular schedule. Let your child see that you eat healthful foods and moderate amounts. As a parent, you should control what foods are brought into the house, and you can be a healthy role model. But you cannot and should not watch over your child's shoulder. The older your children are, the less likely they are to respond positively to such supervision, and they may do exactly the opposite of what you've intended.

It's important to remember that as the parent, you are responsible for putting healthful meals on the table. It is your child's responsibility to eat them. Force-feeding is never the answer. Young children's appetites come and go with different stages of development—often even from day to day. Accept these changes, knowing that your child will probably make up for a lack of appetite today by eating heartily later in the week. If, however, lack of appetite becomes a chronic, long-term problem, talk it over with your child's pediatrician. In older children, especially girls, a chronic lack of appetite could be the sign of an eating disorder. (See Chapter 10, Eating Disorders.)

For younger children, avoid giving food as a reward or withholding it as a form of punishment. Bribery doesn't work. Threatening to withhold ice cream if your child doesn't eat her peas, or not allowing her to watch her favorite television show unless she cleans her plate, will only backfire. Such threats exaggerate the value of the carrot being dangled—in this case, ice cream or television. Moreover, a child who is pressured to eat may end up eating less than one who is allowed to choose what and how much to eat from what's offered.

For older children, unless what they're eating is actually harmful, avoid passing judgment. Doing so will only make matters worse. Your child's latest dietary dos and don'ts may be nothing more than a passing phase.

Lifestyle Logistics

When both parents work outside the home and older children are involved with outside activities such as sports, dance, or scouting, every minute of family time counts. Much of that family time is likely to be mealtime. To make the most of it, don't let television take the place of talking to one another. Nor is a meal the time to read the newspaper or air grievances with other family members. Because family time is precious, try to make the time spent together at meals an opportunity for talking and listening rather than for arguments and confrontations. A peaceful atmosphere increases the chance that your child or teenager will talk about

WE DON'T NEED TO ADD SALT TO FOOD

Table salt is made up of sodium and chloride, 2 chemicals that are essential for health but only in very small amounts. Sodium and chloride occur naturally in many foods and it's not necessary to add them to prepared foods. A balanced diet based on the *Dietary Guidelines for Americans* (www.cnpp.usda.gov/DietaryGuidelines.htm) contains more than enough sodium to meet our daily requirement. Americans on average eat about 1 to 3 teaspoons of salt a day, adding up to between 2,300 and 6,900 mg of sodium. But the average daily sodium *requirement* is much less, ranging from 1,200 g of sodium for 4- to 8-year-old children to 1,500 g for 9- to 18-year-olds. This amounts to about half a teaspoon of salt a day.

We add salt to food from force of habit or because we've learned to like a salty taste. Adding moderate amounts of salt to food for taste is acceptable, but excessive amounts of salt should be discouraged as the child's taste preferences are formed early and large quantities of sodium may lead to high blood pressure later in life. So it's a good idea to train children to avoid unnecessary salt. One way is to keep the saltshaker off the dinner table. Taste food *before* you add salt and other seasonings. At the same time, keep in mind that most of the sodium in our diets does *not* come from salt added at the table or while cooking. Almost 80% of the sodium in our diets comes from processed foods like bread, soups, salty snacks, fast foods, canned foods, or processed meats.

HIGH-SODIUM PACKAGED FOODS	
Serving Size	**Sodium (mg)**
Maruchan Instant Lunch Ramen Noodles with Vegetables, 1 package	1,120
Progresso Classics Hearty Tomato Soup, 1 cup	1,110
Celeste Pizza for One, Original Cheese, 1 pizza	1,090
Giant Spaghetti Rings, 1 cup	970
Oscar Mayer Lunchables Deluxe Ham & Swiss & Cheddar, 1 package	930
Stouffer's Lean Cuisine Macaroni and Cheese Frozen Dinner, 1 package	630

(continued on next page)

WE DON'T NEED TO ADD SALT TO FOOD, *CONTINUED*	
HIGH-SODIUM RESTAURANT FOODS	
Item	**Sodium (mg)**
Cheese fries with ranch dressing	4,890
House Lo Mein	3,460
Denny's Meat Lover's Scramble (2 eggs scrambled with bacon, ham, sausage, and cheddar cheese)	3,180
Beef with broccoli with rice	3,150
Buffalo wings with blue cheese dressing and celery sticks	2,460
Spaghetti with sausage	2,440

Adapted from Center for Science in the Public Interest, www.cspinet.org/salt/hsrestaurant.html and www.cspinet.org/salt/hspackaged.html, accessed June 2, 2011

her day. It also makes it more likely that young children will taste and accept new foods. By doing your best to create a welcoming atmosphere, you'll make mealtimes occasions the whole family looks forward to with pleasure.

Unfortunately, for many families, family mealtime is more an illusion than a reality. When the entire family is in a constant time crunch with no chance to sit down for family meals, nutrition suffers. Fast food and takeout become a habit, especially for evening meals. When both parents work outside the home, teenagers may be responsible for many of their own meals and those of younger siblings. Fast food offers an easy solution. But fast food doesn't have to mean bad food. There are lower-fat, lower-calorie healthier options at many fast-food restaurants. With just a little planning, you can point your family in the direction of these more healthful foods and still get them fed in the limited time available.

If family meals are rare during the workweek at your house, try to make at least one meal on the weekend—say Sunday dinner—a time when everyone is expected to take part. And do your best to set the example you wish you had time for during the week by serving a variety of healthful foods.

Child Care Providers

When Deborah Jackson went back to work 3 days a week, she was lucky to find a kind, active caregiver who looked after her 2 children with grandmotherly concern. The children looked forward to the caregiver's visits. They loved their daily reward of candy "for being good" and the potato chips and chocolate chip cookies she regularly served as after-school snacks.

But when Deborah became aware of these snacks, she approached the problem as if speaking to her own mother. "The children are so happy, they feel they've practically got a new grandma. And I can go back to work with peace of mind. But we have our own way of doing things. I prefer to serve carrots and celery sticks or crackers and cheese for after-school snacks, and we save cookies for special treats. When it comes to being good, a word of praise is enough; they don't need candy. It's fine for a treat once in a while, but I worry about their teeth if they have it every day."

Deborah backed up the discussion by writing daily instructions that always ended with a cheerful note of thanks. If her caregiver privately thought Deborah was a bit misguided, she kept it to herself and went along with Deborah's wishes.

Regardless of whether you're an at-home parent or work outside the home, chances are that at some point in your child's life you'll have to deal with outside influences on what your

MAKING MORE HEALTHFUL CHOICES	
Instead of	**Choose**
Pan-crust pepperoni pizza with extra cheese	Thin-crust vegetarian pizza with a sprinkling of cheese
Cheeseburger with fries	Grilled chicken sandwich with baked potato
Beef burrito with sour cream and cheese	Bean burrito with lettuce, tomato, and salsa
Chicken nuggets with fries	Chicken fajita with salad and low-fat dressing

child eats. That holds true whether it's a live-in nanny, the teenager across the street, or a group care worker who looks after your child. How you handle different influences depends on who's doing the feeding. Your neighbor's teenaged daughter will probably readily take instructions about what your child should and shouldn't eat. If she does not follow instructions well, she probably won't be getting too many more babysitting jobs.

A live-in nanny should also be willing to follow your wishes about feeding your child. But if your care provider is older and has children of her own, or comes from another culture with different ideas about food, it could be more of a challenge to make sure your child gets the foods you want her to have. You and your care provider may agree to disagree about what food is right, but be firm in letting her know how you would like your child's meals prepared. Be specific; the clearer your instructions, the less likely it is you'll have disagreements. If you work full-time, chances are your care provider will feed more meals and snacks to your child than you do. So it's crucial to have open communication to ensure your child's good nutrition and your peace of mind.

What your child eats at a child care center is less within your control. When selecting a care center, look into the food selections and how meals are served. If you're not satisfied with the food provided, speak with the director to find out if changes can be made or your child can brown-bag meals and snacks. If you're able to pack your child's meals and snacks for the day (some places require it, but others don't allow it), include whole-grain breads, cereals, and crackers; a source of protein such as lean meat, fish, or low-fat cheese; and fruits and vegetables.

Family Food Feuds

You work hard at putting food on the table. You read labels, select foods of good quality, and try out new, healthful recipes. So don't let critical comments from visiting family members throw you off balance. Your father may grumble that there's not enough meat on the table, or your mother may insist that your 5-year-old needs whole-fat milk to stay healthy. Remember that they mean well. However, as the parent in charge of the household, you control what's put on the table.

If it's your mother or mother-in-law who's offering feeding advice, the situation may have to be handled with special finesse. After all, these women come with experience and memories of rearing and feeding their own children. As they see it, their children turned out all right, so what's wrong with the way they did things? Don't give a lecture on how times have changed or why your meals are more nutritious and healthful; you'll invite a confrontation, and power struggles over food only create an uncomfortable mood at the dinner table. Feelings may be hurt unless suggestions are made tactfully. Instead of, "Don't force any more food on Tim," it may be more helpful to say, "We've learned that Tim likes to decide for himself how much to eat." Or rather than, "Don't overload Cindy's plate," try, "Cindy has an easier time eating if you only offer one or two foods at a time." Or try recruiting your mother's or mother-in-law's help. "Mom, I need a hand. Could you feed the baby while I finish getting dinner?" If your dad wants more meat on the table, budget your family's fat intake to allow a roast or steak dinner when he visits.

What should you do about comments from other family members? Thank them for their suggestions, chalk them up to differences of opinion, and let it go. You may never truly see eye to eye, but you all have the same goal—to do the best for your children and see them grow up healthy and strong.

Peer Pressure

On weeknights, 3-year-old Stephanie ate earlier than her parents because her father didn't get home from work until close to her bedtime. Stephanie's mother planned meals carefully but sometimes allowed the preschooler a choice for supper. Stephanie set a personal record for consistency by asking for spaghetti with tomato-vegetable sauce every night for

---

LUNCH BOX ALTERNATIVES FOR GOOD NUTRITION

- Whole wheat bread is out? Try a whole-grain, high-fiber white bread.
- They want bologna? Try a low-fat turkey bologna instead of beef.
- The apple is now a thing of the past? Try applesauce or a different fruit.
- Chips are a must? Replace greasy, salty potato chips with low-fat baked snacks, or try a reduced-fat, low-salt brand of potato or vegetable chips.

2 weeks in a row (except on the weekend, when she ate dinner with her parents). On the 15th evening, Stephanie threw a tantrum when she saw her mother reach for the pasta box. "No spaghetti!" she shrieked. "I hate bad worms!"

Stephanie's mother was relieved that the spaghetti craze was over. While it made meals easy, it certainly was boring. When Stephanie calmed down, however, she revealed that her best friend at child care had let her in on a big secret—spaghetti with red sauce was made with worms and blood, and no 3-year-old in her right mind should eat it.

Stephanie's parents bought pasta in different shapes and experimented with different sauces until the great worm scare was forgotten.

As a parent, you should brace yourself for unexpected influences that can affect your children as early as age 2½ years. By this time, most children are talking and beginning to socialize with siblings and neighbors, in play groups, or with others in preschool or child care. Food likes and dislikes among toddlers and school-aged children can vary from day to day. While a food may have been your child's favorite for weeks, even months, don't be surprised if it's suddenly blacklisted. This may simply be a toddler's fickle tastes or the result of another child telling her that it's disgusting.

When she reaches school age, your child's focus will shift away from the home toward friends, teachers, and outside activities. The influences affecting her will grow wider, while what you do will seem somewhat less important.

You may begin to see the effects of peer pressure early on, when your first grader decides she no longer wants whole wheat bread for her sandwiches because her best friend always has white bread. Other children will ask what's in her lunch box and tell her what they think of it. There are ways to make the experience easier on your child while still giving her the good nutrition you want her to have.

In early adolescence and later, your child's friends are likely to have a growing influence on what, when, and how she eats. As with many other aspects of life, from dress to language, adolescents are likely to make food choices with little more in mind than what their friends think. Because adolescents are self-conscious about their changing bodies and may not be completely comfortable with the changes taking place, concern with size and shape can easily cross over into obsession. That makes adolescence a high-risk time for eating disorders such as anorexia nervosa and bulimia. But because our society as whole values thinness, while obesity is often viewed as a character defect rather than a disorder, it is sometimes tough to tell when a teenager's preoccupation has crossed the line. (Also see Chapter 10, Eating Disorders.) While girls' concerns most often center on thinness, boys pay more attention to muscle development. High-priced products such as protein powders and amino acid supplements promise body-builder physiques but deliver little more than unnecessary protein.

While your teenaged boy may amaze you at the sheer quantities of food he can eat in one sitting, try not to become a food monitor. If your teenager is normally active, chances are he'll naturally regulate his own intake. Because weight is such a pressing concern for adolescent girls, parental watchfulness together with warnings of eating too much could have the

SNACKS: THE WELL-STOCKED KITCHEN	
Low-fat yogurt	Low-fat pudding
Fresh fruit	1%-fat or skim milk
High-fiber, unsweetened cereals	Low-fat cottage cheese
Nuts	Dried fruit
Low-fat microwave popcorn	Rice cakes
Reduced-fat cheese	Whole-grain crackers
Peanut butter	Whole wheat bread
Bagels	Pita bread
Low-fat lunch meats, cold cuts	Reduced-fat mayonnaise or fat-free dressings
Pretzels	Baked snack chips
Tofu	Microwaveable, low-fat entrees (eg, enchiladas, burritos, pasta with chunky tomato and vegetable sauce)
Bean dip, chickpea spread (hummus), eggplant dip	Salsa
Low-fat granola bars	
Prepackaged, precut vegetables with low-fat dips	

opposite effect to what you intend. Your teenager may eat more than normal just to prove she is in control.

As your adolescent matures and learns more about food and nutrition from other sources, it's likely she'll begin to develop her own opinions. She may begin to experiment with different food styles, such as vegetarianism. Try not to react negatively. Rather, listen to the reasons behind the decision and try to be supportive. Learn as much as you can about this new eating style so you can help your teenager use it to achieve a nutritionally balanced diet. (Also read about alternative diets and supplements in Chapter 15.) Now is a good time to shift responsibility for some shopping and food preparation to your child, especially if her new eating style is different from that of the rest of the family. However, if the new way of eating seems unhealthy, it is your responsibility to explain why it's *not* a good idea. Round up some reading material that supports what you're saying if your teenager is unwilling to accept your opinions about food fads or even junk foods. It becomes even more important to provide healthful choices when the family eats together because you have less influence on what your adolescent eats outside the home. If your teenager is always on the run, coming in to eat at odd hours long after the table has been cleared, keep the kitchen stocked with nutritious, easy-to-fix foods and snacks that you know she will eat. If you lay a good foundation at home, chances are your teenager will do just fine, in spite of temptations and distractions.

Limit Media Influences

Like it or not, media has a major effect on most of our lives. The Stevens family had a single television set, and when it broke, they never got around to having it fixed. For a year and a half, they lived without television and didn't miss it. But then Naomi Stevens's mother stayed with the family for a few months between the time her house was sold and her new condominium was ready—and she brought her television with her.

"All of a sudden, I found myself alone in the kitchen making dinner every night," Naomi said. "Before, everyone used to help with setting the table and cooking. After dinner, we would sit around the table and talk for a while.

"When that TV came into the house, the kids raced into the den and argued over what show they would watch. I was glad when Mom's condo was finally ready. We could get back to being a family that talked again."

After the family, television and other forms of media, like the computer and Internet, are probably the most important influence on child development and behavior in our society. Children 8 to 18 years old on average spend more than 7 hours a day using media. They commonly use multiple forms of media simultaneously—they may be tweeting or using Facebook, text messaging or talking on their cell phone, and watching television at the same time. Television and the Internet are the forms of media most likely to affect your child's eating habits. More than 4 hours a day is spent watching television. By the time the average teenager graduates from high school, he has spent more time watching television than in the classroom. Not surprisingly, research has shown that young people who use a lot of media are less physically fit; media use takes away from play and other physical activity. In many cases, television exerts a subtle and destructive influence on a family's eating habits and communication around the table.

Set firm limits on television viewing and the time spent on the computer and playing video games. If your child is a video game "addict," encourage use of "active" video games such as *Wii Fit* or *DanceDance Revolution,* and decrease exposure to violent video games. Join your children outdoors and get the whole family moving. For young children, arrange play dates

---

MEDIA TACTICS

The cardinal rule at mealtime is, "Turn off the television." You may want to consider making the table a "phone-free zone" to curb text messaging. As your children grow, meals together become rare and precious opportunities for family interaction. Make the most of them by eliminating as many distractions as possible.

HOW MUCH IS ENOUGH?

The average child watches about 4 hours of television a day; however, 1 to 2 hours a day of quality television programming, videos, movies, computer games, or surfing the Internet is the maximum recommended by the American Academy of Pediatrics.

so they have something to occupy their time besides sitting in front of the television or computer. For older children, encourage extracurricular activities such as tennis, soccer, football, gymnastics, volleyball, swimming, in-line skating, and dance. When possible, make physical activity a family affair by going for walks or bike rides together.

On television, your child sees one sales pitch after another designed to convince them that they want things they don't need. The average child sees more than 40,000 television commercials each year and is increasingly exposed to advertising on the Internet, in magazines, and in school. A large number of these ads are for high-calorie and high-fat foods such as candy, snacks, soft drinks, and presweetened cereals that add excessive fat and calories to the diet. More than 40% of all commercials that children see are for sugared cereals, candy, fatty foods, and toys. Commercials for healthy foods and drinks make up only about 4% of the food ads shown during children's programming, and ads for fruits and vegetables are virtually nonexistent. Because exposure to food advertising influences a child's food preferences, it stands to reason that television would play a role in childhood obesity. Research bears that out—indeed, the risk of being overweight is more than 4½ times greater for children who watch more than 5 hours of television a day compared with children who watch no more than 2 hours a day.

Don't expect your child to be able to resist all those ads for candy and snack foods without your help. When your child asks for a product he saw advertised, explain how the media makes him want things he does not need—even things that could be harmful. Be specific; point out the commercials you're talking about. When a commercial plugging a children's cereal comes on, explain why advertisers chose to buy time during your child's favorite show. Explain that advertisers want people to buy cereal and are not necessarily concerned with your child's well-being. Children often do not understand the purpose of commercials until it is spelled out for them. Your child may nag, whine, cry, and try to cajole you into buying unhealthful foods, but be firm and ignore it as much as you can. Once you begin negotiating over junk food, you've already lost the battle.

Here are some tips for avoiding ads that sell nutritionally poor products to your children.

- Choose public television over commercial television whenever possible.
- Record programs for your children for watching at a later time, and fast-forward through the commercials.
- Build up a family library of child-friendly favorite videos.

Children are particular targets for commercials advertising fast-food restaurants. These chains attract children with promotional tie-ins for toys. The playgrounds at some locations are hard to resist. Some pediatricians have observed, only half-jokingly, that children's ability to recognize chain restaurant logos has become something of a developmental milestone.

How effective are these promotional efforts by fast-food restaurants? If you've had doubts that even very young children are influenced by advertising, a chilling study showed that the effects of advertising might actually be underestimated. In the study, 63 children aged 3½ to 5 years were given 5 different foods—a quarter of a hamburger, a chicken nugget, french fries, milk (or apple juice for those who could not drink milk), and baby carrots. They received the food in a plain wrapper and in a McDonald's wrapper, and were asked which one tasted better. For 4 out of 5 of the comparisons, children reported that the foods in the McDonald's wrappers tasted better, even though they were identical foods.

Children's food preferences can be affected not only by brand names but also by endorsements of these products by cartoon figures or movie personalities. For example, a study by Sesame Workshop, which produces *Sesame Street*, examined the extent to which a *Sesame Street* character could have a positive effect on children's food choices. In this study, almost 80% of children had chosen chocolate as a food that they would want to eat, compared to 20% who chose broccoli. Then, when the character Elmo was shown standing next to some broccoli and waving, and an unknown figure was shown next to chocolate, the percentage of children who indicated that they would choose broccoli increased to 50%. Then a switch was made; Elmo was moved next to the chocolate and the unknown figure was shown next to broccoli—and 90% of the children said they would select chocolate. The findings of this study may carry over into many foods that children say that they want.

If your child is attracted to fast-food restaurants, it's true that most fast-food menu items are relatively low in valuable nutrients such as vitamin C, iron, and vitamin A, and high in saturated fat, cholesterol, and sodium. However, some menus offer more nutritious, low-fat options, such as grilled chicken sandwiches, reduced-fat milk, and salads. If your child never swerves from his choice of a saturated-fat–heavy burger and fries, cut down on trips to fast-food outlets. The clogging of arteries from atherosclerosis, which sets the stage for heart disease, begins in childhood and is influenced by the amount and type of fat in the diet. Keep trips to fast-food restaurants as treats rather than as routine meals. If your family's usual diet is well balanced and low in fat, an occasional burger and fries aren't going to be harmful. But frequently eating high-fat foods, like hot dogs, burgers, and fries, is unhealthy for adults and children alike.

As mentioned earlier, in adolescence your child's friends are likely to have the strongest influence over his choices. Here, too, television is important, and fast-food outlets play a major role in the lives of teenagers. It's not clear whether that is because of the influence of television, friends, or both, but because fast-food restaurants offer affordable fare and a place to sit, they often serve as gathering spots.

To diminish the effect media has on your child, regardless of his age, the best thing you can do as a parent is to set limits on its use. First, be aware of how many hours of media time your child uses. Remember to limit television time to 1 to 2 hours per day. Finally, keep

---

THE UNREAL WORLD OF ADVERTISING

In advertisements, sports figures, supermodels, rock stars, and movie stars push everything from potato chips and fast food to soft drinks and dietary supplements. Slick ads imply that if you drink this soda, eat this food, or take this supplement, you will be as confident, beautiful, slim, and fun loving as the beautiful people in the ads. Because adolescence is a time of intense approval-seeking behavior, teenagers are especially vulnerable to the unspoken promises of self-improvement and acceptance in such ads. While most food ads are appealing, few promote overall healthful eating. In fact, some blatantly encourage overeating. Yet, paradoxically, the overwhelming majority of people in ads and television shows are athletically built and uncommonly slim. Explain to your children that if the actors frequently snacked on the products they promoted, they wouldn't stay slim for long.

ISSUES PARENTS OFTEN RAISE ABOUT OUTSIDE INFLUENCES

My toddler will be starting at a group child care center when I go back to work. I'm worried that she won't get healthful meals the way she does at home.

Look into the food selections and how meals are served. If the center allows you to pack your child's meals and snacks for the day, include whole-grain breads, cereals, and crackers; a source of protein such as lean meat, fish, or low-fat cheese; and fruits and vegetables. (Also see page 253.)

Both of us work full-time, so our teenager often has to get dinner for himself and his younger sister. We often let him order out for fast food. My kids seem to be growing OK, so is fast food as bad as some people say?

Fast food doesn't have to mean bad food. There are lots of lower-fat options, such as thin-crust vegetarian pizza with just a sprinkling of cheese, or chicken fajitas with salad and low-fat dressing. Stock your freezer with low-fat, microwaveable entrees. And if family mealtime is a rarity during the week, try to make at least one weekend meal a family dinner when everyone takes part. (Also see pages 252 and 253.)

My first grader refuses to take whole wheat bread in his lunch box because his best friend always has white bread.

Lunch box contents are inevitably examined and criticized. You can make it easier on your child while still giving him good nutrition. Make sandwiches with whole-grain white bread. If he must have bologna, buy low-fat turkey bologna. Pack flavored applesauce if he won't take an apple. If he must have chips, replace greasy, salty potato chips with baked chips or reduced-fat, low-salt potato or vegetable chips. (For more tips, see page 255.)

I try to keep my family on a healthy, low-fat diet, but when our folks visit, I hear nothing but criticism. "There's not enough meat here to feed a cat!" "These green vegetables are still half-raw." "I always gave you whole milk and you turned out all right."

Don't let family members' comments throw you off balance. They mean well, but this is your family now and you're in charge of what goes on the table. Avoid confrontation; it will only lead to an uncomfortable mood at the dinner table. Listen to their opinions, smile, and then enlist their help, where possible, in dealing with immediate, manageable needs such as playing with the baby or preparing vegetables. (For other tips, see page 254.)

My teenager has just announced she's going vegetarian. What'll I do?

A properly planned vegetarian diet is healthful and well balanced, and it can easily fit with regular family meals. Listen to the reasons behind your teenager's decision. Learn as much as you can so you can help her achieve a nutritionally balanced diet. Round up some reading material to help her plan meals. The whole family may eat more healthfully by incorporating some vegetarian choices. (Also see page 258 and Chapter 15, Alternative Diets and Supplements.)

the media under your control. That means no television or computer in children's rooms. Even though recent statistics reveal that two thirds of young people have televisions in their rooms, be firm. If necessary, install devices or software on family computers and televisions that prevent young people from tuning in to selected channels and Internet sites.

Help your child become physically active. Not only is media use synonymous with inactivity, but snacking while doing so sets the stage for unwanted weight gain. The best approach is to limit television viewing from your children's very earliest years so they don't become dependent on it for entertainment and stimulation. If your child is used to watching a lot of television each day or playing computer games or surfing the 'net, it may take some effort to get him interested in other activities. Don't be surprised if your child rebels and even goes through a sort of withdrawal when you cut back on his media use. And remember, your children look to you for an example. It might be a good idea to take a critical look at your own media habits before you try to revamp those of your children. For example, if you come home and immediately turn on the news before you interact with the rest of the family, you are sending a message that television time is more important than family time.

Keep in mind that magazines aimed at adolescents—especially young girls—also offer nutrition information and advice, together with articles about dieting, alongside food advertising. While some columns and articles are responsible and accurate, others reinforce an adolescent's least healthy inclinations. Perhaps most disturbing are the images of overly thin models pushing products ranging from makeup and clothes to the latest dating advice. While you can't monitor all your adolescent's reading material, be aware that she may be turning to magazines as her main source of information about diet and health, and thus absorbing an unrealistic image of what the "ideal" body should be. Whether your teenager's goal is an ultra-slender figure or the ultimate performance in her chosen sport, help her to be comfortable with herself and her body type through sound information and balanced nutrition.

Chapter 12

Can I Cut My Child's Risk of…?

Heredity is clearly an important risk factor for conditions such as heart disease, cancer, and diabetes. However, researchers are steadily gathering strong evidence about how diet influences the development of diseases. Most research into the diet-health connection has been done in adults, but experts agree that healthy eating habits from an early age can lower the risk of developing several deadly diseases later on. A diet designed to lower the risk of heart disease, diabetes, and other serious diseases is one that benefits the whole family, adults and children alike.

In the course of a well-child visit for 5-year-old Sara, her mother mentioned that Sara's grandmother, 54 years old, had recently been hospitalized for a heart attack. Because of that, Sara's father had his cholesterol level checked and it turned out to be high, about 260 mg/dL. He was now receiving treatment to lower his cholesterol and with it, his risk of heart disease.

Routine cholesterol testing for all young children is not considered necessary. However, given the information about Sara's family, their pediatrician advised a blood test. Sara's results showed no sign of the high blood cholesterol that sometimes runs in families and can appear at a young age. The pediatrician suggested that Sara's mother base family meal planning on the *Dietary Guidelines for Americans* (www.cnpp.usda.gov/DietaryGuidelines.htm) recommendations for a low-fat diet. Such guidelines advise no more than 30% of daily calories in the form of fat, with saturated fat making up no more than one third of total fats. He also suggested that Sara's parents strictly limit her television-viewing time and make time available for active play. When she was older, there'd be time for more structured exercise. Finally, although Sara's cholesterol level was normal, her pediatrician recommended periodic blood tests to catch any change early and provide corrective steps.

Heart Disease

Heart disease is the number one killer of men and women in the United States and most industrialized countries. The chief risk factors are smoking, high blood pressure, diabetes, a high blood level of cholesterol, physical inactivity, and overweight. If members of your family have had heart disease at an early age, your child may be at risk for early-onset heart disease.

American children and adolescents, on average, eat more saturated fat and have higher blood cholesterol levels than young people their age in most other developed countries. The rate of heart disease tends to keep pace with cholesterol levels. One study found early signs of hardening of the arteries (atherosclerosis) in 7% of children between ages 10 and 15 years, and the rate was twice as high between ages 15 and 20. According to the American Heart Association, a heart-healthy diet from an early age lowers cholesterol and if followed through adolescence and beyond, should reduce the risk of coronary artery disease in adulthood.

All children older than 2 years should follow a heart-healthy diet, including low-fat dairy products. For children between the ages of 12 months and 2 years with a family history of obesity, abnormal blood fats, or cardiovascular disease, reduced-fat milk should be considered.

IS THERE A FAMILY HISTORY?

When you and your children first saw your pediatrician, you were probably asked if there was a history of heart or vascular disease in your family. If your children were young, their grandparents were probably relatively young as well and may not have had a heart attack or stroke (even though they may have been headed for one). If heart disease in the grandparents becomes apparent later on, be sure to bring it to your pediatrician's attention at the next checkup.

CHOLESTEROL TESTING FOR ADOPTED CHILDREN

Complete biological family medical histories are not usually available to adopted children and their parents, even for those adopted in open proceedings. To prevent the development of diseases linked to high blood cholesterol levels, adopted children should be screened periodically for blood lipid (fat) levels throughout childhood.

CHOLESTEROL LEVELS IN CHILDREN AND ADOLESCENTS		
Classification	**Total Cholesterol**[a]	**Low-Density Lipoprotein (LDL)**[a]
Acceptable	<170	<110
Borderline	170–199	110–129
High	>200	>130

[a]Milligrams per 100 mL of blood.

Testing Blood Cholesterol Levels

The American Academy of Pediatrics (AAP) recommends cholesterol testing for the following groups of children:

- Those whose parents or grandparents have had heart attacks or have been diagnosed with blocked arteries or disease affecting the blood vessels, such as stroke, at age 55 or earlier in men, or 65 or earlier in women
- Those whose parents or grandparents have total blood cholesterol levels of 240 mg/dL or higher
- Those whose family health background is not known (eg, many adopted children), or those who have characteristics associated with heart disease, such as high blood pressure, diabetes, smoking, or obesity

For children in these categories, their first cholesterol test should be after 2 years but no later than 10 years of age.

A child may have high cholesterol for a variety of reasons such as obesity, diabetes, liver disease, kidney disease, or an underactive thyroid. If an initial test shows high cholesterol, your pediatrician will check your child's blood again at least 2 weeks later to confirm the results. If it is still high, the doctor will also determine if your child has an underlying condition.

A recent government report indicated that there is good evidence that children with cholesterol problems become adults with high cholesterol. So it is important to monitor the cholesterol of children who may have an increased risk of elevated cholesterol.

Diet to Lower Blood Cholesterol Levels

If a second blood test confirms that your child's blood cholesterol is high, a change in diet is the first approach for reducing it. This means embracing foods that can positively affect cholesterol levels—and that are described throughout this book. This approach also includes reducing dietary fat and cholesterol by consuming more fruits and vegetables, fish, whole grains, and low-fat dairy products. For a high-risk child, your pediatrician may recommend that saturated fats stay at 7% of total daily calories, while dietary cholesterol be limited to 200 mg per day. Your blood cholesterol levels may improve further by choosing soft or tub margarine with no trans saturated fat, orange juice, and cereal bars that are fortified with cholesterol-lowering plant stanol and sterols (naturally occurring substances found in fruits, vegetables, and other plant sources). In fact, all family members should adopt these dietary and exercise approaches to support the child with high cholesterol levels.

If you would like further guidance in planning a heart-healthy diet for your child (and most parents are glad to have some guidance), talk with your pediatrician and ask for a referral to a registered dietitian who specializes in children and families. She might suggest a program known as the DASH (Dietary Approaches to Stop Hypertension; see Appendix H) diet. Before you meet with the dietitian, you will probably be asked to keep a record of everything your child eats over the course of several days, to provide an idea of his eating patterns as well as his likes and dislikes.

Despite efforts to educate parents and children about healthy eating, and surveys showing that children and adolescents are eating less fat than they did 25 years ago, Americans of all ages are getting fatter. Obesity can be a cause of abnormal cholesterol levels. Total cholesterol, LDL ("bad") cholesterol, and triglycerides are elevated in obese children and adolescents, and HDL ("good") cholesterol levels are low. As a result, maintaining a healthy weight is crucial to reducing your child's risk of developing atherosclerosis and heart disease. In addition, when children and adolescents lose weight, it improves abnormal cholesterol levels. (For more information on obesity and weight maintenance, see Chapter 8, Nutrition Basics.)

However, you should not try to reduce your child's fat or calorie intake without your pediatrician's or a dietitian's advice. Cutting back too much could negatively affect the number one childhood goal, which is normal growth and development. In particular, fat and cholesterol should not be restricted in children younger than 2 years unless specifically instructed to do so by your pediatrician. Children need the calories from fat during this period of rapid development, when nutritional requirements are intense and restrictions could be harmful. The period beginning with the second birthday is a time of transition when you should decrease the fat and cholesterol content of your child's diet to the recommended levels. So after age 2, he should be drinking skim or low-fat milk and getting no more than 30% of daily calories from fats, with one third or less of fat calories from saturated fats (see chapters 8 and 14).

In addition to these guidelines, the National Cholesterol Education Program Expert Panel on Blood Cholesterol Levels in Children and Adolescents recommends that children eat a wide variety of foods, with enough calories to support normal growth and reach or maintain a healthy body weight.

Fiber and Cholesterol

Fiber comes from parts of plants in the diet that resist digestion. One type of fiber, called *soluble* fiber, is found in beans, fruits, and oat products, and dissolves in water. Another kind of fiber, *insoluble* fiber, which is found in whole-grain products and vegetables, does not dissolve in water. Both types of fiber are important to keep the digestive tract functioning smoothly, and soluble fiber also helps to lower blood cholesterol in adults. Studies have not been performed to see whether these foods lower cholesterol in children. However, in all likelihood, fiber is equally beneficial at every age.

The AAP recommends that children consume fiber equal to ½ g per kg (2.2 lb) of body weight per day, but not more than 35 g. Pediatricians suggest a simpler way to calculate fiber—your child's age plus 5. Thus, for a 7-year-old, daily intake should be no less than 7 + 5 = 12 g, up to a maximum of 35 g up to age 13.

You probably don't have to calculate your child's fiber intake in grams because there should be plenty of fiber in a normal diet that includes the recommended number of daily servings of fruits and vegetables, in addition to whole-grain breads and cereals. For example, all

DAILY RECOMMENDED INTAKE OF FIBER	
Gender/Age	**Fiber (g)**
1–3 y	19
4–8 y	25
9–13 y	26 (female); 31 (male)
14–18 y	26 (female); 38 (male)

OMEGA-3 FATTY ACIDS FROM PLANTS
Oils from plants such as rapeseed or canola, flaxseed, and walnuts are good sources of linolenic acid, a fatty acid that our bodies convert to protective omega-3 fatty acids.

children and adolescents older than 2 years should have 2 or 3 servings a day of fruit. Young children (aged 2 to 6 years) also should consume 3 servings of vegetables, compared with 4 servings of vegetables in older children and teenaged girls, and 5 servings in teenaged boys. At the same time, if your child is constipated or not getting these recommended servings per day, try to increase her fiber intake in other foods. Avoid refined white flour and serve whole-grain breads, crackers, pasta, and cereals instead. For snacks, offer fruit or carrot sticks, celery, and other vegetables.

One Fish…Two Fish….

Adults who eat fish several times a week have a lower risk of heart disease than those who don't. The protective effect has been traced to omega-3 fatty acids, a special kind of fat found in fish.

Researchers haven't yet looked for evidence of comparable protection in children, but it's a good idea to make fish a regular part of your child's diet. Years ago, people called fish "brain food." They did not know how right they were. Not only are the omega-3 fatty acids in fish beneficial for cardiovascular health, but fish also contains high levels of DHA (a type of essential fat in fish), which is good for brain development in children. Fatty fish like salmon, mackerel, and bluefish are especially rich sources of omega-3 fatty acids. When preparing fish, choose low-fat cooking methods such as broiling and steaming; deep-frying in batter only adds unnecessary fat and calories.

But there's an added dimension to the fish story these days. Fish can contain mercury, which can be toxic for children and a developing fetus. How to balance the good and the bad?

A study from Harvard Medical School evaluated about 900 mothers and their children at age 3 years. They found that 2 servings of fish a week during the pregnancy was associated with higher scores in tests of intelligence, vocabulary, spatial and visual acuity, and gross and fine motor skills in the children, compared with those who ate no fish or more than 2 servings a week.

The lesson from this is that a little fish is better than a lot or none. Fish that contain the highest levels of mercury are shark, swordfish, and large tuna sold as sushi and tuna steaks. (See "Mercury and Fish," Chapter 13, page 285.)

Giving supplements with fish oil may not be as effective as having fish in the diet. Getting any nutrient from the natural source of food is always better than artificial supplements, and thus giving children omega-3 supplements may not be the same as eating fish. Besides, the appropriate dose for children has not been established.

Cholesterol-Lowering Medications

Pediatricians can consider using cholesterol-lowering medications in children aged 8 years and older who still have high cholesterol after trying low-fat, low-cholesterol, high-fiber dietary measures for 6 months to 1 year. Specifically, children may be candidates for these cholesterol-reducing medications after 6 to 12 months if they still

- Have a high LDL cholesterol of 190 mg/dL or more
- Have a high LDL cholesterol of 160 mg/dL or more with a family history of early heart disease or 2 or more additional risk factors (eg, obesity, high blood pressure)
- Have a high LDL cholesterol of 130 mg/dL or more if diabetes is also present

The only medications the AAP currently approves for children are colestipol, cholestyramine, and a statin drug. Colestipol and cholestyramine are known as bile acid binders. They attach to molecules of bile acids, which help digest fats. Bile acids are made from cholesterol; when bound to these drugs, bile acids pass out in the stool. Pediatricians prescribe these medications only after trying other nondrug methods, however, because of the small risk associated with using any medication.

Statin drugs are the most popular cholesterol-lowering drug in adults, and the AAP now believes that statins should be considered for some children as well. These medications block the manufacture of cholesterol by the liver.

However, no drug should be prescribed for a child without parents having a discussion with their pediatrician or a pediatric cardiologist about the risks and benefits of these medications, including the limited information on the long-term effects of medications like statins.

Physical Activity

Physical activity is notoriously difficult to measure in children and teenagers. However, reduced physical education programs in schools and fewer opportunities for physical activity as part of everyday life have lowered physical activity levels in many US children and teenagers. Not only is physical activity essential to maintain a healthy weight, but aerobic activities such as soccer, basketball, track, skating, and jumping rope also strengthen the heart and lungs. In addition, physical activity improves a number of risk factors for heart disease such as cholesterol and triglyceride levels, blood pressure, and glucose tolerance (meaning children who exercise are better able to process the sugar in their diets).

In 2008, for the first time, the US Department of Health and Human Services released *Physical Activity Guidelines for Americans.* The guidelines recommend 1 hour of physical activity daily, doing things that are age appropriate, fun, and offer variety. Most of this activity should be moderate- or vigorous-intensity aerobic physical activity. Children should do vigorous physical activity like running or swimming, as well as muscle-strengthening activity and bone-strengthening physical activity, at least 3 days per week.

A recent study of children aged 9, 11, 12, and 15 years showed that almost all 9- and 11-year-old boys and girls met the government's 60-minute recommendations for physical activity on weekdays and weekend days, but by age 15, only 31% met the recommendation on weekdays and only 17% on weekend days.

To keep your child fit, make physical activity a family affair. Regulate television time and arrange for children to play outside. Go for family walks, hikes, and bicycle rides. Gather neighborhood young people for running bases, basketball games, or touch football. Regular physical activity is just as important as a healthy diet in preventing heart disease.

Diabetes

People with diabetes are diagnosed according to whether they require insulin treatment (type 1), or can manage their condition with diet, exercise, and oral medications to control blood glucose levels (type 2). Type 1 diabetics do not produce *insulin,* a hormone made in the pancreas, which helps convert sugar into energy. Type 2 diabetics produce insulin but are resistant to its effects. Although children most often develop type 1 diabetes, type 2 diabetes has increased as a result of the obesity epidemic.

Environmental factors such as viral infections, toxins, and emotional stress may trigger a child's genetic predisposition to type 1 diabetes. It is called an *autoimmune* disease, in which the body mistakes its own tissue as unfamiliar. When that happens, the immune system attacks the pancreas as if it were a foreign invader and interferes with its ability to produce

SYMPTOMS OF TYPE 1 DIABETES
If your child has these symptoms, call your pediatrician at once.
• Weight loss
• Excessive thirst
• Frequent urination
• Dehydration with dry lips, sunken eyes, and no tears when crying

insulin. Those with type 1 diabetes often have family histories of other autoimmune conditions, such as thyroid disorders or rheumatoid arthritis. Some researchers suggest that early exposure to cow's-milk protein may, in some children, trigger destruction of the insulin-producing cells in the pancreas. Though this theory is unproven, the AAP recommends that parents avoid giving cow's milk for the first year for many reasons, including reducing the risk of type 1 diabetes in children. Breastfeeding during the first year may protect against diabetes, in addition to its many other benefits.

Type 2 diabetes now accounts for one-third of all new cases of diabetes, and the greatest number of these cases occur in obese adolescents. Obesity increases the body's need for insulin, and eventually the need for insulin exceeds the body's supply. Family history plays a role, but being overweight is probably the strongest risk factor of all. Reduce your child's risk of type 2 diabetes by helping him maintain a healthy weight with a well-balanced diet and regular exercise. Healthy habits you instill in childhood can help keep risk low in the adult years.

Cancer

As with heart disease, diet throughout life appears to influence the risk of various cancers. While it's not clear which cancers can be linked specifically to fat consumption, there's no doubt that a low-fat diet is associated with a lower overall risk for many diseases, including most types of cancer.

Grilled and Barbecued Foods

Chemicals that cause cancer can form during any cooking process. Some are even produced in the body during digestion. High-heat methods of cooking meat, such as broiling, frying, and barbecuing, produce concentrations of DNA-altering chemicals that are about 50 times greater than those in baked and boiled meats. Hydrocarbons, including benzene, form when meat is broiled, and cancer-causing nitrosamines are produced during cooking and in the digestive tract when processed meats containing nitrite, such as bacon, are eaten.

There's no call for undue alarm, however. As with all foods, moderation and balance are the key. It's a good idea to steam, bake, and braise most of the time, but there's no harm in grilling or barbecuing occasionally. Besides, you can take steps to reduce exposure to potentially harmful compounds.

Do all grilling and barbecuing in a well-ventilated area to reduce exposure to carcinogens in smoke. Use a drip pan with a spatter-proof shield to prevent fat from forming smoke. Reduce

---

DIET TIPS TO PREVENT DENTAL PROBLEMS

A balanced diet, with plenty of calcium and vitamin D to increase calcium absorption, should provide all the nutrients necessary to build strong teeth and keep gums and mouth tissues healthy. Young people can get adequate calcium from 3 or 4 daily servings of dairy foods, as well as from many other sources (eg, calcium-processed tofu, calcium-fortified orange juice, green vegetables such as broccoli).

Fluoride reduces dental decay by making the enamel harder, reducing the ability of bacteria to produce acid that erodes enamel, and by replacing minerals in the teeth after they have been lost. In areas where the natural fluoride content of the water is low and water supplies are not fluoridated, or if your household uses bottled or reverse osmosis filtered water, pediatricians and dentists may advise fluoride supplements (also see Chapter 2, page 49), fluoride toothpaste, or fluoride treatments to strengthen children's tooth enamel against decay. Most bottled water does not contain adequate amounts of fluoride. Home water treatment systems like reverse osmosis and distillation units remove much of the fluoride from tap water. However, carbon or charcoal water filtration systems generally do not remove substantial amounts of fluoride.

One of the complications of too much fluoride is dental fluorosis. Fluorosis ranges from minor white lines that run across the teeth to a chalky appearance of the teeth with brown staining. Fluorosis can be caused by prescribing fluoride supplements in communities with fluoridated water, or young children swallowing fluoridated toothpaste. To avoid this latter problem, children should use no more than a smear of fluoridated toothpaste before age 2, if your child's pediatrician or dentist suggests using fluoridated toothpaste. For children older than age 2, use only a small pea-sized amount of fluoridated toothpaste. Also, your pediatrician or pediatric dentist will know the fluoride content of your local water and can advise you if a supplement is necessary or excessive.

All sugars promote the growth of mouth bacteria that produce acid and cause tooth decay. Unrefined sugars such as honey, maple syrup, and molasses are just as damaging as refined white sugar in this respect. The worst offenders are the sugars in sticky foods that cling to teeth, such as dried fruit leathers and candies. Sodas and sweetened juice drinks leave the teeth awash in sugar. Cereals and other starchy foods, such as popcorn, leave a residue that bacteria rapidly convert to sugar.

BABY BOTTLE TOOTH DECAY

Tooth decay (early childhood caries) is the most common chronic infectious disease of childhood. Tooth decay may also be called *nursing caries* or *baby bottle tooth decay*.

Tooth decay develops when a baby's mouth is infected by acid-producing bacteria. It also develops when the child's teeth and gums are exposed to any liquids or foods other than water for long periods. Natural or added sugars in liquids or foods are changed to acid by bacteria in the mouth. This acid then dissolves the outer part of the teeth, causing them to decay.

The most common way this happens is when parents put their children to bed with a bottle of formula, milk, juice (even diluted), soft drinks, sugar water, or sugared drinks. It can also happen when children are allowed to drink continually from a sippy cup, or suck on a bottle filled with something other than water. To help prevent decay,

- Never put your child to bed with a bottle or food.

- After your child gets teeth, gently wipe the child's mouth with a damp cloth after every feeding to clean the teeth and gums.

- Give your child a bottle or sippy cup filled with something other than water only during meals.

- Teach your child to drink from a regular cup as soon as possible, preferably by 12 to 15 months of age.

- If your child must have a bottle or sippy cup for long periods, fill it with water only.

- Avoid feeding your child meals or snacks that are sticky, or high in sugar or starch.

---

high-heat cooking time—partially bake or parboil foods, then finish off with just a few minutes on the grill to add flavor.

Vitamins C and E block the chemical process that forms nitrosamines in the digestive tract. Phytates in wheat bran bind with nitrite and prevent nitrosamine formation. Bioflavonoids—pigments found in many fruits and vegetables—and other naturally occurring compounds known as phytochemicals are believed to block the action of many cancer-causing substances. So when you have a barbecue, round out the meal with vegetables and fruits, as well as whole-grain breads and salads for fiber, vitamins, and other natural cancer fighters.

However, while fructose, the sugar in fruits, can promote tooth decay, eating fruit also stimulates the flow of saliva, which helps to wash such naturally occurring sugars out of the mouth. The fats in walnuts and certain proteins and fats in cheddar cheese appear to neutralize bacterial acids and may help to counteract their destructive effect. Sweets are likely to be less harmful if eaten as part of a meal.

Encourage children to floss and brush after meals. When brushing is impossible (such as when out on a hike or in school), children should try to end a meal by drinking plain water or chewing on a firm, fibrous snack such as a carrot or celery stick to help remove food scraps and stimulate saliva flow. If all else fails, chewing sugarless gum also stimulates saliva flow, and some brands help cut down on the bacteria that cause cavities.

Balance Is Best

There can be little doubt that childhood diets have an effect on the risk of disease in adulthood. Most evidence of factors that trigger disease is evaluated in statistical terms, as trends in vast numbers of people rather than as changes in individuals. However, evidence points toward a protective effect from a diet rich in grains, vegetables, and fruits, and with low levels of saturated fat. Serve at least one green and one yellow or red vegetable, plus a starchy vegetable or whole grain every dinnertime, and follow a just-one-bite policy. That is, even if your child claims not to like vegetables, ask that he try at least one bite of those on the plate. Serve fruits routinely for dessert, alone or with cheese or yogurt. A habit of eating the recommended daily servings of fruits and vegetables may help reduce your child's risk of developing heart disease, high blood pressure, cancer, diabetes, and other serious ailments later in life.

ISSUES PARENTS RAISE ABOUT FOOD AND HEALTH RISKS

Should children have cholesterol checks just as adults do?

Young children with a strong family history of heart disease or lipid disorders may need to have a cholesterol test (see page 266). These children need to be checked between 2 and 10 years of age. All children should have cholesterol levels checked again later in adolescence. See what are considered acceptable, borderline, and high cholesterol levels on page 267.

Is fiber all it's cracked up to be?

Not only is fiber important to keep the digestive tract functioning smoothly, but it also helps regulate blood cholesterol. Diets rich in soluble fiber—the kind found in grains (especially oats), legumes and other vegetables, and fruits—have been shown to lower cholesterol levels in adults. Studies have not been performed to see whether these foods lower cholesterol levels in children; however, in all likelihood, fiber is equally beneficial at every age. (See page 270.)

There's a lot of diabetes in my wife's family. Does this mean our children will get diabetes?

Family history plays a role in the development of diabetes, but being overweight is probably the strongest risk factor of all. Reduce your children's risk of type 2 diabetes by helping them maintain a healthy weight with a well-balanced diet and regular exercise. Healthy habits you instill in childhood can help keep their risk low in the adult years. (See page 273.)

Chapter 13

Food Safety

According to government estimates, as many as 80 million Americans may suffer at least one bout of food poisoning, or gastroenteritis, every year. Fortunately, most of us, including healthy older children, can shrug off the uncomfortable symptoms of diarrhea, cramps, and perhaps vomiting in a day or two. However, the very young, the elderly, and those with chronic diseases may develop complications unless they receive prompt treatment.

Recent serious outbreaks of food poisoning linked to unusual organisms or treatment-resistant strains of common bacteria are warnings we cannot afford to ignore. *Escherichia coli* O157:H7, which has been found in undercooked beef, unpasteurized cider and fruit juices, contaminated salad greens, and fruits, among other foods, can lead to hemolytic uremic syndrome with kidney failure and death. Infection with *Campylobacter* species, found in undercooked poultry and eggs, can result in painful and bloody diarrhea, as well as Guillain-Barré syndrome, a disease that can cause sudden paralysis in children and adults. *Salmonella*, cryptosporidium, cyclosporiasis, and a variety of other bacteria, viruses, and parasites can infiltrate any stage in the food chain and lead to serious illness. Raw (unpasteurized) milk can also be a source of these infections. (See also "Pasteurized Milk: Myths and Proven Facts," Chapter 15, page 303.)

Food safety practices on farms, in factories, at packing plants, and during transportation are beyond the control of consumers. In any case, these are relatively minor sources of contamination. The vast majority of cases of food poisoning reported to the Centers for Disease Control and Prevention (CDC) are traced to the way food is handled in homes and food service operations such as cafeterias and caterers. Most episodes could be prevented with simple precautions in the choice, storage, and preparation of food. (See Appendix I for food safety resources.)

Preventing Food-Borne Illness

Those caring for children need to know how to guard against food-borne illness. It's never too early to be a good example for children, with proper hand washing, cleanliness, and careful preparation and storage of food. There are 3 basic facts to keep in mind when preparing food.

1. **Bacteria rapidly multiply in foods that are lukewarm or kept at room temperature.** Therefore, keep hot foods hot and cold foods cold.

2. **Bacteria are often present in raw foods.** Thoroughly cook foods of animal origin, and thoroughly wash vegetables and fruits that are eaten raw.

3. **Bacteria and viruses are easily transferred from our bodies to food, and from one food to another.** Wash hands frequently and encourage your children to do the same. Never put a spoon used to taste food back into food without washing it. Keep raw foods and cooked foods separate. Wash knives, cutting boards, and other utensils used for preparing one food before reusing for another.

You can reduce your family's risk of food-borne illness by choosing foods in good condition and following a few simple rules for handling, storage, and preparation.

SYMPTOMS OF FOOD POISONING

The most common symptoms of food poisoning are

- Stomach cramps
- Diarrhea
- Nausea/vomiting
- Fever

While similar symptoms may occur in several conditions, food poisoning is the likely cause if 2 or more members of the household become ill after eating the same dishes. The problem usually clears up if the child avoids eating for a few hours and takes sips of fluid to replace lost fluid as soon as the vomiting stops. If symptoms are still present after 3 to 4 hours for an infant younger than 1 year, or 6 to 8 hours for an older child—or if the child appears ill or drowsy, or has bloody or unusually severe diarrhea—call your pediatrician immediately for advice.

Buying Foods

- If you notice unsatisfactory food handling at markets or restaurants, bring it to the manager's attention.
- Check "Sell by" and "Best before" dates to avoid buying outdated items.
- Don't buy damaged cans or packages.
- Make sure frozen foods are frozen solid, with no ice or water marks indicating the product has been thawed and refrozen.
- Check that foods from the refrigerator case are cold when purchased.
- Inspect eggs and reject any that are dirty, cracked, or unrefrigerated; check freshness dates on the carton.
- Bag meats separately from fresh produce.
- Avoid unpasteurized or raw juices and milk, as well as cheese made from unpasteurized or raw milk.

Storing Foods

- Store foods at correct temperatures. Storage at improper temperatures is the most common cause of outbreaks of food-borne illness. Refrigerate or freeze foods as soon as you unpack them. Wrap raw meat, poultry, and fish so they don't come into contact with other foods, especially foods that are eaten raw.
- Keep refrigerated produce in the crisper. Keep other fruits and vegetables at cool room temperature. Protect potatoes from light (a paper shopping bag works well) to guard against the formation of toxic solanine compounds, which are indicated by a green color. Discard potatoes that have turned green and sprouted.
- Store and use cans and packages in date order.
- Store grains and cereals in cupboards or in opaque containers; their vitamin content deteriorates on exposure to light. Similarly, store oils away from light to prevent them from turning rancid.

Preparing Food

- Wash hands for at least 10 to 20 seconds with soap and warm water before preparing foods, and wash again periodically as necessary. If children are helping, tell them to wash long enough to sing their ABCs slowly. If you wear rubber gloves, wash your hands with the gloves on.
- Follow the safe-handling labels on prepackaged raw meat and poultry.
- Defrost frozen foods in the refrigerator or under running cold water, not on the countertop or in a bowl of water at room temperature.
- Use separate cutting boards for preparing raw meats and raw produce.
- After using a cutting board or a knife for raw meat, fish, or poultry, wash it with soap and hot water. Rinse the cutting board with a mild bleach solution (¼ cup of bleach to a gallon of water) before reusing it for any food. Wash plastic cutting boards in the dishwasher, if you have one. Cook meat to the recommended temperature and use a meat thermometer if you have difficulty judging when meat is done. Beef and lamb can be eaten rare to medium, provided the internal temperature has reached 140°F, which will kill most bacteria.

MAKING IMPORTED FOODS SAFER

Approximately 44% of fresh fruits and 16% of fresh vegetables that Americans eat are grown in other countries. Concern about the rising incidence of germs traceable to imported produce (eg, *Cyclospora* on raspberries from Guatemala, hepatitis A on strawberries from Mexico, cholera in coconut milk from Thailand) led government food authorities to devise a new method of inspecting production sites abroad just as thoroughly as suppliers are monitored in the United States.

According to the new procedures, produce will be banned if farms and processors in the country of origin fail to meet our safety standards. Under the old way of doing things, suspect foods were seized only after they reached the US port of entry. The far-reaching approach gives the Food and Drug Administration the authority to oversee the growing, processing, shipping, and selling of all foods intended for the American market. It covers all agricultural practices, including the use of pesticides, manures and fertilizers, and water for irrigation.

The World Health Organization estimates that for every reported case of food-borne illness worldwide, as many as 350 go unreported. By improving food growing and handling abroad, the new system may reduce the incidence of food-borne illness not only in the United States but also in other countries.

- Don't serve hamburgers rare. Unlike germs on the surface of meat, bacteria transferred into ground meat during processing may escape sterilization by the heat of cooking. Cook hamburgers until brown in the center or until the meat thermometer registers 160°F. Reheat ground beef leftovers to 165°F.
- Cook poultry until the thigh joints move easily and the juices run clear; cook poultry pieces such as breasts to 165°F or until the flesh springs back to the touch and no pink color remains.
- If you stuff poultry, cook it immediately or better yet, bake the stuffing in a separate dish.
- Cook pork until it reaches a temperature of 145°F to prevent the spread of trichinosis parasites. Some pink color may remain even after the meat has reached this temperature.
- Rinse salad greens—including prepackaged, prewashed salads—in at least 2 changes of water.
- Refrigerate leftovers as soon as possible, no longer than 2 hours after serving, to cut down on the time during which bacteria can multiply.

Getting Rid of Pesticides

Regular monitoring of commercial food sources by the Food and Drug Administration (FDA) shows that pesticides are almost always well below the highest levels legally allowed. However, it's a good idea to wash fruits and vegetables anyway to get rid of any residues.

- Wash food in a large amount of cold or tepid tap water.
- Scrub with a brush if necessary, preferably under running water.
- Discard the outer leaves of leafy vegetables, such as lettuce and cabbage.
- When present in foods of animal origin, pesticides tend to be concentrated in the fatty tissues; therefore, trim all visible fat from meat and trim fat from poultry.

For more information about pesticides, see "Organic Foods" on page 287.

Safe Drinking Water

Children drink much more water for their size than adults. Most of this water comes from the tap, and the quality of this water is regulated by standards instituted by Congress, included in the Safe Drinking Water Act of 1974. Subsequent laws have set drinking water standards for chemicals that were known to be in some water supplies. Today the drinking water in the United States is among the safest in the world, although problems can occur from time to time. Violations in water safety standards are most likely to occur in small systems that serve fewer than a thousand people. Also, keep in mind that private wells are not federally regulated and should be tested for nitrates and other environmental toxins if appropriate.

To ensure that you're consuming safe drinking water, you can check the water quality by contacting the county health department, the state environment agency, or the Environmental Protection Agency Safe Drinking Water Hotline (800/426-4791). Local water companies are mandated to report what is in the water on an annual basis. Well water should be tested yearly.

RECYCLE SENSIBLY

Recycling is praiseworthy but should not be carried to extremes. It's not a good idea, for instance, to turn plastic bread bags or other branded plastic bags inside out and use them to store food or pack lunches. The inks used to print the bags can contain lead, which may leach into food. When bags are used as intended, with the printing on the outside, there is no risk to health.

SUSHI, SHELLFISH, SEVICHE

Any animal protein eaten raw or only partly cooked is more likely to cause illness than thoroughly cooked food. When it comes to fish and seafood, the main sources of illness are bacteria and viruses in water polluted by human waste. There are also harmful marine bacteria that are unrelated to human pollution. They are commonly found in fish and shellfish taken from estuaries, where seas and rivers mingle. In addition, freshwater and saltwater fish may be colonized by parasites that can transfer to human hosts unless destroyed by freezing or thorough cooking. In susceptible people—especially children, the elderly, and those with chronic illnesses or immune disorders—disease-causing organisms from raw or undercooked fish can cause serious illness. Children should not eat raw fish and shellfish, including dishes prepared like seviche, which uses soaking in an acidic citrus marinade to "cold cook" the protein. Sushi made with cooked fish, however, is safe.

Other guidelines include

- **Use cold water for cooking and drinking.** Contaminants can accumulate in hot water heaters.
- **Drinking water that may be contaminated should be boiled and then allowed to cool before drinking.** Boil for no more than one minute. However, it is important to remember that boiling water only kills bacteria and other germs; it does *not* remove toxic chemicals. If you don't like the taste or smell of your tap water, filters made with activated carbon will remove the taste or smell. Such filters will also remove undesirable chemicals without removing fluoride that prevents tooth decay.

Mercury and Fish

Mercury is released in the form of gas from the Earth's crust and oceans, or as an industrial by-product. It dissolves in water, where it is transformed by bacterial action into methyl mercury, a more toxic form. When fish absorb methyl mercury from the water and from feeding on smaller life-forms, the metal builds up in their tissues. The larger the fish, the greater the intake and buildup. In humans, mercury poisoning can damage the brain and nervous system.

Although contamination is widespread, methyl mercury levels don't reach the FDA limit for human consumption of 1 part per million (ppm) except in a very few species, such as shark, swordfish, and the large tuna sold as steaks and sushi. The smaller tuna used for canning have much lower levels. Freshwater fish may have high mercury levels, especially in areas where environmental levels are high. The FDA recommends that sport fishers check with state or local government offices for up-to-date information about mercury and other contaminants in local waters and fish. Cooking does not reduce mercury content. Women who are pregnant or planning to get pregnant shouldn't eat shark, swordfish, king mackerel, or tilefish. Eating up to 12 ounces (2 average meals) a week of a variety of fish and shellfish that are lower in mercury is fine. There's no risk of methyl mercury poisoning from eating top-selling species, which include canned tuna, shrimp, pollack, salmon, cod, catfish, clams, crabs, and scallops. If you have questions about methyl mercury or other fishy issues, call the 24-hour FDA seafood hotline, 800/FDA-4010 (332-4010).

BIOTECHNOLOGY AND PESTICIDES

One of the goals of scientists involved in biotechnology is the production of plants with improved resistance to diseases and pests, enabling farmers to harvest crops with much lower residues of herbicides and pesticides. These plants will satisfy consumers' demands for high-quality produce and lower levels of synthetic chemicals.

Bioengineered Foods

Bioengineering has pushed farmers beyond the age-old practice of selective breeding, whereby one animal or plant strain was crossed with a related one to bring out desirable characteristics and suppress less useful ones. Now, scientists can manipulate genes and create new strains out of unrelated species. Foods, ingredients, and additives produced by bioengineering must meet the same FDA safety standards as traditional products. The total acreage of bioengineered crops is still small, but it represents a growing practice.

Food producers are responsible for ensuring that the foods they sell are safe. The US Department of Agriculture has the authority to remove meat, poultry, and egg products produced in federally inspected plants, and the FDA has the authority to remove all other foods from the market if they pose a risk to public health.

One area of concern related to the transfer of genetic material is the possibility that proteins introduced from one food into another could cause allergic reactions in people sensitive to the first food. For example, a tomato bred to produce a protein normally found in peanuts could cause potentially life-threatening symptoms when eaten by someone allergic to peanuts. For this reason, the FDA requires clear scientific proof of safety from developers working with foods to which people are commonly allergic, such as milk, eggs, wheat, fish, tree nuts (eg, walnuts, pecans), and legumes (eg, beans, peanuts). It's impossible to predict allergic reactions to proteins derived from plants or other sources if they are not recognized causes of allergy. Nevertheless, scientists can test a bioengineered protein to see whether its structure resembles that of a known allergen. If it does, further tests show whether an allergic cross-reaction is likely.

Organic Foods

Many people prefer to buy organic produce and meat out of concerns for their health and the environment (also see Chapter 15, Alternative Diets and Supplements). Purchasers generally assume that foods marketed as organic have been grown without synthetic fertilizers and pesticides and have not been treated with antibiotics, hormones, or synthetic additives such as dyes and preservatives. Even foods raised organically, however, may contain pesticides and other contaminants carried by wind, water, or soil residues. In addition, while free of certain contaminants, organic products are not necessarily more nutritious or more flavorful than other foods. Retailers generally demand higher prices for organic foods, but such produce may spoil faster because it is not treated against insects and bacteria.

So is buying organic worth the price?

A small study in 2008 measured levels of pesticide in the urine of children prior to the study. There were detectable but low levels of some pesticides in the urine of most children before the study began. Their diets were then limited to organic fruits and vegetables, and some corn- and wheat-based products such as pasta and cereal. Because meats and dairy products do not contain significant levels of pesticides, they were not changed in the diet. The result? After a week of eating only organic products, urinary pesticide levels decreased significantly.

Does this mean that the increased cost and decreased shelf life of organic foods are justified for all children? The answer is maybe. Children are exposed to pesticides in other ways such as playing on grass in a park that has been sprayed for insect control or drinking water into which pesticides have leaked.

Measures such as washing and peeling all produce before serving it, buying only domestically grown produce rather than imported, buying from local farmers' markets, and participating in a community garden using organic farming methods can reduce the risk. Keep in mind, however, that locally grown produce is not always pesticide-free, so look for a label that states that it is organic to minimize pesticide content. If you live in an agricultural area and drink well water, testing it for pesticide content may be helpful as well.

Even if pesticides are present, they are often not the major environmental threat to children's health that they once were because of advances in pest management that have lowered that risk considerably. For example, substances that disrupt the growth only of a certain insect that can attack a crop but not harm humans in the process are used in some situations. Another approach is the use of a particular pheromone (a chemical secreted by animals) that disrupts the mating of some insects. Breeding plants that resist diseases and careful monitoring of residues in soil before planting have also contributed to a reduction in risk.

Irradiation

Irradiated food is exposed to low levels of x-rays and other forms of ionizing radiation. The process does not make food radioactive but it kills molds, bacteria, and insects that cause spoilage. It can delay the ripening of fruits, thus extending their shelf life, and it inhibits sprouting of potatoes, onions, garlic, and other foods so they stay fresh longer.

Though consumers have been slow to accept irradiation of food, experts believe it may be a safer means of preservation than many additives. Resistance to irradiated foods seems to be based on persistent but groundless fears of nuclear fallout and radiation sickness. The FDA, which classifies irradiation as an additive, allows its use in wheat, flour, potatoes, spices, and many fresh foods. Products that have been irradiated must be labeled and must bear an international symbol.

Food Hazards and Scares

For children and adults alike, it's good to eat a wide variety of foods. Not only does variety promote a healthful intake of nutrients, but it also lowers the risk of exposure to potentially harmful substances that may be concentrated in 1 or 2 foods.

In recent years, parents have been besieged with reports of contaminated food (as well as toys and baby products) that may contain harmful chemicals. Infants are particularly sensitive to chemicals and contamination. For example, perfluorooctanoic acid used in packaged food such as microwave popcorn or frozen pizza to prevent food from sticking to the package is a cancer-causing chemical—yet there are no requirements to label products that contain this substance.

BISPHENOL A (BPA)

In recent years, bisphenol A, or BPA, has emerged as a widely used plastic chemical—and a controversial one at that. Can children be safely exposed to it? Should parents try to limit that exposure?

Bisphenol A is in many food and liquid containers made of a strong plastic called polycarbonate, or lined with an epoxy containing BPA. This chemical is used to harden plastics to reduce the risk of breakage and to prevent food contamination from bacteria. Children are most often exposed to BPA when it leaches from hard-plastic baby bottles, sippy cups, and metal cans containing food and infant formula.

Concerns over possible harmful effects of exposure to plastics, and specifically to BPA, have focused particularly on infants and children during development. Some animal studies have shown that BPA exposure can affect the endocrine system (ie, hormones, glands). In animals dosed with BPA during pregnancy, there have been negative hormonelike effects on their fetus' reproductive system, as well as injury to the nervous system. However, more research is necessary to determine if these same health effects occur in humans.

As research continues, many parents are taking steps to reduce their child's exposure to plastics and BPA. Breastfeeding is an excellent alternative to using BPA-containing products like baby bottles. The American Academy of Pediatrics recommends exclusive breastfeeding in the early months of life, and then continuing at least through 12 months of age in combination with solid foods.

Other precautionary measures include the following:

- If you're using plastic bottles, consider those certified or identified as BPA free. Avoid clear plastic containers that are imprinted with the #7 recycling code and the letters PC. These bottles and containers may contain BPA.

- Choose bottles that are opaque plastic. They are made of polyethylene or polypropylene and do not contain BPA.

- Although glass bottles are another alternative, keep in mind that there is a risk of injury to your baby if the bottle is dropped or breaks.

- Heat can trigger the release of BPA from plastics. For that reason, do not boil liquids in polycarbonate plastic bottles or heat these bottles or containers in the microwave oven. Polycarbonate bottles and containers should not be washed in the dishwasher either.

- Limit the use of canned foods because BPA may be used in the linings of these cans. Rely more often on fresh or frozen foods.

So how can you evaluate food and product information and food scares without becoming afraid of everything?

✔ **First, consider the source.** Some reports—for example, a recent study that found that using lotions and wipes was correlated with high levels of phthalates (chemicals used in plastics) in infants' urine—are poorly done and their results are open to questions. Some reports are sponsored by companies that want to sell you an alternative product. Your pediatrician can be a resource for these judgments.

✔ **Fully inform yourself.** In 2008, there were reports of *E coli* contamination of some tomatoes. But this contamination turned out to affect only specific tomatoes—and then probably jalapeños and not even tomatoes, and only those from a specific area. In spite of that, millions of families stopped eating tomatoes and crops were plowed under unnecessarily. Most bacterial outbreaks affect only a small number of people and are contained quickly.

✔ **Know how to avoid risks.** As mentioned earlier, wash fruits and vegetables thoroughly, even before putting them away. Patronize local farmers' markets where you know the source of the food. Ask farmers about their methods.

✔ **Consult reputable authorities.** The CDC (www.cdc.gov) usually has up-to-the-minute reports on problems in the food supply. Your pediatrician can help, but realize that if you heard something on the morning news, your pediatrician may not even be aware of it yet. Doctors are usually better informed after a day or two.

ISSUES PARENTS RAISE ABOUT FOOD SAFETY

It's not unusual for one or another of my children to have a bout of vomiting and diarrhea after eating something. How can I tell when it's more serious than a touch of food poisoning?

If symptoms are still present after 3 to 4 hours for an infant younger than 1 year, or 6 to 8 hours for an older child—or if the child appears ill or drowsy, or has bloody or unusually severe diarrhea—call your pediatrician immediately for advice. (See page 280.)

I'm not sure how long I need to wash my hands to get them really clean for food preparation.

Wash your hands for at least 10 to 20 seconds with soap and warm water before preparing foods, and wash again periodically as necessary. (See page 282.)

With all the new bioengineered foods coming onto the market, who is overseeing safety, especially for people who are allergic to certain foods?

One concern related to bioengineering is the possibility that proteins introduced from one food into another could cause allergic reactions in people sensitive to the first food. For this reason, the FDA requires proof of safety from developers working with foods to which people are commonly allergic. It's impossible to predict allergic reactions to proteins if the sources are not recognized causes of allergy; still, scientists can test a bioengineered protein to see if it resembles a known allergen. If it does, further tests can show whether a cross-reaction is likely. (See page 286.)

Does irradiating food make it radioactive?

Experts believe irradiation may be a safer means of preserving food than many additives. The process does not make food radioactive or change it in any way. However, consumers have been slow to accept irradiated foods on the basis of groundless fears of nuclear fallout and radiation sickness. (See page 288.)

Chapter 14

Food Additives

Additives, in general, have had a bad reputation, but that is not necessarily appropriate. Unless you grow your own food and bake your own bread, getting food to your supermarket requires that it stay fresh and unspoiled. Even skin creams and lotions must have preservatives to keep them from harboring dangerous germs.

Chemicals that the Food and Drug Administration (FDA) considers safe may be added to food and other products but only at the minimum levels necessary. Of course, the more fresh fruits and vegetables and unprocessed food in your family's diet, the fewer of these additives you will have to contend with.

Food additives, properly used, allow us to enjoy a variety of wholesome foods in every season. Many people, wary of additives, believe that they are toxic chemicals brewed up in laboratories. Such fears are groundless. The great majority of the 3,000 or so additives allowed by the FDA are foods or normal ingredients of foods. Additives help keep our food healthful in at least 5 important ways.

- They retard spoilage.
- They improve or maintain nutritional value.
- They make breads and baked goods rise.
- They enhance flavor, color, and appearance.
- They keep flavors and textures consistent.

Additives listed on food labels under their chemical names seem less intimidating when you know their everyday equivalents. For example, salt is sodium chloride, vitamin C is ascorbic acid, and vitamin E is alpha-tocopherol. Not every additive has a familiar name, but it's reassuring to remember that all food is made up of chemicals, just as our bodies are. Regulations known as good manufacturing practices limit the amounts of additives that may be used in foods. Manufacturers use only as much of an additive as is needed to achieve the desired result.

The additives most widely used are salt, sugar and corn syrup, vitamin C, vitamin E, and butylated hydroxyanisole (BHA) and butylated hydroxytoluene (BHT). These substances prolong shelf life, stop fats and oils from turning rancid, and prevent discoloration and changes in texture. Additives are also used in packing materials and must be approved for this purpose.

ADDITIVES THAT ENRICH AND FORTIFY

Additives used for enriching and fortifying foods are particularly beneficial. Enrichment restores essential nutrients that are lost during the processing of raw materials. For example, white flour and rice are enriched with B vitamins that are removed when the grains are milled. As a public health measure, certain foods are fortified with important nutrients to make sure people consume enough to stay healthy. Vitamin D, for example, is added to milk; vitamin A to margarine; and iron and folic acid to flours and cereals.

ADDITIVES DON'T APPEAR TO INFLUENCE HYPERACTIVITY

Years ago, Dr Benjamin Feingold, a pediatric allergist, claimed that the behavior of hyperactive children improved dramatically when they followed a diet that eliminated additives, including artificial colors and flavors, as well as naturally occurring salicylates in fruits and vegetables. But when tested scientifically, the Feingold diet had no favorable effect. Some children, however, appeared to benefit from the extra parental attention.

In other cases, belief in the diet's efficacy seemed to bring about an improvement similar to the placebo effect sometimes seen with medical treatments. In one study, the behavior of a small group of children with more severe hyperactivity changed for the worse when they were given food spiked with huge doses of artificial colors. However, the doses were many times greater than children would normally consume, and the findings, therefore, do not apply to usual situations.

Nevertheless, it is possible that a child may be unusually sensitive to a particular ingredient or food. If you are convinced there's a connection between your child's behavior and his diet, talk to your pediatrician, who may perform sensitivity testing or recommend cutting out an offending food and finding alternative sources if essential nutrients are involved (also see chapters 15 and 16).

SULFITES: A SENSITIVE ISSUE

According to Food and Drug Administration (FDA) estimates, about 1 person out of every 100 has allergic symptoms after exposure to *sulfites,* chemical additives widely used in the food industry. Asthma adds to the risk; sulfites cause serious symptoms in about 5% of people with asthma.

Sulfites are added to prolong the shelf life of many fruits, vegetables, and shellfish; to halt the growth of bacteria in wines; and to whiten food starches and condition dough. They are also used as preservatives in some medications. Although once freely allowed under the FDA category of "generally regarded as safe" (GRAS), sulfite use has been more closely regulated in the past couple of decades after being linked to numerous health problems, including allergic symptoms ranging in severity from hives and difficulty breathing to fatal anaphylactic shock. While sulfites are indeed harmless to the great majority, they can cause potentially life-threatening reactions in some people with asthma and others who are sensitive to the compounds. Scientists haven't yet determined the smallest amount needed to trigger a reaction. Current methods cannot detect sulfite concentrations below 10 parts per million (ppm) in food, although many experts believe that a sulfite-sensitive person may experience symptoms at even lower concentrations. To reduce the risk, the FDA has imposed the following restrictions:

- Sulfites may not be used on fruits and vegetables intended to be eaten raw, such as in supermarket produce departments or restaurant salad bars.

- Product labels must list sulfites in concentrations of 10 ppm or higher, or any sulfites that have been used in processing, regardless of the concentration. In addition, labels must specify the purpose for which sulfites were used.

If you suspect that exposure to sulfites has triggered hives, chest tightness, difficulty breathing, or other symptoms in your child, call your pediatrician to determine whether a sensitivity is present (also see Chapter 16, Is My Child Allergic?).

WATCH THE SALT!

Almost 80% of the salt in our diet comes as an additive in processed foods like bread, soups, snacks, fast foods, canned foods, or processed meats. It may be one of the most common additives, but it's important to choose and prepare foods with as little of it as possible. (For more information on salt, see Chapter 11, What Do I Do About Outside Influences?)

Nitrites and Nitrosamines

Nitrites are chemicals used to cure meats such as bacon and ham and prevent the growth of *Clostridium botulinum,* the bacterium that causes botulism. Nitrites are nothing new; they've been used in one form or another for at least a couple of thousand years. After they reach the digestive tract, some of these chemicals are transformed into nitrosamines, which are potentially carcinogenic, or cancer causing. To keep the risk as low as possible, meat processors are allowed to use only the lowest amount of nitrites needed to stop *C botulinum.* In addition, cured meats, by law, must contain vitamin C, an antioxidant that blocks the formation of nitrosamines.

FACTS ABOUT TRANS FATS

Nutrition experts have long encouraged consumers to replace saturated fats—animal fats and others that stay firm at room temperature—with unsaturated vegetable oils. To create an acceptable substitute for butter, which is a saturated fat, unsaturated liquid fats are hydrogenated so they will stay firm and resist spoilage through oxidation. After they are partially hydrogenated, these fats are called trans fats and appear to take on not only the firmness but perhaps other, less desirable properties of butter as well. Trans fats adversely affect blood cholesterol levels by lowering levels of the protective HDL cholesterol and raising the level of the harmful LDL cholesterol, and are now felt to be major contributors to coronary heart disease. These concerns about trans fat led the Food and Drug Administration in 2006 to require that trans fat content be added to food package labels.

Experts caution, however, that we should not leap to the conclusion that butter is better. Dairy products and meat also contain small amounts of trans fats, but the benefits of the other nutrients that dairy products contain more than balance the risks of their trans fat content. Consumption of low-fat or no-fat milk minimizes naturally occurring trans fats in milk. A substantial decrease in coronary heart disease over the past 30 years is partly due to the substitution of unsaturated vegetable fats—including trans fats—for saturated fats. A number of cities have banned trans fat in restaurants, and the voluntary reduction in trans fat in processed foods has already reduced trans fat in the food supply. Keep reducing your child's intake of saturated fats, and at the same time, eliminate his trans fat intake by using only products that contain zero trans fats.

Fat Substitutes

To guard against the health risks linked to long-term consumption of a high-fat diet, all Americans older than 2 years are urged to limit their fat intake to 30% or less of daily calories and to keep saturated fat to no more than one third of total fat, or 10% of calories. The period between 2 and 5 years is one of gradual transition to a low-fat diet. Food producers have responded to the fat-reduction trend by developing reduced-fat and nonfat products that often contain fat substitutes.

The FDA allows egg-white– and dairy-protein–based fat substitutes as "generally regarded as safe" (GRAS), meaning that they can be used without restriction in food manufacturing.

For more information about fat consumption, see "Heart Disease" in Chapter 12 (page 266).

ISSUES PARENTS RAISE ABOUT FOOD ADDITIVES

I've heard that artificial colors and flavors can affect children's attention. My child is having problems in school, but it is hard to avoid all additives.

A diet that includes a minimum of processed foods and concentrates on fresh fruits, vegetables, whole grains, and lean meat is better for everyone. There is no evidence that artificial colors and flavors contribute to attention or other problems. (See page 294.)

My family has a history of high blood pressure. How do I reduce the amount of sodium in my child's diet?

Most of the sodium we consume is from salt in processed foods. You can find the sodium content on the Nutrition Facts panel on the back of food packages. Easy ways to lower sodium intake is to read food labels and chose lower sodium products and to minimize the amounts of processed foods in your child's diet. (See page 295.)

What's the difference between an enriched food and a fortified one?

Enrichment puts back essential nutrients that are lost during the processing of raw materials. White flour and rice are enriched with B vitamins that are lost when the grains are milled. As a public health measure, certain foods are fortified with important nutrients to make sure people consume enough to stay healthy. These nutrients, such as vitamin D in milk and iron in flours and cereals, are not usually present in the food to begin with. (See page 294.)

Chapter 15

Alternative Diets and Supplements

People adopt alternative diets for many reasons—cultural, religious, health, ethical, and environmental concerns, to mention a few. The diets themselves range from age-old vegetarianism to short-lived fads. While some alternative diets can be just as healthful as more traditional fare, when it comes to feeding children, special care is needed to make sure they are well nourished.

Maria Baretta took great pride in serving her family the tasty Italian dishes she had learned from her mother and grandmothers. She looked forward to continuing the tradition by teaching her 12-year-old daughter, Anita, the fine art of Italian cooking. But those plans came to a screeching halt when Anita announced that she was becoming a vegetarian, largely because of her concern for animals, plus the fact that her best friend had also decided to become a vegetarian.

"At first, I refused to take her seriously," Maria recalls. "I continued to make my favorite meat dishes, but no amount of pleading or threatening could make Anita eat them."

Finally, Maria consulted her pediatrician. She had expected the doctor to agree that Anita's refusal to eat meat was unhealthy. Instead, the pediatrician assured Maria that a vegetarian diet—especially one like Anita's, which included dairy products and eggs—was just as healthful as one centered on meat dishes. The doctor suggested a couple of books on healthy vegetarian diets, and Maria also bought an Italian vegetarian cookbook. Although many of the Barettas' meals still include a meat dish, Maria also now serves vegetarian alternatives. And instead of hurt feelings or angry dinnertime outbursts over Anita's refusal to eat meat, mealtimes in the Baretta household are peaceful again.

A Growing Movement

Only a few years ago, many Americans looked on vegetarianism with suspicion, often mixed with disdain. Today, a vegetarian diet is almost mainstream compared with the many other alternative diets that are being adopted by a growing number of Americans. Many of these diets make outlandish claims, promising everything from painless weight loss to increased brain power or sports ability. When the diet fails to deliver the promised magic, the person is likely to revert to former eating habits or try the next fad. Obviously, such faddish or overly restrictive alternative diets should not be forced on growing children. Still, many alternative diets can be just as healthful as a mainstream diet. For children, this means that the diet must provide all of the vitamins, minerals, protein, and energy needed for appropriate growth and development. Any alternative diet that falls short of meeting children's basic nutritional needs should be modified or avoided. Likewise, a conventional diet that provides lots of meat, fatty foods, and sweets while skimping on vegetables, fruits, and grains and other starches can lead to serious nutritional problems. Regardless of the type of diet you or your child select, you won't go wrong if you follow the basic rules of variety, moderation, and balance (see Chapter 6, Is My Child Overweight?).

Vegetarian Diets

In general, a vegetarian is a person who eats mostly plant foods and excludes meat, poultry, and fish from the diet. However, there are many shades of vegetarianism, ranging from *partial vegetarians,* who eat dairy products, eggs, and perhaps fish or poultry, to *vegans,* who are strict vegetarians who shun all animal products, including milk and eggs (see "Variations on the Vegetarian Theme" on page 306).

Although some people still worry that a vegetarian diet is unhealthful, numerous studies have found just the opposite. In general, vegetarians have a reduced risk of obesity, heart disease, high blood pressure, type 2 (non–insulin-dependent) diabetes, certain digestive disorders, and some cancers. It is not clear, however, whether these health benefits are due solely to following a vegetarian diet or to a combination of other factors that often go hand in hand with a vegetarian lifestyle. In 2009, the American Academy of Pediatrics Committee on Nutrition stated in its *Pediatric Nutrition Handbook:*

Vegetarian diets can meet the nutritional needs of children and adolescents if appropriately planned and monitored by a health care professional or nutritionist.

Health Benefits

Diets based mostly on plant foods are low in cholesterol and saturated fats and high in fiber. Most also provide fewer calories than diets loaded with meat and high-fat dairy products. These factors may account for the lower rates among vegetarians of obesity, heart disease, diabetes, gall bladder disease, and certain cancers.

Plant foods also are rich in vitamins, minerals, and other compounds called *antioxidants,* substances that protect body cells against the damage that naturally occurs when the body burns oxygen. Antioxidants are believed to help prevent some of the cell changes that lead to premature aging and cancer.

Vegetarians often point to other benefits unrelated to health. For example, vegetarian diets tend to be less costly than diets that include meat. Pound for pound, beans and grains are much cheaper sources of protein than meat.

There are also important environmental benefits. It takes many more acres of farmland or pounds of grain to produce an equivalent amount of human plant food. Grains are by far the world's leading foodstuff, and the United States leads the world in per capita grain use. But unlike people in other grain-consuming nations, Americans actually eat very little of this grain themselves. Instead, it is fed to animals to produce meat, eggs, and dairy products.

Finally, many people—especially children and adolescents—become vegetarians because of their concern for animals.

Possible Problems

Nutritionists caution that a healthful vegetarian diet for children takes more planning and knowledge about nutrition than does a diet featuring meat and other animal products. The task is relatively easy, if the diet allows eggs or milk and other dairy products. But a strict vegetarian or vegan diet is another story. Particular challenges for a vegan diet include

- **Calories.** A growing child may not be able to eat enough plant foods to get the energy needed for proper growth and normal activities, especially in early childhood.
- **Protein,** which is needed to build muscle and other body tissue, must be obtained by balancing foods, such as grains and legumes, to get the range of amino acids that make up high-quality, or complete, proteins.
- **Vitamin B$_{12}$,** which can be absorbed only from animal products, must be obtained from supplements or fortified foods.
- **Vitamin D,** which is found in egg yolks, fish and fish liver oil, and fortified milk and butter, may be lacking. The body also makes vitamin D when the skin is exposed to sunlight, but children in northern climates may have difficulty getting enough sun.

ORGANIC? NATURAL? HEALTH FOODS?

Although these terms are often used interchangeably, they have different meanings.

- Organic foods are grown without artificial pesticides, fertilizers, or herbicides. Organic meat, eggs, and dairy products are obtained from animals that are fed natural feed and not given hormones or antibiotics.
- Natural foods are free of synthetic or artificial ingredients or additives.
- "Health foods" is a general term that may be applied to natural or organic foods, or to regular foods that have undergone less processing than usual, such as stone-ground whole-grain flours.

Although some have claimed that organic foods have a higher concentration of some nutrients, the evidence is mixed. The nutritional content of foods also varies greatly according to when the food was harvested and how it has been stored or processed. Unless they are fresher, there is also no evidence that organic, natural, or health foods taste better than regular foods. However, taste is determined by plant genetics, rather than by whether the crop is organically or conventionally grown. Harvesting and handling also affect taste. A peach or tomato that is picked when it is too green will never develop the full taste of fruit that is allowed to ripen on the tree or the vine.

Although the type of fertilizer may not affect taste or nutrition, it does have an effect on the environment. Many people prefer to pay premium prices for organic foods because their production does not cause environmental damage from pesticides and herbicides, and composted fertilizers help restore soil and are not as damaging to the environment as artificial fertilizers. However, simply stating "organic" does not protect the food from being contaminated from field to market.

(For more information on organic foods, see "Organic Foods," Chapter 13, page 287.)

PASTEURIZED MILK: MYTHS AND PROVEN FACTS

Pasteurization is a process that kills harmful bacteria by heating milk to a specific temperature for a set period. Some people continue to believe that pasteurization harms milk and that raw milk is a safe, healthier alternative.

Raw milk can harbor dangerous microorganisms, such as *Salmonella, Escherichia coli,* and *Listeria,* that can pose serious health risks, and children are particularly susceptible to the potential infections of unpasteurized or raw milk.

Here are some common myths and proven facts about milk and pasteurization.

- Raw milk DOES NOT kill dangerous pathogens by itself.
- Pasteurizing milk DOES NOT cause lactose intolerance and allergic reactions. Raw and pasteurized milk can cause allergic reactions in people sensitive to milk proteins.
- Pasteurization DOES NOT reduce milk's nutritional value.
- Pasteurization DOES NOT mean that it is safe to leave milk out of the refrigerator for an extended time, particularly after it has been opened.
- Pasteurization DOES kill harmful bacteria.
- Pasteurization DOES save lives.

Courtesy of FoodSafety.com. Source: www.foodsafety.gov/keep/types/milk

- **Calcium,** whose best sources are milk and milk products, must be obtained from plant sources or supplements.
- **Zinc,** whose best sources are beef, liver, and yogurt, may be lacking.

Social Issues

Vegetarianism and other alternative diets can be a major source of conflict unless they are a family affair. Even if parents are strict vegetarians, they might allow their child to eat the foods his friends enjoy, such as an occasional hamburger or roast chicken. However, if the entire family follows a vegetarian diet, the child will grow up accepting it as normal and will also be less likely to feel set apart when he eats foods that are different from what his friends enjoy at school or social gatherings.

THE EGG AND YOU: WHAT SHOULD YOU CHOOSE?

All eggs sold in stores are grade A, so the "choice" of grade is a no-brainer. But these days, you'll find plenty of other labels on eggs, intended to make you buy one particular product or another. Because the choices can be dizzying and unclear, it can be difficult to know what is best for your family. To help you sort things out, here are some terms and a little information about what each means—or doesn't mean.

Organic. If an egg is US Department of Agriculture–certified organic, the hens have not been given antibiotics and their feed is free of pesticides, fertilizers, and other chemicals. But if the organic label carries a state agency's name, the standards may be different.

No Antibiotics. The Food and Drug Administration (FDA) does not allow routine use of antibiotics, but they can be used if the chicken is ill. No antibiotics have been used if the eggs are part of the National Organic Program.

No Hormones. This terminology is meaningless because the FDA does not allow any hormone products in egg production. Every egg should already be hormone-free.

Natural or **Naturally Raised.** This label has no meaning other than what egg producers want it to mean.

Cage-free. Hens that provide these eggs are kept out of cages. They have access to food and water but are not necessarily allowed outdoors.

Free Range. These birds have access to the outdoors but still may be allowed only on concrete areas.

Pasture-raised. Hens in this category get part of their food from outdoor sources (eg, bugs, greens), which may increase some vitamins and omega-3 fatty acids and reduce saturated fats. There is no regulation on the use of this term.

Vegetarian-fed. The hens are fed only vegetarian foods. Chickens are not naturally vegetarian; they enjoy the occasional grub or caterpillar.

Pasteurized Eggs. These eggs are heated just enough to destroy bacteria but not hot enough to cook them. They are increasingly found in supermarkets and are a good choice for people who are susceptible to infection (such as those undergoing chemotherapy or who have AIDS) or who like their eggs undercooked. Remember that the risk of infection from eggs these days is quite small and is almost completely eliminated if they are cooked adequately before eating.

Omega-3 Eggs. Producers of eggs carrying this label claim that their product has higher levels of omega-3 fatty acids, which may be beneficial for heart health and brain development. However, they are not inspected by the FDA for their omega-3 content unless there is a complaint.

> ### THE EGG AND YOU: WHAT SHOULD YOU CHOOSE? *CONTINUED*
>
> **Animal Welfare Approved.** This term is given to independent farmers whose hens are in small flocks of fewer than 500, spend all of their time outside in pesticide-free pastures, and are not fed animal by-products.
>
> **American Humane Certified.** This category is similar to the previous one, but these hens also are not subjected to forced molting, which increases egg production.
>
> **United Egg Producers Certified.** This term is applied to a coalition of egg producers with lower standards, such as each hen being provided space only equivalent to a letter-sized piece of paper.

The example of the Baretta family at the beginning of this chapter is very typical of what happens when a somewhat older child insists on becoming a vegetarian in a meat-eating family. The switch often occurs during adolescence, a time when many families are strained by a teenager's growing independence. Still, children as young as 6 years may become lifelong vegetarians when they become sensitive to the relationship between humans and animals.

A 6-year-old patient of Dr Stern's once asked his mother what he was eating. His mother said, "Fish sticks."

He had a pet goldfish. "Fish? Like my fish?" he asked.

When his mother said "Yes," he replied, "That's *disgusting!*" He has not eaten fish (or meat) since, and it has been many years since the incident. A child's continued refusal to eat what parents perceive as foods essential for health sets the stage for mealtime conflicts. Very often, the vegetarian child adopts an irritating moral stance: "You may not care about animals (or the environment), but I do!"

Although adolescents of both sexes become vegetarians, the switch is more common among girls, and concern for animals is by far the most common reason that young people shun meat. In contrast, adults are more likely to cite health reasons for adopting vegetarianism or another alternative diet.

VARIATIONS ON THE VEGETARIAN THEME	
All vegetarian diets allow grains, vegetables, and fruits, but they vary considerably when it comes to animal products.	
Partial vegetarian	Diet allows dairy products, eggs, seafood, and perhaps poultry, but not meat and sometimes not poultry.
Lacto-ovo vegetarian	Diet allows dairy products and eggs but not meat, seafood, or poultry.
Lactovegetarian	Diet allows milk and milk products but not eggs, meat, seafood, or poultry.
Ovovegetarian	Diet allows eggs but not meat, seafood, poultry, or milk or other dairy products.
Vegan	No animal products—no dairy products, eggs, meat, seafood, or poultry.

Other Alternative Diets

There are dozens of different alternative diets, but they have certain common themes. Most are built on philosophical, religious, or other personal convictions. Many promise unlikely benefits, such as rapid and painless weight loss or increased brain power. Some are promoted as treatments (usually unproven) for diseases ranging from childhood hyperactivity to cancer.

Because many of these diets eliminate entire groups of foods, they carry a risk of nutritional deficiencies, especially for children. Some of the most popular alternative diets, summarized in "Overview of Other Alternative Diets" on page 312, are described in more detail as follows:

Whole-Foods Diet

This diet is based on the belief that foods should be eaten in their entirety and in as natural a state as possible. The premise is that whole foods provide a balance of nutrients and energy that is lacking in fragmented or processed foods. Thus, in a whole-foods diet, eating a whole baked potato with its skin would be preferable to potatoes that are peeled and cut. In addition to fresh fruits and vegetables, other examples of whole foods include unrefined grains, beans and other legumes, seeds, sea vegetables, and eggs. Fragmented foods, such as sugar, flour, polished rice, and peeled vegetables, are avoided as much as possible. When fragmented foods are eaten, they are balanced with complementary fragments to form a whole. Thus, flour might be balanced with wheat germ and bran to mimic what is found in the whole grain.

Although many people who follow a whole-foods diet are vegetarians, some are not. And some animal products, such as fertilized eggs, are whole foods. A soft-shell crab is also considered a whole food because the entire crab, shell and all, is eaten.

Living Foods Diet

This diet is based on the notion that raw foods are more healthful than cooked ones because they contain enzymes that aid in digestion and, more importantly, they contain the life force or natural energy of the plant. Proponents of a living foods diet believe that heating foods destroys these enzymes and also changes the molecular structure of food to make it toxic—an assertion that simply is not true. Cooking certainly does not make foods toxic. And even if foods are eaten raw, the enzymes will be broken down during digestion.

The diet allows all organically grown fruits, vegetables, sprouts, nuts, seeds, grains, and sea vegetables. Grains and seeds may be soaked so that they are soft enough to eat, but they are not cooked. Beverages include fresh juices and coconut milk. This diet is not recommended for children or adolescents, and adults who follow it are likely to need supplements of vitamin B_{12}, iron, calcium, and zinc. Followers also have an increased risk of food-borne illnesses from eating possibly contaminated uncooked foods.

Variations of the living foods diet include sproutarian, a diet based mostly on sprouted seeds and grains, and juicearian, in which the living foods are put through a juicer. These variations have the same shortcomings as the basic living foods diet.

Fruitarian Diet

This is another extreme variation of a living foods diet that is limited to organically grown fruit, seeds, nuts, and grains. The idea is to avoid killing a plant for food. Thus, carrots and other vegetables are excluded because eating the edible part kills the plant. In contrast, picking an apple or peach does not kill the tree. This diet is potentially dangerous for children and adults; it lacks adequate protein, vitamins B_{12} and D, calcium, iron, zinc, and other trace minerals.

Macrobiotic Diets

Closely related to Zen Buddhism, macrobiotic diets are largely vegetarian and rooted in Eastern philosophy. All foods are classified as yin (female) or yang (male), and meals seek to balance these so-called opposing natural forces. Thus, yang foods—meat, seafood, seeds, and grains—are served with yin foods—vegetables, fruits, juices, and dairy foods. An individual diet is tailored to the specific yin or yang needs of the person. If a person falls ill with a yang disease, yin foods in the diet should be increased to try to restore the balance of yin and yang. In addition, foods should be seasonal, locally grown, and prepared in a specific manner with wooden cooking utensils.

The extreme macrobiotic diets that were popular in the United States during the 1960s created a lot of misunderstanding of macrobiotics and the underlying philosophy. These extreme diets, which are no longer widely practiced, were limited mostly to brown rice and other grains, legumes, and teas. Following such a restrictive diet for very long can cause severe nutritional deficiencies, and some deaths were attributed to these macrobiotic regimens. The traditional macrobiotic diet, however, emphasizes variety and balance and can be healthful, but it requires time to learn and to prepare.

Crash Weight-Loss Diets

It seems that every few months, yet another "miracle" weight-loss diet comes along. Although the specifics vary, all promise that you'll quickly and easily shed unwanted pounds. And those who follow these diets for even a few weeks do, indeed, lose weight. But as soon as they stop dieting, the lost weight returns, often with a few extra pounds added. The main reason

(continued on page 312)

SAMPLE VEGETARIAN MENUS

The following menus follow the principles of various diets, with suggestions for supplements or fortified foods to fill nutritional gaps:

PARTIAL VEGETARIAN

Breakfast

Whole-grain cereal with low-fat or skim milk

Sliced banana

English muffin

Beverage

Lunch

Tomato and mozzarella salad

Vegetarian bean soup

Whole-grain crackers

Fresh fruit

Low-fat milk

Dinner

Mixed green salad

Baked potato with grated Parmesan cheese

Green beans

Poached fish fillet

Frozen yogurt with oatmeal cookie

Snacks

Low-fat milk, cheeses, or yogurt

Air-popped popcorn

Hummus with pita bread

Choice of fresh fruit or raw vegetables

Supplements: None needed; diet provides proper variety and balance of nutrients.

LACTOVEGETARIAN

Breakfast

½ grapefruit

Oatmeal with mixed dried fruit

Skim or low-fat milk

Lunch

Green salad

Vegetarian chili and rice

Skim or low-fat milk

Dinner

Leek and potato soup

Vegetable lasagna made with cheese

Rice pudding made with low-fat milk

Snacks

Whole-grain crackers

Low-fat yogurt

Fresh fruits or vegetables

Supplements: None needed; diet provides proper variety and balance of nutrients.

(continued on next page)

SAMPLE VEGETARIAN MENUS, *CONTINUED*

LACTO-OVO VEGETARIAN	OVOVEGETARIAN
Breakfast	*Breakfast*
Orange juice or sliced orange	Fresh orange
Scrambled egg	Poached egg
Whole wheat toast	Whole wheat toast
Skim or low-fat milk	Calcium-fortified soy milk
Lunch	*Lunch*
Minestrone soup	Lentil salad
Fruit salad and cottage cheese	Peanut butter sandwich
Date bread	Fresh fruit
Low-fat fruit yogurt	*Dinner*
Dinner	Pasta and bean soup
Chopped vegetable salad	Steamed broccoli
Pasta with marinara sauce	Vegetarian garden burgers
Low-fat cheese and poached pear	Tofu ice cream with fresh berries
Skim or low-fat milk	*Snacks*
Snacks	Trail mix, soy milk, fresh fruit shake
½ toasted bagel or bran muffin	
Choice of fresh fruit, low-fat cheese,	
or vegetables	

Supplements: None needed; diet provides proper variety and balance of nutrients.

Supplements: None needed; diet provides proper variety and balance of nutrients.

SAMPLE VEGETARIAN MENUS, *CONTINUED*

VEGAN

Breakfast
Calcium-fortified orange juice
Iron-fortified cereal with dates and
soy milk
Fresh fruit

Lunch
Spinach and tomato salad
Vegetarian barley and vegetable soup
Applesauce
Calcium-fortified soy milk

Dinner
Fruit cup
Steamed Chinese vegetables and
bean sprouts
Red beans and rice
Fresh berries and sorbet

Snacks
Trail mix, fresh fruit, or vegetables
Calcium-fortified orange juice or soy milk

Supplements: Multiple vitamin-mineral pill to provide vitamin
B_{12}, iron, extra calcium, and zinc. Extra snacks or servings may
be needed to provide adequate calories.

OVERVIEW OF OTHER ALTERNATIVE DIETS	
Whole foods	Diet is based on belief that foods should be eaten in their whole, natural state. Followers include vegetarians and meat eaters.
Living foods	Diet allows only organic plant foods that are not cooked, heated, pasteurized, or processed.
Macrobiotic	Diet, part of an Eastern philosophic approach to life, is based mostly on locally grown organic grains, vegetables, legumes, sea vegetables, and soups, although seafood and animal products may be eaten occasionally.
Fruitarian	Diet is based mostly on raw and dried fruits, seeds, sprouted seeds and grains, and nuts; excludes processed and cooked foods, vegetables, and all animal products.
Sproutarian	Variation of living foods diet that consists mostly of sprouts.
Juicearian	Variation of living foods diet based mostly on fresh juices.
Feingold	Diet designed by an allergist to treat hyperactivity; it is promoted as a treatment for attention-deficit/hyperactivity disorder.
Crash weight loss	These are generally restrictive, low-calorie diets designed to produce rapid weight loss, which is usually temporary.

these diets fail is that they don't address the underlying reason for being overweight—faulty eating habits, lack of exercise, and perhaps hereditary and metabolic factors. So when you go off such a diet and return to your normal eating habits, you again gain weight.

There are many types of crash diets; examples include liquid-protein diets, low-carbohydrate diets, herbal diets, and diets based on 1 or 2 foods (eg, grapefruit, cabbage). All of these pose special hazards for children (see Chapter 8, Nutrition Basics).

DIETS TO TREAT DISORDERS

Folk medicine is filled with dietary remedies to treat various diseases, and research shows that some of these may be helpful. For most medical conditions, however, modern medicines are more effective and easier to control than dietary remedies. Extra caution is needed when using a diet to treat a childhood disorder. Two prominent examples are the ketogenic diet to treat epilepsy and the Feingold diet to treat attention-deficit/hyperactivity disorder.

The Ketogenic Diet

This diet is used to treat epileptic seizures that cannot be controlled with medication. It is a low-calorie diet that is made up mostly of high-fat foods—lots of cream, butter, and cheese—with a limited amount of protein and vegetables and no sugar or starch. Studies by Johns Hopkins neurologists show that seizures in 70% of children who are put on a ketogenic diet improve, and most can go off the diet in 2 or 3 years.

The ketogenic diet is designed to mimic the metabolism that occurs during fasting. Instead of burning mostly glucose for energy, the body is forced to burn mostly fat. Even ancient healers observed that fasting could halt seizures, but fasting cannot be a long-term treatment for epilepsy. Although there are some widely publicized success stories of children whose epilepsy was brought under control by the ketogenic diet, doctors stress that it's not a do-it-yourself solution. The diet must be very carefully structured for the individual child and then followed exactly. It is essential to make sure that the child obtains enough protein. Frequent checkups are necessary to make sure the child is growing normally and not suffering any adverse effects.

The Feingold Diet

This diet, developed by the late Dr Benjamin Feingold, is designed to treat childhood hyperactivity that may be caused by food allergies. It calls for eliminating all foods that contain artificial colors, flavors, and 3 common preservatives—BHA, BHT, and TBHQ. Also eliminated are aspirin and foods that contain natural salicylates, compounds found in aspirin. These include apples, apricots, berries, cherries, cucumbers, currants, grapes, green peppers, tomatoes, nectarines, oranges, peaches, plums, prunes, and tangerines, as well as tea and coffee.

If any of these foods contributes to hyperactivity, an improvement should be noted after a few weeks on the diet. To further identify the offending foods, those in the salicylate group can be reintroduced, one at a time, every 5 or 6 days. After each food is reintroduced, the child should be watched to see if symptoms recur. If so, the food should be eliminated from the diet. If not, it can be assumed to be safe, and the child can go on to the next food on the list.

Studies have shown that the Feingold diet fails to control hyperactivity. Some parents, however, insist that the diet helps. (For more information about the Feingold diet, see "Additives Don't Appear to Influence Hyperactivity," Chapter 14, page 294.)

THE QUESTION OF SUPPLEMENTS

Nutritionists agree that most healthy people, adults and children, who consume a varied diet based on the *Dietary Guidelines for Americans* (www.cnpp.usda.gov/DietaryGuidelines.htm) do not need vitamin and mineral supplements. However, millions of Americans persist in taking a daily multiple vitamin pill "to be on the safe side." Although the pill may not be needed, it probably will not do any harm so long as it does not exceed 100% of the recommended dietary allowance for any vitamin or mineral.

There are instances, however, in which higher doses of a specific vitamin or mineral may be needed. Children who cannot properly absorb fats in the diet may need supplements of fat-soluble vitamins A, D, E, and K. An adolescent girl with very heavy periods may require extra iron to keep from becoming anemic. Children on a strict vegetarian diet or those with rare metabolic disorders may also need supplements. In such cases, you should rely on your pediatrician to prescribe the nutrient and its dosage. Vitamin D cannot be overemphasized because of epidemiologic data that now demonstrates that a great proportion of the American population consumes less than recommended intakes and that low intake of vitamin D has lifelong consequences.

Serious problems can develop when vitamins or minerals are given in very large amounts or megadoses. When given in megadoses, vitamins and minerals take on the property of drugs, and like all drugs, they carry a risk of negative side effects. Unfortunately, many people try to self-treat various conditions—everything from the common cold to childhood mental illnesses—with megadoses of vitamins and minerals. This is referred to as orthomolecular therapy, a term coined by the late Dr Linus Pauling to describe the treatment or prevention of disease with megadose vitamins.

There have been a number of reports of children with autism, psychoses, hyperactivity, and dyslexia and other learning disorders improving when using orthomolecular therapy. Unfortunately, none of these findings has been proved in controlled scientific studies. Indeed, one study of high-dose vitamin therapy to treat hyperactivity found no benefit, but 42% of the children were found to have potentially serious nutritional imbalances. So when it comes to giving high doses of any vitamin or mineral, always check with your pediatrician first. Unless your child has a rare nutritional deficiency or a specific disorder, your pediatrician is likely to advise against high-dose vitamins.

ISSUES PARENTS RAISE ABOUT ALTERNATIVE DIETS AND SUPPLEMENTS

My teenaged son has told me he won't eat meat from now on. He's still growing, and I'm concerned that he'll get too little protein if he eats nothing but nuts and berries.

A vegetarian diet can be healthful and nutritionally balanced when based on the *Dietary Guidelines for Americans* (www.cnpp.usda.gov/DietaryGuidelines.htm). Your son can get more than enough protein from grains and legumes, especially if his diet includes animal foods such as dairy products and eggs. A vegetarian diet can be economical too. In fact, pound for pound, grains and beans are much cheaper sources of protein than meat. Regardless of the diet your son adopts, he won't go wrong if he follows the basic rules of variety, moderation, and balance. (See also page 300.)

Do children on vegetarian diets need supplements to make up for missing nutrients?

Children on properly planned vegetarian diets that include some animal foods, such as eggs, milk and other dairy foods, or fish, are unlikely to need supplements. However, a strict vegan diet that excludes all animal products may be lacking in vitamins B_{12} and D, as well as the minerals calcium and zinc (see page 311). If your family follows a vegan lifestyle, ask your pediatrician for advice to make sure that your children are getting the full range of nutrients together with the calories they need for growth.

Are organic foods and health foods better for you than regular foods from the market?

There's no evidence that organic, natural, or health foods are more nutritious than regular foods. The nutritional content of food varies according to when it was harvested and how it has been stored or processed. However, many people prefer foods from crops that have been raised without artificial pesticides, fertilizers, and herbicides or, in the case of meat, eggs, and dairy products, from animals raised on natural feed and not given hormones or antibiotics. Many people also prefer to pay more for organic foods because their production causes less damage to the environment. (See page 302.)

Chapter 16

Is My Child Allergic?

While many foods can cause allergic reactions, true food allergies are less common than you might think. Currently, they affect 2% of the general population and 6% to 8% of children. While food allergies cause only mild symptoms in many cases, they can trigger more serious reactions in some children, and in very rare instances even be life threatening. And while any food can trigger a food allergy, several cause the vast majority of cases in children.

Shortly after his fourth birthday, Leshawn's sweet temperament turned sour. He was often irritable and complained of a stomachache. His appetite dropped off and he frequently had loose, watery stools and a lot of gas. Because Leshawn usually developed the symptoms about an hour after meals and didn't have any other problems such as a fever or headache, his mother wondered if he might have an allergy. However, she couldn't trace the symptoms back to any one food.

After listening to her describe the symptoms, Leshawn's pediatrician had his mother eliminate milk and milk products from his diet for 2 weeks. When milk was reintroduced, his symptoms returned. The exercise proved that Leshawn was sensitive to milk; however, he was not allergic. His symptoms were caused by *lactose intolerance,* an inability to digest lactose, the natural sugar in milk and some other dairy products. Symptoms followed meals because he usually drank milk at mealtimes. The pediatrician referred Leshawn and his mother to a registered dietitian, who guided them in the use of lactase enzyme supplements, which break down lactose to an easily digested form. She also recommended lactose-free milks and other dairy foods with reduced lactose levels. In addition, she suggested calcium-rich nondairy foods as alternative sources of calcium.

Allergy Versus Adverse Reactions

Most symptoms caused by foods in young children are not allergic reactions. In an allergy, the immune system mistakenly tries to defend the body against certain food proteins as if they were invading germs. During this "attack," the immune system can cause problematic symptoms such as skin rashes, trouble breathing, vomiting, and diarrhea. Some allergies can be life threatening.

By contrast, there are a number of adverse reactions to foods that do not involve the immune system. For example, spoiled food has overgrowth of bacteria, and chemicals from the bacteria can cause food poisoning with symptoms such as vomiting, stomach pain, and diarrhea. Sometimes chemicals in foods can cause adverse reactions. For example, caffeine in soda may increase a child's activity or increase arousal, making bedtime difficult. Some people with asthma are sensitive to sulfites used to preserve certain foods and experience more wheezing when exposed to them. Some adverse reactions result from a reduced ability to digest specific types of sugars. These are called *intolerances.* However, *gluten intolerance* or *gluten sensitivity* are terms used to describe celiac disease, a lifelong condition in which the immune system reacts to the gluten in certain grains. If people with celiac disease ingest gluten they experience damage to the gut, resulting in diarrhea, poor growth, and other symptoms.

Food Allergy

In an allergic person, the immune system reacts to protein in a specific food. On exposure to the food, the body produces an antibody (immunoglobulin E) to the protein. Substances that cause allergies are called *allergens.*

It may take weeks, months, or years before antibody builds up, but once it does, a repeat exposure to the food triggers the release of histamine, causing allergic symptoms that may include runny nose, itchy eyes, diarrhea, rash, or wheezing; swelling of the lips, tongue, or mouth; itching; and tightness in the throat. Symptoms may appear immediately—that is, within a few minutes and up to 2 hours after eating. Some types of food allergies result in chronic symptoms such as persistent rashes or gut symptoms.

The number of young people with food or digestive allergies increased 18% between 1997 and 2007, according to a report from the Centers for Disease Control and Prevention (CDC).

FOODS AND INGREDIENTS TO AVOID IF YOUR CHILD IS ALLERGIC TO MILK		
Buttermilk	Cream	Powdered milk
Calcium caseinate	Evaporated milk	Sherbet (if made with milk)
Casein	Ice cream, ice milk, frozen yogurt	Sodium caseinate
Cheese, cottage cheese	Margarine	Whey
Condensed milk	Milk chocolate	Yogurt
Cow's milk	Milk solids	

ANAPHYLAXIS, A LIFE-THREATENING ALLERGIC REACTION

Anaphylaxis is a severe allergic reaction. Symptoms of anaphylaxis include

- Swelling in the mouth and throat
- Difficulty breathing
- Collapse/shock

Anaphylaxis is a life-threatening emergency and requires immediate medical attention. Call emergency medical services (911) at once. This type of food allergy can kill. Caring for a child who has anaphylactic sensitivity to food can be difficult. Young children cannot fully understand dietary restrictions, and their older siblings must be taught how serious food allergy is. The food allergen should be eliminated from the home; when this is impossible, warning stickers may be placed on foods containing the allergen. It is particularly important to inform your child's teachers, friends, fellow students, and neighbors about the dangers. Children should be warned never to test whether claims of allergies are true by hiding the allergen in another child's food.

In 2007, approximately 3 million US children and teenagers younger than 18 years (nearly 4% of that age group) had a food or digestive allergy in the previous 12 months, compared with just over 2.3 million (3.3%) in 1997.

The only way to manage allergies is to strictly avoid the offending food. Although allergies cannot be cured, most children eventually outgrow allergies to foods such as milk, egg, wheat, and soy. Nevertheless, according to the CDC, children seem to be taking longer now to outgrow milk and egg allergies than in past decades. Allergies to foods such as peanuts, tree nuts (eg, walnuts, pecans, cashews), fish, and shellfish are more likely to persist. About 20% of young children outgrow a peanut allergy by school age.

Common Causes of Food Problems

Cow's milk is the most common cause of food allergy in young children. Cow's-milk allergy affects 2 or 3 out of every 100 young children. Fortunately, most outgrow the allergy and can tolerate milk by age 4. Some of the proteins in cow's milk can be transmitted to babies in breast milk. If your breastfed baby develops recurrent diarrhea, spitting up, blood in the stool, and gas after you have consumed milk or other dairy foods, eliminating such foods from your diet may relieve the baby's symptoms. This is usually caused by a condition called allergic colitis in which the baby's intestinal tract is irritated by cow's milk proteins in human milk. Be sure to seek your pediatrician's advice and find alternative sources of calcium as long as you are breastfeeding.

If your bottle-fed infant appears to be allergic to cow's-milk formula, your pediatrician may recommend another. Although most infants with milk allergy tolerate soy, your pediatrician may recommend an alternative depending on your infant's symptoms because there are increased risks of soy allergy in children with a milk allergy. For babies who have difficulty tolerating the usual kinds of formulas, pediatricians generally recommend a formula made with predigested protein that is unlikely to trigger a reaction. These formulas are quite expensive but if it is vital to your child's health, insurance or Medicaid may cover the cost.

When you introduce solid foods, check labels to make sure that products are free of cow's-milk protein, which may appear under various names (see "Foods and Ingredients to Avoid if Your Child Is Allergic to Milk" on page 319). Tell your child's caregivers about the seriousness of the allergy and the importance of avoiding products containing cow's-milk protein.

Eggs are another common allergen. Specifically, it's the protein-rich egg white that is allergenic. However, if your child has a confirmed egg allergy, avoidance of egg yolk and white is typically advised. Some vaccines, such as the annual flu vaccine and the vaccine for yellow fever, have egg protein, so talk to your pediatrician about allergy risks. The measles-mumps-rubella vaccine is *not* considered a risk for children with egg allergy.

Wheat allergy (not to be confused with gluten intolerance or celiac disease; see page 323) is the most common grain allergy. In addition to breads and baked goods, wheat can be found in a wide variety of foods including salad dressings, processed (American) cheese, and breaded fish sticks and chicken nuggets. Wheat is also a hidden ingredient in many commercial food products such as canned soups and stews. Read labels carefully. If you want to offer breads and cereals but avoid wheat, try pure oat or rye breads; corn tortillas; oat, rice, or rye crackers; and cereals made with oats, corn, or rice.

Soy allergies sometimes emerge when an infant is given a soy-based formula. If your child is allergic to soy, read all food labels carefully because soy products are used in many processed foods. Code words that may indicate the presence of soy include textured vegetable protein, emulsifiers, flavorings, stabilizers, lecithin, shortening, and vegetable oil.

Peanuts, tree nuts (eg, walnuts, cashews, Brazil nuts), fish, and shellfish are allergens that are more often associated with severe allergic reactions and more persistent allergies. Peanuts are actually legumes from the pea and bean family, not true nuts. Therefore, some children who are allergic to peanuts have no problems with tree nuts such as pecans and

---

REACTIONS TO DYES AND PRESERVATIVES

Allergic reactions to chemical dyes and preservatives are rare. Some natural colors, from annatto seed or cochineal (a red coloring extracted from insects), for example, may rarely trigger allergy. Sulfites, which are used to prolong the shelf life of some fruits and vegetables, shellfish, and certain medications, as well as to whiten food starches and condition dough (see Chapter 14, Food Additives), may trigger wheezing in some sensitive children with asthma.

FOOD ALLERGY SYMPTOMS IN INFANTS

Signs and symptoms of a possible food allergy in infancy include the following:

- Skin rash/eczema
- Vomiting most or all food after feeding; loose, watery stools 8 or more times a day
- Bloody diarrhea

walnuts. Similarly, those who are allergic to tree nuts may tolerate peanuts. Most children with a peanut allergy tolerate beans such as string beans, peas, and navy beans.

Avoiding Food Allergens

In the United States, labeling laws require that specific common allergens, namely milk, egg, soy, wheat, peanut, tree nuts, fish, and crustacean shellfish (eg, shrimp, lobster but not clams, mussels), must be declared in plain English words on the label. For example, a label may use the term "casein," which is a milk protein, but it must also have the word "milk" on the label. Virtually any food can trigger an allergic reaction in some sensitive children, but labeling laws currently only apply to the foods or food groups mentioned herein. For example, garlic or sesame might not be disclosed in an ingredient list but may be included under a broader, nonspecific term such as "spices." Advisory labeling terms such as "may contain peanut" or "in a facility that processes peanut" are currently not regulated and the exact risks are not known, so avoidance is necessary for sensitive children.

Avoiding an allergen requires carefully reading food labels on packages, discussing ingredients with others (friends, family, and restaurants), and understanding how to avoid cross contact with an allergen. Cross contact means that an allergen can contaminate an otherwise safe food through contact during preparation. Thus, care about using shared utensils, fryers, and cookware is needed. Using a knife in the peanut butter jar and then in the jelly jar can leave peanut residue in the jelly, making it unsafe for a child with peanut allergy.

COMMON SYMPTOMS OF FOOD ALLERGY
At any age, food allergy may trigger • Respiratory tract symptoms such as runny nose, sneezing, wheezing, and coughing • Gastrointestinal symptoms such as bloating, stomachache, cramping, nausea, and diarrhea • Skin symptoms such as hives, a rash, and itching If the symptoms are triggered by an allergy, your child will not have a fever.

Diagnosing Food Allergies

Diagnosing food allergies starts with discussing your suspicions with your pediatrician. If there was a sudden allergic reaction, your pediatrician will need to know the exact symptoms, how much time went by between when the food was eaten and the symptoms appeared, and details of the exposure to the possible culprit foods. Usually, a careful review of the circumstances and some confirmatory testing can determine the cause. Do not feed your child the suspected food until you speak further with your doctor. When persistent symptoms such as atopic dermatitis or gut symptoms occur, it is trickier to determine what, if any, food may be a trigger. In this circumstance, your pediatrician may suggest eliminating some suspect foods for a period to see if symptoms improve.

If your child has symptoms that suggest a food allergy but the cause is not clear, your pediatrician will probably provide a referral to a pediatric allergist for skin or blood tests. Unfortunately, these tests often cannot, by themselves, be depended on to determine culprit foods. For example, one cannot order a battery of tests and know exactly what foods are or are not allergens for your child (the test is not that accurate and may fail to identify or may misidentify an allergen). These tests must be interpreted in the context of your child's experience (medical history) with exposure to the possible culprit foods. In some cases, an allergy cannot be confirmed by the tests and it may be necessary to have your child eat the food gradually under doctor supervision, a test called a *food challenge.*

Food Intolerance and Celiac Disease

Food intolerance is an abnormal, nonallergic response to a food or additive. The most common is lactose intolerance. People who are lactose intolerant, like 4-year-old Leshawn, produce insufficient amounts of lactase, the enzyme needed to digest lactose, the natural sugar in milk. Most people of Asian, African, and Native American ancestry gradually lose the ability to digest lactose starting at about age 4 or 5. In contrast, those of Northern European descent can usually digest milk and other dairy foods throughout their lives.

Undigested lactose is broken down by bacteria in the large intestine, producing gas and discomfort. Symptoms such as cramping, bloating, flatulence, and diarrhea occur about 30 minutes to 2 hours after consuming lactose. If there is a question, the diagnosis can be

---

COMMON ALLERGY TRIGGERS

Any food has the potential to trigger an allergy or intolerance, although certain foods are more likely than others to cause problems. The most common food allergy triggers are cow's milk and other dairy products, egg, peanut, fish, shellfish, wheat, tree nuts, and soy.

LACTOSE IN COMMERCIAL FOODS

Milk is the only natural source of lactose, but milk sugar is often added to commercial products such as the following:

- Bread and other baked goods
- Candies and snacks
- Instant potatoes, soups, and breakfast drinks
- Margarine
- Medications (as filler)
- Mixes for pancakes, biscuits, and cookies
- Nondairy creamers
- Non-kosher lunch meats and hot dogs
- Processed breakfast cereals
- Salad dressings

---

confirmed by measuring the amount of hydrogen in a person's breath after consuming a lactose-containing food, with the guidance of a pediatric gastroenterologist.

Lactose intolerance is uncomfortable, but unlike some allergies, it is not life threatening. Lactose-intolerant people vary greatly in their ability to digest lactose. Many can eat at least some yogurt and cheese because most of the lactose is broken down in processing. Some can drink a little milk as long as it is accompanied by food. Often the small amount of lactose included in some of the foods mentioned herein may not be a problem. If a child cannot drink milk or eat dairy products, it is important to make sure that her diet includes plenty of calcium.

There are many other choices for those who are lactose intolerant. Lactose-free milk and dairy products are available; chewable lactase supplements can be taken before lactose-containing foods are eaten to aid lactose digestion; and lactase enzyme drops can be added to regular milk to predigest the lactose.

Nondairy options that are lactose free include milks made from soy, rice, oats, or almonds, in addition to tofu beverages and calcium-fortified orange juice; however, most have less calcium than real milk. You can also replace dairy cheese with cheese substitutes made from rice, tofu, almond, or soy. Bear in mind, however, that while these products are lactose free, some may contain milk proteins that are off-limits for those who are allergic to milk.

Temporary lactose intolerance may follow a bout of infectious diarrhea in a baby. The symptoms disappear as the condition clears up. Your pediatrician may recommend a lactose-free formula for a week or two.

Gluten enteropathy, also called *celiac disease* (as well as *gluten intolerance* or *celiac sprue),* is an inability to tolerate gluten, a protein found in many grains such as wheat, barley, and rye (also see Chapter 9, Spitting Up, Gagging, Vomiting, Diarrhea, and Constipation). In children with this condition, exposure to gluten causes an immune system response that damages the folds or fingerlike protrusions (villi) of the small intestinal lining, which prevents the absorption of many nutrients, including protein, carbohydrates, fats, and fat-soluble

HIDDEN GLUTEN	
• Alcohol-based flavorings (eg, vanilla extract)	• Hydrolyzed vegetable protein
• Brown rice syrup	• Imitation seafood
• Canned broth	• Malt or malt flavoring
• Caramel flavor	• Maltodextrin
• Distilled vinegar (an ingredient in condiments such as ketchup, pickles, mayonnaise, salad dressings, and barbecue sauce)	• Modified food starch
	• Self-basting poultry
	• Vegetable gum
• Flour and cereal products	• Vegetable protein

vitamins. While the cause of celiac disease is not known, in some cases it may be a hereditary abnormality in part of the immune system involving the intestine. Typical symptoms, such as irritability, diarrhea or constipation, abdominal pain or distension, stunted growth, delayed puberty, or poor weight gain or weight loss, usually occur after an affected baby is introduced to wheat-containing cereal. In some children, the only symptom is stunted or delayed growth caused by undernutrition related to the malabsorption of nutrients during important years in a child's development.

The intestinal damage in celiac disease may lead to lactose intolerance and a loss of electrolytes (eg, sodium, potassium, chloride). Poor vitamin absorption may cause complications such as softening of the bones (osteomalacia), rickets, muscle spasms, night blindness, abnormal blood clotting, and anemia. A child (or adult) with celiac disease must strictly follow a gluten-free diet, avoiding cereals, breads, pasta, and any other foods made with grains containing gluten. Your pediatrician will provide dietary advice and refer your child to a dietitian for guidance. The number of gluten-free products in grocery stores continues to increase, and some restaurants have gluten-free menus. After a gluten-free diet is started, the intestinal tract will begin to repair and heal itself and symptoms will subside. These improvements often start just days after the new diet is adopted (although some problems such as short stature may not be reversed). However, this diet must be followed for life. If your child eats gluten, the symptoms will recur.

Can Food Allergies Be Prevented?

If allergies run in your family, chances are higher that your child will have them. Some studies indicate that for babies with a family history of allergy, exclusive breastfeeding for at least 4 months might reduce the risk of milk allergy. However, studies are otherwise too few or inconclusive to know whether specific diets prevent food allergies. There is no current clear evidence that avoiding allergens during pregnancy or having otherwise healthy infants avoid allergens beyond 6 months of age influences allergy outcomes such as atopic dermatitis (eczema) or asthma. There is not much evidence that if mothers avoid allergens while they are nursing that they will prevent atopic dermatitis.

PREVENTING ALLERGIES IN BABIES AT HIGH RISK	

According to the American Academy of Pediatrics, there is evidence suggesting that the following can prevent or delay allergies in babies at high risk (such as those with a family history):

- Breastfeeding exclusively for at least 3 to 4 months (4 to 6 months is recommended) may reduce atopic dermatitis, milk allergy, and early wheezing.

- If not exclusively breastfeeding, using certain extensively or partially hydrolyzed milk-protein–based formulas (compared with standard milk or soy formulas) may delay or prevent atopic dermatitis.

Give your baby just one new food at 2- to 3-day intervals. If symptoms such as diarrhea, rash, or vomiting appear, stop giving the food in question until you've talked to your pediatrician. Follow the recommendations in Chapter 2 for introducing foods and expanding your baby's diet.

Large amounts of fruit or juice can make a baby's stool acidic and irritating to the skin. The resulting painful red rash is sometimes mistaken for an allergic reaction. Cutting down on fruit and diluting juice half-and-half with water or omitting juice altogether may help get rid of the irritation. Remember that small infants should not drink more than 4 oz per day of juice (see "No Liquid Lunches," Chapter 3, page 63).

Allergies and Hyperactivity

Parents often blame candies and other high-sugar foods when children get unruly. Some insist that sugar triggers hyperactivity. However, when put to the test, the sugar-behavior link does not hold up. In a carefully controlled study of preschool and school-aged children, researchers found no effect on behavior or ability to concentrate when sugar intake was far above normal, even among those whom parents identified as "sugar sensitive." Another study found that sugar had the opposite effect to what was expected—when boys whose parents believed them to be sugar reactive were each given a large dose of sugar, they were actually less active than before. Finally, several studies comparing blood glucose levels have found that children with attention-deficit/hyperactivity disorder (ADHD) have exactly the same response to sugar consumption as do children without ADHD. There is no scientific basis for claims that sugar and other sweeteners influence behavior or cause ADHD, even at levels many times higher than in a normal diet. The overactivity children show after a birthday party or Halloween may be due more to the stimulation of the event than the sugar.

Special diets for hyperactivity are based on the belief that allergies or reactions to foods cause undesirable behavior. The diets typically target artificial additives, sugar, or the commonly allergenic foods (ie, corn, nuts, chocolate, shellfish, and wheat). However, there is no evidence that links foods and behavior. Some studies show that chemical preservatives or dyes, presumably through a drug rather than allergic mechanism, might contribute to these problems, but the evidence is weak and not widely accepted by experts. Therefore, the American Academy of Pediatrics does not recommend special diets for treating hyperactivity. If your child behaves oddly or has unusual symptoms after eating a particular food, it will do no harm to avoid it, provided his diet includes other choices from the same food group.

Asthma and Allergies

A family history of any type of allergy increases the risk that a child may develop asthma. Children with asthma and food allergies are at increased risk for anaphylaxis, a severe allergic reaction, even when their asthma is well controlled.

For children with known food allergies, especially those who also have asthma, parents should be thoroughly familiar with food ingredients. If their child has anaphylactic reaction to foods, they should also carry an emergency dose of epinephrine at all times and make sure there is some with the child care provider and at school. Epinephrine, a drug that stops or slows down anaphylaxis, is available in spring-loaded self-injectable syringes. Though not a cure, a dose of epinephrine administered soon after symptoms begin should stall severe symptoms long enough to get necessary medical attention by calling emergency medical services (911).

Sulfites, which are used to stop discoloration, overripening, and spoiling, are known to trigger asthma attacks. These additives are found in processed beverages and foods, including fruit juices, soft drinks, cider vinegar, potato chips, dried fruits and vegetables, maraschino cherries, and wines. Numerous reports of allergic reactions—mostly among people with asthma—and of deaths associated with sulfite ingestion have led the Food and Drug Administration to ban the use of sulfites in fresh fruits and vegetables (also see Chapter 14, Food Additives). Sulfites may be used in certain processed foods, provided they are listed on labels in quantities higher than 10 parts per million, or when used at all in manufacturing. Processed potatoes and some canned foods may contain sulfites. If your child has asthma or is sensitive to sulfites, be cautious about any processed or prepared food.

ISSUES PARENTS RAISE ABOUT FOOD ALLERGIES

What's the difference between a food allergy and an intolerance, like lactose intolerance?

In an allergic person, the immune system reacts to protein in a certain food. This is not the case for someone with food intolerance, who usually does not make enough of a certain enzyme required for digesting some part of a food. (Also see page 323.)

My 18-month-old has eczema and when our pediatrician tested him, she found he was sensitive to cow's milk. Does this mean he can't eat dairy foods for the rest of his life?

In many cases, children outgrow sensitivities to cow's milk and other foods, often by age 3 or 4 years. Lifelong food allergies are quite rare. Ask your pediatrician for guidance about which foods your child should avoid and for how long. (Also see page 320.)

Lots of members of my husband's family are allergic to different foods. Is there any way to lower my baby's risk of being allergic?

If allergies run in the family, the risk is higher than average that your child will also develop allergies. However, it is possible to delay or prevent some allergies by exclusive breastfeeding for 4 to 6 months. If not breastfeeding during that period, allergy reduction may be possible by choosing specific formulas that are extensive hydrolysates of casein or partial whey hydrolysates that were studied and showed reduced atopic dermatitis compared with standard milk formula. (Also see page 326.)

What Caregivers Need to Know: A Checklist

Parents should provide caregivers with specific instructions about feeding children—not only about what to serve but also when, where, and how. Most new teenaged caregivers and those new to the household need more details than extended-family members and the usual caregivers do. Parents may need to be tactful with older family members, as the practices they are comfortable with do not necessarily suit a new generation.

If you are leaving a picky eater in the care of a caregiver, pass on any necessary information out of the child's hearing and avoid giving overly detailed instructions. Many picky eaters will eat without a fuss when sharing a meal with other children or caregivers. The less attention paid to their demands, the easier meals can be.

For Babies and Young Children

- If a new caregiver will be caring for babies, infants, and toddlers, arrange a time before the actual date of care for the caregiver to visit your home during a meal to observe and help feed the children. In this way, the caregiver will be familiar with the routine before taking on the job alone, the children will be more comfortable with the caregiver, and the parents can be more confident that mealtimes will go smoothly.

For Newborns and Infants

- If you are breastfeeding and if you usually express and refrigerate breast milk for times when you must be away from your baby, show your caregiver how to properly warm and store the bottles.
- For a bottle-fed newborn or infant, mix and refrigerate several bottles of formula before going out.

- Show the caregiver how to warm a bottle by standing it in a pitcher of warm water or placing the bottle under running, warm tap water, and how to flick a few drops on to the wrist to test that the temperature is no hotter than lukewarm. Remind the caregiver to mix the formula carefully to distribute the heat evenly.
- Warn the caregiver never to heat bottles in the microwave.

For Toddlers and Older Children

- If the children's food is already prepared and needs only to be heated, leave written instructions about oven temperatures and timing. Show the caregiver how to use the oven, microwave, and other appliances.
- When you expect the caregiver to prepare the meal, leave all the ingredients and utensils ready together with clear, written instructions.
- Let the caregiver know exactly what appropriate finger foods are and be clear about those that your child is still too young to manage (see "Unsafe for Toddlers," Chapter 3, page 68).
- If you prefer that your child not have cookies, candies, and other sugary foods, make sure the caregiver is aware of your concerns and provide other choices for treats.

For Children With Special Needs

- If your child has a chronic condition that requires a special diet, such as diabetes, cystic fibrosis, or gluten enteropathy (celiac disease), provide written, step-by-step procedures for all meals and snacks. Also provide clear instructions about how to protect a child with cystic fibrosis against excessive salt loss and dehydration in warm weather.
- Be sure to leave a list of permitted treats as well as a list of foods that the child absolutely cannot eat.
- If your child has diabetes, leave written instructions about the importance of regular meals and snacks and what foods may be eaten. Many people have the mistaken impression that children with diabetes can never eat sweets or candy. This is not so. While foods with added sugar should be consumed sparingly, they are not forbidden for diabetic children. Sweet foods have a place in a balanced and nutritious diet plan. In your written instructions, include a list of allowable exchanges and emphasize that any sugary food the

child consumes must be included in the overall carbohydrate allowance for a given meal or snack.

- In the case of food allergy or sensitivity in your child, go over the list of foods that must be avoided because they may contain the food or ingredient that causes the allergy but in hidden forms.

- To help the caregiver to be ready for problems and to be able to find help when necessary, write out a list of symptoms that may be related to food, such as vomiting, diarrhea, wheezing, rash, hives, swelling, and difficulty breathing.

- Leave the list of symptoms next to the numbers to call in case of emergency (pediatrician, Poison Help, 911, close neighbor).

For All Children

- Give the caregiver a written schedule of doses for any medicine your child must take while you are gone, including the times when the medicine should be taken.

- Make sure the caregiver knows how to deal with a choking infant and how to perform the Heimlich maneuver for an older child who is choking (see Appendix F).

Food-Medication Interactions

Medical treatments can affect the way children digest and absorb food. By the same token, what children eat can influence the effects that medications have on the body. For example, griseofulvin, an antifungal medication, needs to be taken with a fatty meal to be absorbed properly. Iron supplements for anemia are best taken with a mild acid like orange juice; if taken with milk they may not be well absorbed. Medications affect nutrition in 4 main areas—they can stimulate or suppress the appetite; they can alter the amount of nutrients absorbed and the rate of absorption; they affect the way the body breaks down and uses up nutrients; and finally, they can slow down or speed up the rate at which food passes through the digestive tract.

Always ask your pediatrician, pharmacist, and other specialists involved in your child's medical care to explain whether medication should be taken with meals or on an empty stomach. Several antibiotics can cause stomach pain or upset unless taken with food. Also find out whether taking medication with a specific food, such as a glass of milk or grapefruit juice, can make the treatment more or less effective, and ask what foods, if any, should be avoided during treatment.

There are thousands of possible drug-food interactions. The following list represents commonly used medications and foods, and guidelines for preventing such interactions or keeping the effects to a minimum. Be sure to check every prescription with the pharmacist and read the package insert.

MEDICATION	INTERACTIONS WITH NUTRIENTS	DIETARY GUIDELINES
Antacids		
Nonprescription indigestion remedies	Foods lessen effects.	Take 1 hour after eating.
Antibiotics		
In general	Reduce intestinal production of biotin (a B vitamin), pantothenic acid (vitamin B_5), and vitamin K; can speed up passage of food through intestine, decreasing availability for absorption.	Eat a well-balanced diet, including plenty of vegetables, grains, and cereals, to ensure adequate intake of all vitamins.
• Amoxicillin	Food slows absorption but does not alter dose effect.	None needed.
• Erythromycin stearate • Penicillin	Food decreases absorption.	Take 1 hour before or 2 hours after meals.
• Clarithromycin • Erythromycin estolate/succinate	Food improves absorption; fruit juice or carbonated beverages interfere with absorption.	Take with meals.
• Tetracycline	Binds calcium and iron so that neither antibiotic nor mineral can be absorbed.	Take 2 hours before or after meals and other medications such as iron supplements or calcium-based antacids.

MEDICATION	INTERACTIONS WITH NUTRIENTS	DIETARY GUIDELINES
Iron Supplements		
Various brands in liquid or tablet form	Milk may interfere with absorption.	Should be taken with water or slightly acidic drinks like fruit juice to improve absorption.
Antifungal		
• Griseofulvin	Can interfere with effectiveness of birth control pills.	Take with fatty meal.
Anticonvulsant/Antiepileptic Medications		
• Phenobarbital • Phenytoin • Primidone	Interfere with vitamin D metabolism and thus with calcium absorption; also alter absorption of folic acid.	A good intake of vitamin D (found in fortified milk, egg yolks, oily fish, sunlight), calcium (dairy foods, leafy greens, broccoli, canned fish with bones), and folic acid (fresh fruits, vegetables, grains) should offset medication effects; ask your pediatrician about vitamin D and calcium supplements if your child is on long-term epilepsy treatment; folic acid supplements should not be used because overly high blood levels may decrease anticonvulsant efficacy.
• Phenytoin	Better absorbed with food or milk.	Take with a meal or a glass of milk.
Thyroid Medications		
• Levothyroxine		Take on an empty stomach.

MEDICATION	INTERACTIONS WITH NUTRIENTS	DIETARY GUIDELINES
Nonsteroidal Anti-inflammatory Medications		
• Aspirin (acetylsalicylic acid)	Interferes with storage of vitamin C; may cause iron loss through bleeding in digestive tract.	Do not give aspirin to children unless your pediatrician specifically prescribes it because it has been associated with Reye syndrome, a rare but serious disease affecting the brain and liver following viral infections; use acetaminophen or ibuprofen.
Antituberculosis Medications		
• Isoniazid	Interferes with vitamin B_6 (pyridoxine) metabolism.	Eat a well-balanced diet, including sources of vitamin B_6 such as grains, spinach, sweet and white potatoes, bananas, watermelon, and prunes.
Corticosteroids		
• Prednisone • Hydrocortisone	May promote excretion of potassium and calcium.	Reduce salt intake; eat foods high in potassium (fresh fruits and vegetables) and calcium (low-fat dairy foods) to counter loss of these minerals; take with food to lessen stomach upset.
Laxatives		
• Mineral oil	Interferes with the absorption of fat-soluble vitamins in the first part of the intestine.	Provide a diet rich in vegetables and fruits for fiber and encourage your child to drink plenty of water; if constipation is a problem, ask your pediatrician's advice; when mineral oil is prescribed, it should be given at bedtime, after most of the day's food has passed through the first part of the intestine.

MEDICATION	INTERACTIONS WITH NUTRIENTS	DIETARY GUIDELINES
Oral Contraceptives		
Various brands	Alter blood cholesterol levels; increase need for folic acid and vitamin B_6.	Use another form of contraception if there is a family history of high blood cholesterol or heart disease; consume plenty of fresh fruits and vegetables, grains and cereals, potatoes, and other sources of folic acid and vitamin B_6; take with food to prevent nausea; antibiotics may decrease the effectiveness of oral contraceptives.

Standard Growth Charts

Growth charts consist of a series of percentile curves that illustrate the distribution of selected body measurements in children. Pediatric growth charts have been used by pediatricians, nurses, and parents to track the growth of infants, children, and adolescents in the United States since 1977.

In 2006, the World Health Organization (WHO) released new international growth standards for term newborns from birth to 2 years of age based on data from 6 countries. In September 2010, the Centers for Disease Control and Prevention issued a recommendation that health care professionals use the new WHO growth standards to monitor growth for newborns, infants, and children aged 0 to 2 years in the United States.

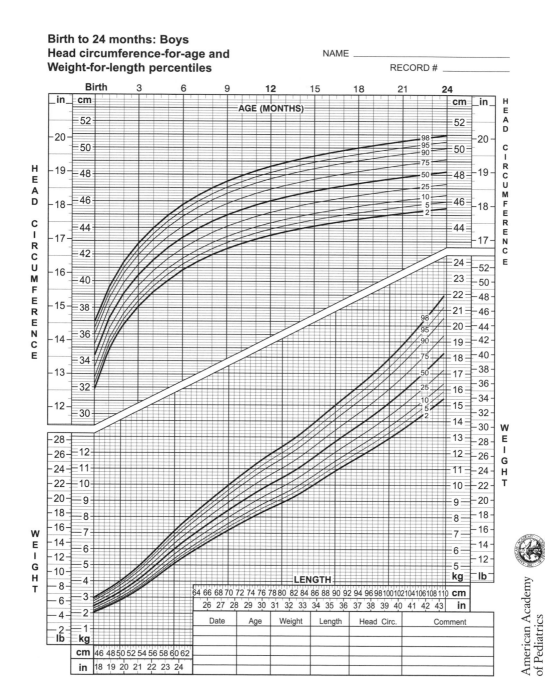

Birth to 24 months: Boys
Head circumference-for-age and
Weight-for-length percentiles

NAME _____

RECORD # _____

Published by the Centers for Disease Control and Prevention, November 1, 2009
SOURCE: WHO Child Growth Standards (http://www.who.int/childgrowth/en)

Reprinted by the American Academy of Pediatrics

The recommendations in this publication do not indicate an exclusive course of treatment or serve as a
standard of medical care. Variations, taking into account individual circumstances, may be appropriate.
© 2011 American Academy of Pediatrics   9-283

Additional copies are available for purchase in quantities of 100.

To order, contact:
American Academy of Pediatrics
141 Northwest Point Blvd
Elk Grove Village, IL 60007-1098
Web site—http://www.aag/org. Minimum order 100.
HE0510

American Academy
of Pediatrics

DEDICATED TO THE HEALTH OF ALL CHILDREN™

Birth to 24 months: Boys
Length-for-age and Weight-for-age percentiles

NAME _____

RECORD # _____

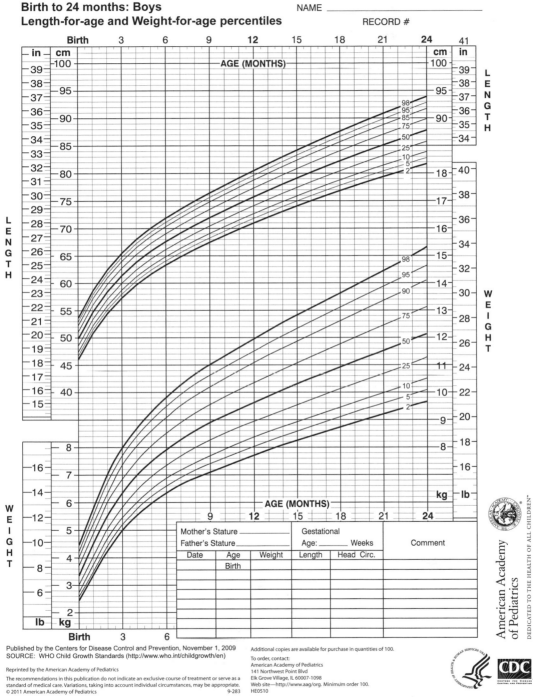

Published by the Centers for Disease Control and Prevention, November 1, 2009
SOURCE: WHO Child Growth Standards (http://www.who.int/childgrowth/en)

Reprinted by the American Academy of Pediatrics

The recommendations in this publication do not indicate an exclusive course of treatment or serve as a standard of medical care. Variations, taking into account individual circumstances, may be appropriate.
© 2011 American Academy of Pediatrics   9-283

Additional copies are available for purchase in quantities of 100.

To order, contact:
American Academy of Pediatrics
141 Northwest Point Blvd
Elk Grove Village, IL 60007-1098
Web site—http://www.aag/org. Minimum order 100.
HE0510

American Academy of Pediatrics

DEDICATED TO THE HEALTH OF ALL CHILDREN®

Birth to 24 months: Girls
Head circumference-for-age and
Weight-for-length percentiles

NAME _____

RECORD # _____

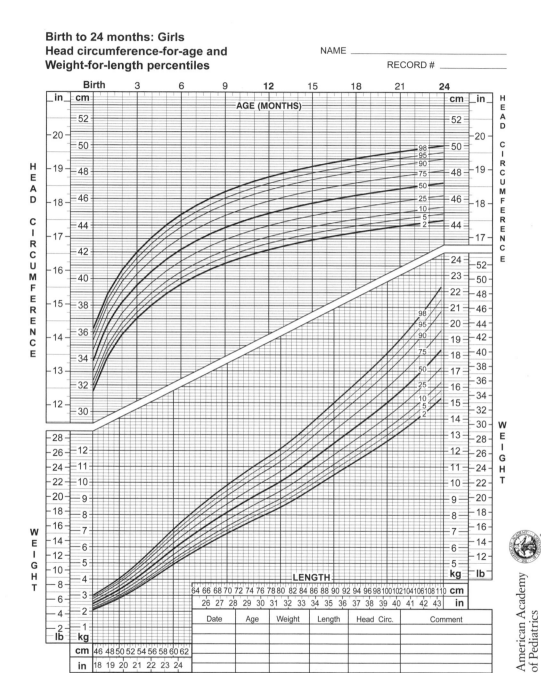

Published by the Centers for Disease Control and Prevention, November 1, 2009
SOURCE: WHO Child Growth Standards (http://www.who.int/childgrowth/en)

Reprinted by the American Academy of Pediatrics

The recommendations in this publication do not indicate an exclusive course of treatment or serve as a
standard of medical care. Variations, taking into account individual circumstances, may be appropriate.
© 2011 American Academy of Pediatrics   9-284

Additional copies are available for purchase in quantities of 100.

To order, contact:
American Academy of Pediatrics
141 Northwest Point Blvd
Elk Grove Village, IL 60007-1098
Web site—http://www.aag/org. Minimum order 100.
HE0511

American Academy
of Pediatrics

DEDICATED TO THE HEALTH OF ALL CHILDREN™

Birth to 24 months: Girls
Length-for-age and Weight-for-age percentiles

NAME _____

RECORD # _____

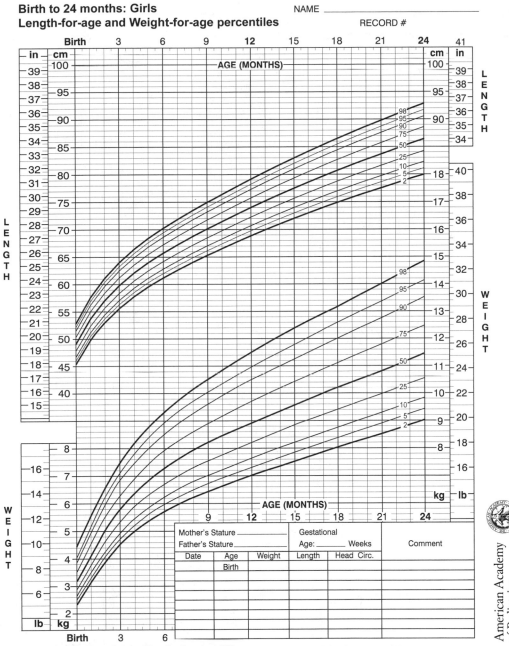

AGE (MONTHS)

LENGTH

WEIGHT

Mother's Stature _____	Gestational	
Father's Stature _____	Age: _____ Weeks	Comment
Date	Age	Weight	Length	Head Circ.	
	Birth				

Published by the Centers for Disease Control and Prevention, November 1, 2009
SOURCE: WHO Child Growth Standards (http://www.who.int/childgrowth/en)

Reprinted by the American Academy of Pediatrics

The recommendations in this publication do not indicate an exclusive course of treatment or serve as a standard of medical care. Variations, taking into account individual circumstances, may be appropriate.
© 2011 American Academy of Pediatrics   9-284

Additional copies are available for purchase in quantities of 100.

To order, contact:
American Academy of Pediatrics
141 Northwest Point Blvd
Elk Grove Village, IL 60007-1098
Web site—http://www.aag/org. Minimum order 100.
HE0511

American Academy of Pediatrics

DEDICATED TO THE HEALTH OF ALL CHILDREN™

Boys, 2 to 20 years

Name _____

STATURE FOR AGE AND WEIGHT FOR AGE PERCENTILES

Record # _____

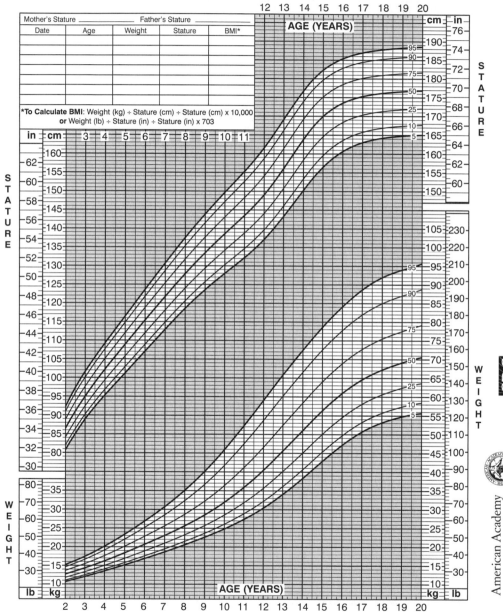

Mother's Stature _____ Father's Stature _____

Date	Age	Weight	Stature	BMI*

*To Calculate BMI: Weight (kg) ÷ Stature (cm) ÷ Stature (cm) x 10,000
or Weight (lb) ÷ Stature (in) ÷ Stature (in) x 703

American Academy of Pediatrics
DEDICATED TO THE HEALTH OF ALL CHILDREN™

Source: Developed by the National Center for Health Statistics in collaboration with the
         National Center for Chronic Disease Prevention and Health Promotion (2000).
         http://www.cdc.gov/growthcharts

Reprinted by the American Academy of Pediatrics

The recommendations in this publication do not indicate an exclusive course of treatment or serve as a
standard of medical care. Variations, taking into account individual circumstances, may be appropriate.

©2000 American Academy of Pediatrics

Additional copies are available for purchase in quantities of 100.

To order, contact:
American Academy of Pediatrics
141 Northwest Point Blvd
Elk Grove Village, IL 60007-1098
Web site — http://www.aap.org
Minimum order 100.

Girls, 2 to 20 years

Name _____

STATURE FOR AGE AND WEIGHT FOR AGE PERCENTILES

Record # _____

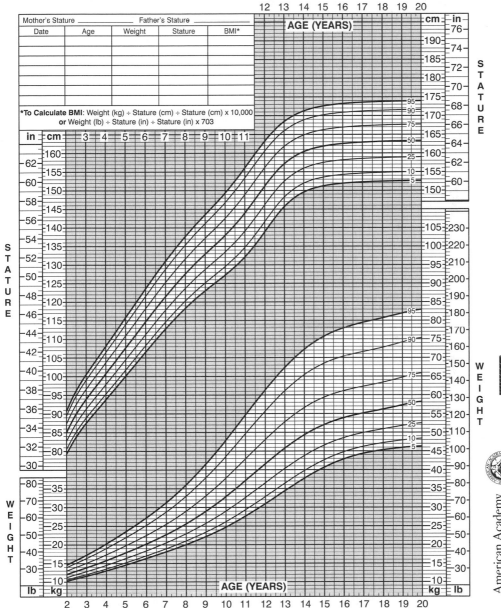

Source: Developed by the National Center for Health Statistics in collaboration with the National Center for Chronic Disease Prevention and Health Promotion (2000). http://www.cdc.gov/growthcharts

Reprinted by the American Academy of Pediatrics

The recommendations in this publication do not indicate an exclusive course of treatment or serve as a standard of medical care. Variations, taking into account individual circumstances, may be appropriate.

©2000 American Academy of Pediatrics

Additional copies are available for purchase in quantities of 100.

To order, contact
American Academy of Pediatrics
141 Northwest Point Blvd
Elk Grove Village, IL 60007-1098
Web site — http://www.aap.org
Minimum order 100.

Body Mass Index Charts

Body mass index (BMI) is a formula used to calculate a child's body weight in relation to her height. Use the following formula or charts to determine your child's BMI:

- Multiply your child's weight (in pounds) by 703. (We'll refer to this as A.)
- Multiply your child's height (in inches) by itself. (We'll refer to this as B.)
- Dividing A by B gives you your child's BMI.

The graphic below specifies what the BMI percentile represents for children and teens aged 2 through 19 years.

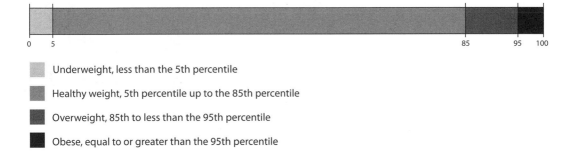

Underweight, less than the 5th percentile

Healthy weight, 5th percentile up to the 85th percentile

Overweight, 85th to less than the 95th percentile

Obese, equal to or greater than the 95th percentile

Boys, 2 to 20 years

Name _____

BODY MASS INDEX-FOR-AGE PERCENTILES

Record # _____

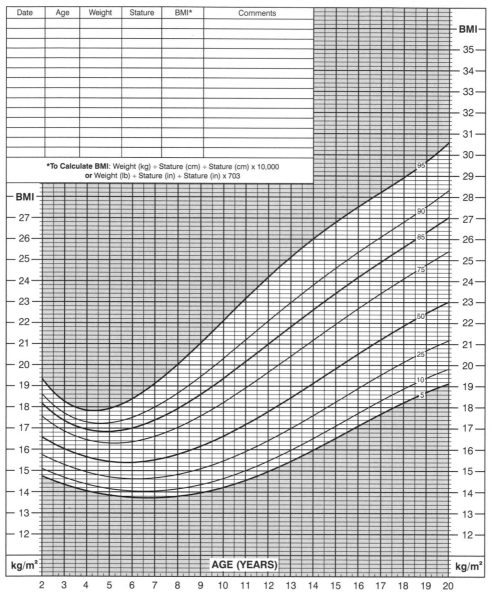

Date	Age	Weight	Stature	BMI*	Comments

*To Calculate BMI: Weight (kg) ÷ Stature (cm) ÷ Stature (cm) x 10,000
or Weight (lb) ÷ Stature (in) ÷ Stature (in) x 703

BMI

95
90
85
75
50
25
10
5

AGE (YEARS)

kg/m²

2 3 4 5 6 7 8 9 10 11 12 13 14 15 16 17 18 19 20

American Academy of Pediatrics

DEDICATED TO THE HEALTH OF ALL CHILDREN™

Source: Developed by the National Center for Health Statistics in collaboration with the
National Center for Chronic Disease Prevention and Health Promotion (2000).
http://www.cdc.gov/growthcharts

Reprinted by the American Academy of Pediatrics

The recommendations in this publication do not indicate an exclusive course of treatment or serve as a
standard of medical care. Variations, taking into account individual circumstances, may be appropriate.

©2000 American Academy of Pediatrics, Revised—5/01

9-8/REP1107

Additional copies are available for purchase in quantities of 100.

To order, contact:
American Academy of Pediatrics
141 Northwest Point Blvd
Elk Grove Village, IL 60007-1098
Web site — http://www.aap.org
Minimum order 100.

HE0304

Girls, 2 to 20 years

Name _____

BODY MASS INDEX FOR AGE PERCENTILES

Record #_____

Date	Age	Weight	Stature	BMI*	Comments

*To Calculate BMI: Weight (kg) ÷ Stature (cm) ÷ Stature (cm) x 10,000
or Weight (lb) ÷ Stature (in) ÷ Stature (in) x 703

AGE (YEARS)

Source: Developed by the National Center for Health Statistics in collaboration with the National Center for Chronic Disease Prevention and Health Promotion (2000).
http://www.cdc.gov/growthcharts

Reprinted by the American Academy of Pediatrics

The recommendations in this publication do not indicate an exclusive course of treatment or serve as a standard of medical care. Variations, taking into account individual circumstances, may be appropriate.

©2000 American Academy of Pediatrics, Revised—5/01

9-10/REP1107

Additional copies are available for purchase in quantities of 100.

To order, contact
American Academy of Pediatrics
141 Northwest Point Blvd
Elk Grove Village, IL 60007-1098
Web site — http://www.aap.org
Minimum order 100.

HE0306

Food Substitutions

IF YOUR CHILD WON'T EAT	SUBSTITUTE
Fruit	Vegetables, raw or cooked; if your child won't eat fresh fruits, try dried fruits such as apricots, pears, raisins, cherries, mango, pineapple, and bananas, and gradually introduce fresh fruits; make pureed sauces for yogurt with fresh or frozen fruit and gradually introduce chunks of whole fruit; serve applesauce instead of whole fruit. If your child refuses citrus fruits, offer alternative sources of vitamin C (eg, strawberries, cantaloupe, vitamin C-enriched juices, broccoli and other cruciferous vegetables, watermelon, potatoes); try mixing fruits such as blueberries, chopped apples, and bananas in muffin, quick bread, and waffle batters.
Meat	Fish, poultry, eggs, tofu, legumes (dried beans, chickpeas, and peas) and grains, and peanut butter; use chopped vegetable mixtures instead of ground meat or poultry to make pasta sauces, taco fillings; breads, crackers, and pasta made with iron-fortified flour.
Milk	Cheeses, yogurts, and other dairy foods made with cow's, goat's, or sheep's milk; soy- and rice-based substitutes for milk and cheese (ask your pediatrician whether your child should be taking supplements of vitamins B_{12} and D); canned fish with bones (salmon, sardines, herring) for calcium and vitamin D; good vegetable sources of calcium such as broccoli; safe exposure to sunlight for vitamin D.
Vegetables	If your child refuses green leafy vegetables, try dark-yellow and orange vegetables (carrots, squash, sweet potatoes) for vitamin A and folic acid, fruits and fruit juices for vitamin C, as well as folic acid; a child who turns down cooked vegetables may enjoy raw vegetable sticks and salads; offer low-sodium vegetable juice instead of fruit juice; children who balk at plain vegetables may enjoy Asian-style stir-fried vegetables; make pasta and taco sauces with finely chopped vegetables instead of, or in addition to, meat.
Whole-grain breads	High-fiber white bread; whole wheat and rye crackers; whole wheat pasta.

Choking/CPR

CHOKING/CPR

**LEARN AND PRACTICE CPR (CARDIOPULMONARY RESUSCITATION).
IF ALONE WITH A CHILD WHO IS CHOKING...
1. SHOUT FOR HELP. 2. START RESCUE EFFORTS. 3. CALL 911 OR YOUR LOCAL EMERGENCY NUMBER.**

START FIRST AID FOR CHOKING IF	DO *NOT* START FIRST AID FOR CHOKING IF
• The child cannot breathe at all (the chest is not moving up and down). • The child cannot cough or talk, or looks blue. • The child is found unconscious/unresponsive. (Go to CPR.)	• The child can breathe, cry, or talk. • The child can cough, sputter, or move air at all. The child's normal reflexes are working to clear the airway.

FOR INFANTS YOUNGER THAN 1 YEAR

INFANT CHOKING

If the infant is choking and is unable to breathe, cough, cry, or speak, follow these steps. Have someone call 911.

INFANT CPR

To be used when the infant is **UNCONSCIOUS/UNRESPONSIVE** or when breathing stops. Place infant on flat, hard surface.

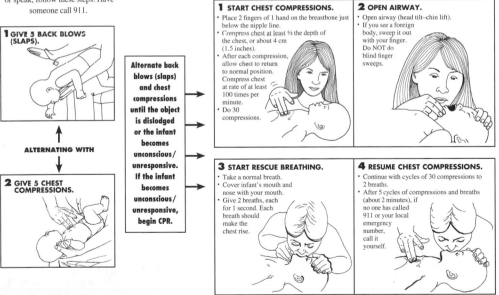

1 GIVE 5 BACK BLOWS (SLAPS).

ALTERNATING WITH

2 GIVE 5 CHEST COMPRESSIONS.

Alternate back blows (slaps) and chest compressions until the object is dislodged or the infant becomes unconscious/ unresponsive. If the infant becomes unconscious/ unresponsive, begin CPR.

1 START CHEST COMPRESSIONS.
• Place 2 fingers of 1 hand on the breastbone just below the nipple line.
• Compress chest at least ⅓ the depth of the chest, or about 4 cm (1.5 inches).
• After each compression, allow chest to return to normal position. Compress chest at rate of at least 100 times per minute.
• Do 30 compressions.

2 OPEN AIRWAY.
• Open airway (head tilt–chin lift).
• If you see a foreign body, sweep it out with your finger. Do NOT do blind finger sweeps.

3 START RESCUE BREATHING.
• Take a normal breath.
• Cover infant's mouth and nose with your mouth.
• Give 2 breaths, each for 1 second. Each breath should make the chest rise.

4 RESUME CHEST COMPRESSIONS.
• Continue with cycles of 30 compressions to 2 breaths.
• After 5 cycles of compressions and breaths (about 2 minutes), if no one has called 911 or your local emergency number, call it yourself.

If at any time an object is coughed up or the infant/child starts to breathe, stop rescue breaths and call 911 or your local emergency number.

Ask your pediatrician for information on choking/CPR instructions for children older than 8 years and for information on an approved first aid or CPR course in your community.

CHOKING/CPR

LEARN AND PRACTICE CPR (CARDIOPULMONARY RESUSCITATION).
IF ALONE WITH A CHILD WHO IS CHOKING...
1. SHOUT FOR HELP. 2. START RESCUE EFFORTS. 3. CALL 911 OR YOUR LOCAL EMERGENCY NUMBER.

START FIRST AID FOR CHOKING IF	DO *NOT* START FIRST AID FOR CHOKING IF
• The child cannot breathe at all (the chest is not moving up and down). • The child cannot cough or talk, or looks blue. • The child is found unconscious/unresponsive. (Go to CPR.)	• The child can breathe, cry, or talk. • The child can cough, sputter, or move air at all. The child's normal reflexes are working to clear the airway.

FOR CHILDREN 1 TO 8 YEARS OF AGE

CHILD CHOKING (HEIMLICH MANEUVER)

Have someone call 911. If the child is choking and is unable to breathe, cough, cry, or speak, follow these steps.

1. Perform Heimlich maneuver.
   - Place hand, made into a fist, and cover with other hand just above the navel. Place well below the bottom tip of the breastbone and rib cage.
   - Give each thrust with enough force to produce an artificial cough designed to relieve airway obstruction.
   - Perform Heimlich maneuver until the object is expelled or the child becomes unconscious/unresponsive.
2. If the child becomes UNCONSCIOUS/UNRESPONSIVE, begin CPR.

CHILD CPR

To be used when the child is **UNCONSCIOUS/UNRESPONSIVE** or when breathing stops. Place child on flat, hard surface.

1 START CHEST COMPRESSIONS.
- Place the heel of 1 or 2 hands over the lower half of the sternum.
- Compress chest at least ⅓ the depth of the chest, or about 5 cm (2 inches).
- After each compression, allow chest to return to normal position. Compress chest at rate of at least 100 times per minute.
- Do 30 compressions.

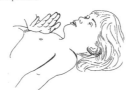

1-hand technique

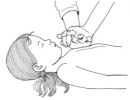

2-hand technique

2 OPEN AIRWAY.
- Open airway (head tilt–chin lift).
- If you see a foreign body, sweep it out with your finger. Do NOT do blind finger sweeps.

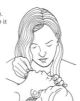

3 START RESCUE BREATHING.
- Take a normal breath.
- Pinch the child's nose closed, and cover child's mouth with your mouth.
- Give 2 breaths, each for 1 second. Each breath should make the chest rise.

4 RESUME CHEST COMPRESSIONS.
- Continue with cycles of 30 compressions to 2 breaths until the object is expelled.
- After 5 cycles of compressions and breaths (about 2 minutes), if no one has called 911 or your local emergency number, call it yourself.

If at any time an object is coughed up or the infant/child starts to breathe, stop rescue breaths and call 911 or your local emergency number.

Ask your pediatrician for information on choking/CPR instructions for children older than 8 years and for information on an approved first aid or CPR course in your community.

Dietary Reference Intakes

The following table was taken from
Pediatric Nutrition Handbook, 6th Edition,
American Academy of Pediatrics, 2009,
and updated as of June 2011.

Dietary Reference Intakes: Recommended Intakes for Individuals, Food and Nutrition Board, Institute of Medicine

	Infants 0–6 mo	Infants 7–12 mo	Children 1–3 y	Children 4–8 y	Males 9–13 y	Males 14–18 y	Females 9–13 y	Females 14–18 y	Pregnancy ≤18 y	Lactation ≤18 y
Carbohydrate (g/day)	60*	95*	130	130	130	130	130	130	175	210
Total Fiber (g/day)	ND	ND	19*	24*	31*	38*	26*	26*	28*	29*
Fat (g/day)	31*	30*	ND	ND	ND	ND	ND	ND	ND	ND
n-6 Polyunsaturated Fatty Acids (g/day) (Linoleic Acid)	4.4*	4.6*	7*	10*	12*	16*	10*	11*	13*	13*
n-3 Polyunsaturated Fatty Acids (g/day) (α-Linolenic Acid)	0.5*	0.5*	0.7*	0.9*	1.2*	1.6*	1.0*	1.1*	1.4*	1.3*
Protein (g/kg/day)	1.52*	1.05*	0.95*	0.95*	0.95*	0.85*	0.95*	0.85*	1.1*	1.3*
Vitamin A μg/day†	400*	500*	300	400	600	900	600	700	750	1200
Vitamin C mg/day	40*	50*	15	25	45	75	45	65	80	115
Vitamin D μg/day‡§	10*	10*	15	15	15	15	15	15	15	15
Vitamin E mg/day‖	4*	5*	6	7	11	15	11	15	15	19
Vitamin K μg/day	2.0*	2.5*	30*	55*	60*	75*	60*	75*	75*	75*
Thiamin (mg/day)	0.2*	0.3*	0.5	0.6	0.9	1.2	0.9	1.0	1.4	1.4
Riboflavin (mg/day)	0.3*	0.4*	0.5	0.6	0.9	1.3	0.9	1.0	1.4	1.6
Niacin (mg/day)¶	2*	4*	6	8	12	16	12	14	18	17
Vitamin B$_6$ (mg/day)	0.1*	0.3*	0.5	0.6	1.0	1.3	1.0	1.2	1.9	2.0
Folate (μg/day)#	65*	80*	150	200	300	400	300	400**	600††	500

Dietary Reference Intakes: Recommended Intakes for Individuals, Food and Nutrition Board, Institute of Medicine

	Infants 0–6 mo	Infants 7–12 mo	Children 1–3 y	Children 4–8 y	Males 9–13 y	Males 14–18 y	Females 9–13 y	Females 14–18 y	Pregnancy ≤18 y	Lactation ≤18 y
Vitamin B₁₂ (mg/day)	0.4*	0.5*	0.9	1.2	1.8	2.4	1.8	2.4	2.6	2.8
Pantothenic Acid (mg/day)	1.7*	1.8*	2*	3*	4*	5*	4*	5*	6*	7*
Biotin (µg/day)	5*	6*	8*	12*	20*	25*	20*	25*	30*	35*
Calcium (mg/day)	200*	260*	700	1000	1300	1300	1300	1300	1300	1300
Choline## (mg/day)	125*	125*	200*	250*	375*	550*	375*	400*	450*	550*
Chromium (µg/day)	0.2*	5.5*	11*	15*	25*	35*	21*	24*	29*	44
Copper (µg/day)	200*	220*	340	440	700	890	700	890	1000	1300
Fluoride (mg/day)	0.01*	0.5*	0.7*	1*	2*	3*	2*	2*	3*	3*
Iodine (µg/day)	110*	130*	90	90	120	150	120	150	220	290
Iron (mg/day)	0.27*	11	7	10	8	11	8	15	27	10
Magnesium (mg/day)	30*	75*	80	130	240	410	240	360	400	360
Manganese (mg/day)	0.003*	0.6*	1.2*	1.5*	1.9*	2.2*	1.6*	1.6*	2.0*	2.6*
Molybdenum (µg/day)	2*	3*	17	22	34	43	34	43	50	50
Phosphorus (mg/day)	100*	275*	460	500	1250	1250	1250	1250	1250	1250
Selenium (µg/day)	15*	20*	20	30	40	55	40	55	60	70
Zinc (mg/day)	2*	3	3	5	8	11	8	9	13	14
Potassium (g/day)	0.4*	0.7*	3.0*	3.8*	4.5*	4.7*	4.5*	4.7*	4.7*	5.1*
Sodium (g/day)	0.12*	0.37*	1.0*	1.2*	1.5*	1.5*	1.5*	1.5*	1.5*	1.5*
Chloride (g/day)	0.18*	0.57*	1.5*	1.9*	2.3*	2.3*	2.3*	2.3*	2.3*	2.3*

Dietary Reference Intakes: Recommended Intakes for Individuals, Food and Nutrition Board, Institute of Medicine

This table (taken from the DRI reports; see http://www.iom.edu/CMS/3788/21370.aspx) presents Recommended Dietary Allowances (RDAs) in **bold type**, and Adequate Intakes (AIs) are in ordinary type followed by the symbol (*). ND indicates not determined.

* RDAs and AIs may both be used as goals for individual intake. RDAs are set to meet the needs of almost all (97%–98%) individuals in a group. For healthy breastfed infants, the AI is the mean intake. The AI for other life stage and gender groups is believed to cover needs of all individuals in the group, but lack of data or uncertainty in the data prevent being able to specify with confidence the percentage of individuals covered by this intake.

† As retinol activity equivalents (RAEs). 1 RAE = 1 µg retinol, 12 µg β-carotene, 24 µg α-carotene, or 24 µg β-cryptoxanthin in foods. The RAE for dietary provitamin A carotenoids is twofold greater than retinol equivalents (RE), whereas the RAE for preformed vitamin A is the same as RE.

‡ As cholecalciferol. 1 µg cholecalciferol = 40 IU vitamin D.

§ In the absence of adequate exposure to sunlight.

|| As α-tocopherol. α-Tocopherol includes RRR-α-tocopherol, the only form of α-tocopherol that occurs naturally in foods, and the 2R-stereoisomeric forms of α-tocopherol (RRR-, RSR-, RRS-, and RSS-α-tocopherol) that occur in fortified foods and supplements. It does not include the 2S-stereoisomeric forms of α-tocopherol (SRR-, SSR-, SRS-, and SSS-α-tocopherol), also found in fortified foods and supplements.

¶ As niacin equivalents (NEs). 1 mg of niacin = 60 mg of tryptophan; 0–6 mo = preformed niacin (not NEs).

As dietary folate equivalents (DFEs). 1 DFE = 1 µg food folate = 0.6 µg of folic acid from fortified food or as a supplement consumed with food = 0.5 µg of a supplement taken on an empty stomach.

** In view of evidence linking folate intake with neural tube defects in the fetus, it is recommended that all women capable of becoming pregnant consume 400 µg from supplements or fortified foods in addition to intake of food folate from the diet.

†† It is assumed that women will continue consuming 400 µg from supplements or fortified food until their pregnancy is confirmed and they enter prenatal care, which ordinarily occurs after the end of the periconceptional period—the critical time for formation of the neural tube.

‡‡ Although AIs have been set for choline, there are few data to assess whether a dietary supply of choline is needed at all stages of the life cycle, and it may be that the choline requirement can be met by endogenous synthesis at some of these stages. 2004.

The DASH (Dietary Approaches to Stop Hypertension) Diet

The DASH diet eating plan is a diet rich in fruits, vegetables, and low-fat or nonfat dairy. It also includes grains, especially whole grains; lean meats, fish, and poultry; and nuts and beans. It is a plan that follows US guidelines for sodium content. The DASH eating plan lowers cholesterol and makes it easy to lose weight. It is a healthy way of eating, designed to be flexible enough to meet the lifestyle and food preferences of most people. And it contains all the healthy foods from the Mediterranean diet.

Specifically, the DASH diet plan includes

TYPE OF FOOD	NUMBER OF SERVINGS FOR 1,600- TO 3,100-CALORIE DIETS	SERVINGS ON A 2,000- CALORIE DIET
Grains and grain products (include at least 3 whole-grain foods each day)	6–12	7–8
Fruits	4–6	4–5
Vegetables	4–6	4–5
Low-fat or nonfat dairy foods	2–4	2–3
Lean meats, fish, poultry	1½–2½	2 or less
Nuts, seeds, and legumes	3–6 per week	4–5 per week
Fats and sweets	2–4	limited

SOURCE: http://dashdiet.org/what_is_the_dash_diet.asp. Accessed June 3, 2011.

Health and Nutrition Resources

Allergies and Asthma

Allergy & Asthma Network Mothers
  of Asthmatics
8201 Greensboro Dr, Ste 300
McLean, VA 22102
800/878-4403
www.aanma.org

Asthma and Allergy Foundation of America
8201 Corporate Dr, Ste 1000
Landover, MD 20785
800/7-ASTHMA (727-8462)
www.aafa.org

Food Allergy & Anaphylaxis Network
11781 Lee Jackson Hwy, Ste 160
Fairfax, VA 22033-3309
800/929-4040
www.foodallergy.org

National Heart, Lung, and Blood Institute
Health Information Center
Attention: Web Site
PO Box 30105
Bethesda, MD 20824-0105
301/592-8573
www.nhlbi.nih.gov

National Institute of Allergy and Infectious
  Diseases
Office of Communications and Government
  Relations
6610 Rockledge Dr, MSC 6612
Bethesda, MD 20892-6612
866/284-4107
www.niaid.nih.gov

Breastfeeding

La Leche League International
957 N Plum Grove Rd
Schaumburg, IL 60173
800/LALECHE (525-3243)
www.llli.org

Diabetes

Juvenile Diabetes Research Foundation
  International
26 Broadway, 14th Floor
New York, NY 10004
800/533-CURE (2873)
www.jdrf.org

Digestive Disorders

Crohn's & Colitis Foundation of America
386 Park Avenue S, 17th Floor
New York, NY 10016
800/932-2423
www.ccfa.org

National Digestive Diseases Information
    Clearinghouse
2 Information Way
Bethesda, MD 20892-3570
800/891-5389
http://digestive.niddk.nih.gov

Eating Disorders

National Eating Disorders Association
603 Stewart St, Ste 803
Seattle, WA 98101
800/931-2237
www.nationaleatingdisorders.org

Food Safety

Centers for Disease Control and Prevention
    Food Safety
www.cdc.gov/foodsafety

Fight BAC! Keep Food Safe From Bacteria
www.fightbac.org

FoodSafety.gov: Your Gateway to Federal
    Food Safety Information
www.foodsafety.gov

US Department of Agriculture Food Safety
    and Inspection Service
www.fsis.usda.gov/help/FAQs/index.asp

US Department of Agriculture Food
    Safety and Inspection Service Safe Food
    Handling
www.fsis.usda.gov/Fact_Sheets/
    Safe_Food_Handling_Fact_Sheets

US Department of Agriculture National
    Agricultural Library
http://fsrio.nal.usda.gov

US Food and Drug Administration for
    Consumers
www.fda.gov/ForConsumers

General Nutrition Information for Children and Families

American Academy of Pediatrics
    HealthyChildren.org
www.HealthyChildren.org

American Dietetic Association
120 S Riverside Plaza, Ste 2000
Chicago, IL 60606-6995
800/877-1600
www.eatright.org

Gluten Enteropathy/ Celiac Disease

Celiac Disease Foundation

13251 Ventura Blvd, Ste 1

Studio City, CA 91604

818/990-2354

www.celiac.org

Celiac Sprue Association

PO Box 31700

Omaha, NE 68131-0700

877/CSA-4CSA (272-4272)

www.csaceliacs.org

Gluten Intolerance Group of North America

31214 124th Ave SE

Auburn, WA 98092

253/833-6655

www.gluten.net

Index